Caring for Your School-Age Child

This invaluable volume was prepared under the editorial direction of pediatrician Shelly Vaziri Flais, MD, FAAP, and draws on the contributions and practical wisdom of more than one hundred pediatric experts. Written in a warm, accessible style, this book gives you the information you need to safeguard your child's most precious asset: his or her health.

In *Caring for Your School-Age Child* you'll find:

- Age-specific advice for children ages 5 to 7 years, 8 to 10 years, and 11 to 12 years of age throughout the book
- Enhanced and extended information on medical, mental health, and behavior conditions
- Parent advice to help children develop resilience and life skills as they grow
- New media chapter with valuable parenting advice regarding use of screen time, electronic devices, internet use and safety, and more
- New chapter on emergency preparedness, hospital care, and money management skills for your child

Parents will also find:

- A guide to your child's personal, physical, behavioral, and social development, including the stages of puberty
- Guidance for parents on being involved in your child's schooling, from starting school to developing good homework habits and reinforcing learning
- Practical suggestions for dealing with sibling rivalry, bed-wetting, and temper tantrums
- Current AAP policy on important child health issues
- The best ways to encourage good nutrition and physical fitness
- Advice on effective discipline and optimal nurturing

Plus reliable information on:

- Choosing child care and when your child wants to babysit
- Safety and injury prevention, plus handling emergency situations
- Learning disabilities, attention deficit hyperactivity disorder, and stuttering
- Common medical problems, from colds to swimmer's ear
- Chronic conditions and diseases, including asthma and diabetes

Additional Parenting Books from the American Academy of Pediatrics

COMMON CONDITIONS

Allergies and Asthma: What Every Parent Needs to Know

The Big Book of Symptoms: A–Z Guide to Your Child's Health

Mama Doc Medicine: Finding Calm and Confidence in Parenting,
Child Health, and Work-Life Balance

My Child Is Sick! Expert Advice for Managing Common Illnesses and Injuries

Sleep: What Every Parent Needs to Know

Waking Up Dry: A Guide to Help Children Overcome Bedwetting

DEVELOPMENTAL, BEHAVIORAL, AND PSYCHOSOCIAL INFORMATION

ADHD: What Every Parent Needs to Know

Autism Spectrum Disorders: What Every Parent Needs to Know

CyberSafe: Protecting and Empowering Kids in the Digital World of
Texting, Gaming, and Social Media

Mental Health, Naturally: The Family Guide to Holistic Care for
a Healthy Mind and Body

NEWBORNS, INFANTS, AND TODDLERS

Baby Care Anywhere: A Quick Guide to Parenting on the Go

Baby & Toddler Basics: Expert Answers to Parents' Top 150 Questions

Caring for Your Baby and Young Child: Ages Birth to Five*

Dad to Dad: Parenting Like a Pro

Guide to Toilet Training

Heading Home with Your Newborn: From Birth to Reality

New Mother's Guide to Breastfeeding*

Raising Twins: Parenting Multiples from Pregnancy Through the School Years

RetroBaby: Cut Back on All the Gear and Boost Your Baby's Development with More Than 100 Time-Tested Activities

Understanding the NICU: What Parents of Preemies and Other Hospitalized Newborns Need to Know

Your Baby's First Year*

NUTRITION AND FITNESS

Achieving a Healthy Weight for Your Child: An Action Plan for Families

Food Fights: Winning the Nutritional Challenges of Parenthood Armed with Insight, Humor, and a Bottle of Ketchup

Nutrition: What Every Parent Needs to Know

Sports Success Rx!: Your Child's Prescription for the Best Experience

SCHOOL-AGE CHILDREN AND ADOLESCENTS

Building Resilience in Children and Teens: Giving Kids Roots and Wings

Raising Kids to Thrive: Balancing Love with Expectations and Protection with Trust

---

FOR ADDITIONAL PARENTING RESOURCES,

VISIT THE HEALTHYCHILDREN BOOKSTORE AT

SHOP.AAP.ORG/FOR-PARENTS/.

---

* This book is also available in Spanish.

Caring for Your School-Age Child

Ages 5 to 12

Shelly Vaziri Flais, MD, FAAP

EDITOR-IN-CHIEF

Pediatric Health Associates
Naperville, Illinois

Assistant Professor of Clinical Pediatrics
Northwestern University, Feinberg School of Medicine
Chicago, Illinois

BANTAM BOOKS
New York

Published in the United States by Bantam Books, an imprint of Random House,
a division of Penguin Random House LLC, New York.

BANTAM BOOKS and the HOUSE colophon are registered trademarks of
Penguin Random House LLC.

This work was originally published in
the United States in hardcover in 1995,
and a revised edition was published in 1999
by Bantam Books, an imprint of Random House,
a division of Penguin Random House LLC.

ISBN 978-0-425-28604-3

Printed in the United States of America on acid-free paper

randomhousebooks.com

2 4 6 8 9 7 5 3 1

Third Edition

Reviewers and Contributors

EDITOR-IN-CHIEF
Shelly Vaziri Flais, MD, FAAP

AAP BOARD OF DIRECTORS REVIEWER
Lisa Anne Cosgrove, MD, FAAP

AMERICAN ACADEMY OF PEDIATRICS

CEO/*Executive Vice President (Interim)*
Mark Del Monte, JD

Chief Product and Services Officer/SVP,
Membership, Marketing, and Publishing
Mary Lou White

Vice President, Publishing
Mark T. Grimes

Manager, Consumer Publishing
Kathryn Sparks

Editor, Consumer Publishing
Holly Kaminski

AMERICAN ACADEMY OF PEDIATRICS
REVIEWERS AND CONTRIBUTORS
Committee on Bioethics
Committee on Drugs
Committee on Injury Violence
Committee on Nutrition
Committee on Psychosocial Aspects of
    Child and Family Health
Committee on Substance Use and
    Prevention
Council on Child Abuse and Neglect
Council on Children with Disabilities
Council on Communication and Media
Council on Early Childhood
Council on Environmental Health
Council on Foster Care, Adoption, and
    Kinship Care
Council on Injury, Violence, and Poison
    Prevention
Disaster Preparedness Advisory Council
Council on School Health
Council on Sports Medicine and Fitness
Section on Allergy and Immunology
Section on Cardiology and Cardiac Surgery
Section on Dermatology
Section on Developmental and Behavioral
    Pediatrics
Section on Hospice and Palliative Medicine
Section on Lesbian, Gay, Bisexual and
    Transgender Health and Wellness
Section on Neurology
Section on Ophthalmology
Section on Orthopaedics
Section on Otolaryngology—Head and
    Neck Surgery
Section on Pediatric Pulmonology and
    Sleep Medicine

Acknowledgments

We thank Edward L. Schor, MD, FAAP, and the countless contributors and reviewers for their work on the first two editions of *Caring for Your School-Age Child: Ages 5 to 12*. A generation of school-age children is in your debt.

Illustrations

All illustrations are by Jeanne Brunick except for illustrations featured on pages 55, 312, and 340. Those were created by Anthony Alex LeTourneau.

PLEASE NOTE

The information contained in this book is intended to complement, not substitute for, the advice of your child's pediatrician. Before starting any medical treatment or medical program, you should consult with your own physician, who can discuss your individual needs with you and counsel you about symptoms and treatment.

The information and advice in this book apply equally to children of both sexes (except where noted). To indicate this, we have chosen to alternate between masculine and feminine pronouns throughout the book.

~ ~ ~

The American Academy of Pediatrics constantly monitors new scientific evidence and makes appropriate adjustments in its recommendations. For example, future research and the development of new childhood vaccines may alter the regimen for the administration of existing vaccines. Therefore, the schedule for immunizations outlined in this book is subject to change. These and other potential situations serve to emphasize the importance of always checking with your pediatrician for the latest information concerning the health of your child. For additional information on caring for your child, their needs and well-being, visit HealthyChildren.org.

This book is dedicated to
all the people who recognize that children
are our greatest inspiration in the present
and our greatest hope for the future

Contents

PART VIII
Medical, Mental Health, and Behavior Issues
525

Foreword

The American Academy of Pediatrics (AAP) welcomes you to the third edition of *Caring for Your School-Age Child: Ages 5 to 12*.

The American Academy of Pediatrics is an organization of 67,000 primary care pediatricians, pediatric medical subspecialists, and pediatric surgical specialists, dedicated to the health, safety, and well-being of infants, children, adolescents, and young adults. This updated edition of *Caring for Your School-Age Child: Ages 5 to 12* is part of the Academy's ongoing education efforts to provide parents and caregivers with high-quality information on a broad spectrum of children's health issues.

What distinguishes this book on the middle years of childhood from others in bookstores and on library shelves is that it has been developed and extensively reviewed by physician members of the American Academy of Pediatrics. An eight-member editorial board developed the initial material with the assistance of more than one hundred contributors and reviewers. Because medical information is constantly changing, every effort has been made to ensure that this book contains the most up-to-date findings. Readers can visit the AAP's official website for parents at healthychildren.org to keep current on the latest information related to child health and guidance on parenting.

It is the Academy's hope that this book will become an invaluable resource and reference guide for parents and caregivers. We believe it is the best comprehensive source of information on matters of children's health and well-being. We are confident that parents and caregivers will find the book extremely valuable, and encourage its use along with the advice and counsel of our readers' own pediatricians, who will provide individual guidance and assistance related to the health of their children.

Colleen A. Kraft, MD, FAAP
President
American Academy of Pediatrics

Introduction

Your School-Age Child

WHEN CHILDREN REACH the middle years of childhood, many parents breathe a sigh of relief. The infancy, toddlerhood, and preschool years—a busy time when children grow so dramatically and require constant attention—have passed. At the same time, adolescence seems far off in the future. Yet the school years are formative years of great growth and transition for kids. During these middle years of childhood, the child learns more about navigating the outside world, yet still requires a stable, nurturing home environment. As parents, our job is to help nurture our kids' self-empowerment, resilience, and life skills, all the while providing a secure home base to return to.

The middle years of childhood are years of enormous social growth. Between the ages of 5 and 12, children's intellectual competence develops dramatically, and they become noticeably better at logical thinking, reasoning, and problem-solving. With these skills in hand, they begin to try out in the outside world what they have learned at home. These years offer children opportunities to see how the skills, behavior, beliefs, and values that serve them at home can work in the company of new friends and social situations.

The middle years are complex years, when children's self-esteem is tested and is reinforced daily. Children must "find themselves" and become more independent, while simultaneously gaining acceptance among their friends and retaining a secure place within their families.

The habits and behavior patterns that children develop during these years will strongly influence their long-term health and well-being, success at school and work, and future relationships. This book is written to assist parents, caregivers, teachers, and others to help children take advantage of the experiences these years provide—to build a firm foundation of healthy behavior, emotional well-being, and academic and social skills for their adolescence and their adult lives. The role of a parent is not to anticipate and solve all our children's problems for them; rather, our role is to help nurture those skills within our children so that they have the tools to resolve issues themselves.

Since you have chosen to read this book, you already have some of the characteristics necessary to guide a child through the middle years—namely, awareness and interest. Children have an innate desire to explore, to learn, to grow, and to do their best, whatever the situation. Parents have that same determination as they go about raising their children, but just like their children, parents need information, advice, and encouragement in order to succeed. There is no one-size-fits-all approach to parenting; rather, a lot of parenting skills develop through trial and error and by learning from experience.

The information in this book is provided by pediatricians, members of the American Academy of Pediatrics, who are national experts in their fields. They have studied child health and development, watched and learned from the tens of thousands of families for whom they have cared, and are parents themselves.

Families Today

Everyone knows that a child's experience within his or her family today continues to evolve. Grandparents, cousins, uncles, and aunts are as likely to be many miles away as they are to be living around the corner. Today, some children live with both of their parents, some live with only one parent, and some live in households with stepparents. Daily routines are dictated as much by the work schedule of the parents as by the needs and wishes of the family, and there seems to be less time just to be a family—spending time together simply to enjoy each other's company. Also vying for family time is the prevalence of screens (smartphones, tablets, and the like); while technology seemingly makes connections easier than ever before, it can interfere with connections within the family.

Growing Up in a Family

The changes and complexities in family life demand that we pay attention to families, for they remain the place where children grow up. During the preschool years families are like incubators, providing children with a safe place where they can feel loved and cared about and discover who they are. In the middle years families provide a working model in which children can observe and practice relationships with other people. Families also provide a supportive environment in which children can find help in understanding, coping with, and finding their place in the world around them.

Children's relationships with their parents evolve during these years. You and your child will spend many fewer of your waking hours together now. Monitoring your child's activities and behavior, and teaching him new skills, will become more of a hands-off process for you, and your child must develop strategies for managing his own behavior.

Increased Independence

During the middle years, children first venture into the world alone, physically unaccompanied by their families. Schools are a place of great importance in the lives of children. They are the site of new social contacts with both adults and other children, as well as new expectations for the child. By participating in school activities and organizations, children develop friendships that for the first time are unrelated to their families. They will form new connections with others, but will also face unfamiliar social behaviors.

To succeed and grow amid shifting interests and allegiances, children must learn about themselves as players in a social game and must discover how best to get along in this new arena. Their expanding self-awareness becomes increasingly stable and comprehensive. They develop standards and expectations for their own behavior, and become more independent and self-sufficient. While they try on new roles and attitudes in order to learn about themselves, they still will need to be able to turn to their families, especially to their parents, for guidance and stability.

Recurring Themes

There is much that parents can do and say that will help their children nurture the tools they need as future adults. First and foremost, parents need to model the values and behavior they wish their children to adopt, and direct their children into situations that reinforce and reward them. Whether it is responding to people less fortunate than themselves or choosing what foods to eat, children's behavior is in part an imitation of behavior they have observed.

Second, parents need to learn how to communicate with their children and to find opportunities to practice these skills. Simply *listening* is a fundamental communication skill. Parents must listen to their children, actively trying to hear what messages they are attempting to convey. The better that parents understand their children, the better able they will be to work together to meet challenges and solve problems when they arise. Good parents are those who have made the effort to know their children well, and have succeeded. Children whose parents know and understand them will have fewer personal and social problems.

In addition to active listening, successful communication is based on mutual respect, shared experiences, and open expression of thoughts and feelings. By paying attention to each child's personal skills and uniquely individual character, parents will find much to admire and respect.

Third, parents must support their children and be an advocate for them in many settings. Parents should be involved in their children's worlds and should help them learn resilience and problem-solving skills for themselves.

Throughout this book, we offer advice on how these parenting skills can be acquired and applied.

How to Use This Book

Sometimes you simply want to understand your child (or someone else's child) better, or to feel reassured that you are doing all right. At other times you want help with a specific problem. The better you understand child development generally, and your child specifically, the better equipped you will be to work together on a problem.

This book has different kinds of chapters to meet these different needs. Some chapters provide background information about school-age children, their development, behavior, health, schools, and the social issues they confront. These chapters take a little longer to read, but the information they contain can be applied to many situations. By reading them, you also will learn about expected child growth, development, and behavior. Other chapters address specific problems that commonly occur during a child's middle years. You can turn to these for advice about a problem you and your child (or you and your student) are facing. In addition, you can find more information about medical conditions in Part VIII, "Medical, Mental Health, and Behavior Issues."

Parenting is a natural process that can be enhanced by learning about your child and understanding your own feelings and inclinations. No two children are alike, and there is no one-size-fits-all parenting strategy. It is our hope that the information and advice in this book will assist your family to support the health and well-being of your child.

PART I

· · · · · · · · · · · ·

Nutritional
and
Physical Fitness

~ 1 ~

Maintaining Your Child's Health

YOU, YOUR CHILD, and your child's pediatrician have equally important roles to play in maintaining your child's health, preventing illness and injury during childhood, and helping establish habits that will promote health and well-being for a lifetime.

Choosing a Pediatrician

When seeking quality medical care for your children, where should you turn? Most parents rely on a pediatrician, a physician (MD, DO) who completed four years of medical school and then three years of residency training in general pediatrics, specializing in the care of children. Pediatricians have special training in the health and illnesses of children through the age of adolescence, and most are certified by the American Board of Pediatrics after passing an initial comprehensive examination covering all areas of health related to infants, children, and young adults, as well as continuing their medical education to maintain board certification.

By your child's middle years, you probably have already found a pediatrician with whom you are happy. However, the occasion may arise where you need to find a new doctor—perhaps you have moved to a new city, or your pediatrician has retired.

In circumstances like these, try to obtain a referral from your present pediatrician. He or she may know a colleague in the city where you are moving, or one who is taking over the retiree's practice. Friends and family members might also recommend one or more pediatricians for you to consider.

There are other good sources of names of qualified pediatricians:

- Find a pediatrician or pediatric specialist at HealthyChildren.org, the official parenting website of the American Academy of Pediatrics.

- Most local/county medical societies provide referral services to pediatricians in their area who are taking new patients.

- If you are located near a major medical center, community hospital, or teaching hospital, contact its department of pediatrics for the names of doctors in your area.

Interviewing Pediatricians

With a list of doctors in hand, you can learn more about your options by investigating the website of each pediatrician's practice. You should be able to learn more about the doctor's background and training, as well as general office procedures. If you are impressed with what you hear, arrange for an interview during which you can meet the doctor and ask some additional questions. It may be more convenient to do this interview by telephone. Here are some things to consider when choosing a pediatrician:

- What medical school did the pediatrician attend, and where did he or she undergo postgraduate and residency training?

- What are the doctor's present hospital appointments? If it becomes necessary for your child to be hospitalized, where would he be admitted? Would your pediatrician be managing your child's hospital stay, or does the hospital use in-house pediatric hospitalists (hospital specialists)?

- Is the pediatrician's office conveniently located? Is it easily accessible by car or public transportation? Is there accessible parking?

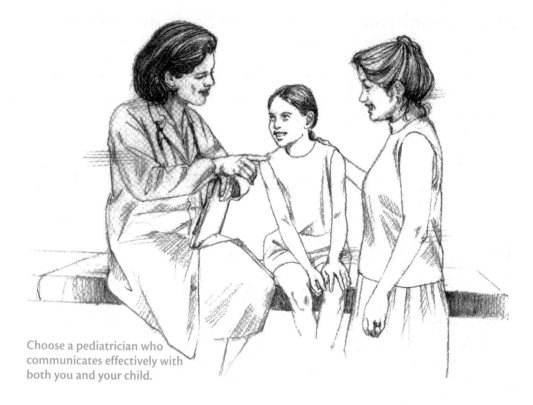

Choose a pediatrician who communicates effectively with both you and your child.

- Are the office hours convenient for your own schedule? If you are a working parent, you may desire evening or weekend hours.

- What is the doctor's policy on taking and returning phone calls? Is there a nurse in the office who can answer routine questions? Who answers emergency calls after hours—for example, overnight or on weekends?

- Is the doctor in a group practice with other physicians? Does another physician cover for the doctor at times?

- How often will the pediatrician see your child for checkups and immunizations?

- Do you sense a genuine interest by the doctor in the problems of *your* child, including particular health disorders he may have?

- Do both the physician and the office staff appear amicable and courteous? Do they demonstrate compassion and patience? Or do you feel rushed in the office, as though the doctor is eager to move on to the next patient?

Recommendations for Preventive Pediatric Health Care (RE9939)
Committee on Practice and Ambulatory Medicine

Each child and family is unique; therefore, these **Recommendations for Preventive Pediatric Health Care** are designed for the care of children who are receiving competent parenting, have no manifestations of any important health problems, and are growing and developing in satisfactory fashion. **Additional visits may become necessary** if circumstances suggest variations from normal.

AGE[5]	PRENATAL[1]	NEWBORN[2]	2-4d[3]	By 1mo	2mo	4mo	6mo	9mo	12mo	15mo	18mo	24mo	3y	4y
				INFANCY[4]						**EARLY CHILDHOOD[4]**				
HISTORY Initial/Interval	●	●	●	●	●	●	●	●	●	●	●	●	●	●
MEASUREMENTS Height and Weight		●	●	●	●	●	●	●	●	●	●	●	●	●
Head Circumference		●	●	●	●	●	●	●	●	●	●	●		
Blood Pressure													●	●
SENSORY SCREENING Vision		S	S	S	S	S	S	S	S	S	S	S	O[6]	O
Hearing		O[7]	S	S	S	S	S	S	S	S	S	S	S	O
DEVELOPMENTAL/ BEHAVIORAL ASSESSMENT[8]		●	●	●	●	●	●	●	●	●	●	●	●	●
PHYSICAL EXAMINATION[9]		●	●	●	●	●	●	●	●	●	●	●	●	●
PROCEDURES—GENERAL[10] Hereditary/Metabolic Screening[11]		◄—	●	—►										
Immunization[12]		●		●	●	●	●	●	—►	●	●	●	●	●
Hematocrit or Hemoglobin[13]								—	—►	★				
Urinalysis														
PROCEDURES—PATIENTS AT RISK Lead Screening[16]								★—	—►			★		
Tuberculin Test[17]									★	★	★	★	★	★
Cholesterol Screening[18]												★	★	★
STD Screening[19]														
Pelvic Exam[20]														
ANTICIPATORY GUIDANCE[21] Injury Prevention[22]	●	●	●	●	●	●	●	●	●	●	●	●	●	●
Violence Prevention[23]	●	●	●	●	●	●	●	●	●	●	●	●	●	●
Sleep Positioning Counseling[24]	●	●	●	●	●	●	●	●						
Nutrition Counseling[25]	●	●	●	●	●	●	●	●	●	●	●	●	●	●
DENTAL REFERRAL[26]											◄—			

1. A prenatal visit is recommended for parents who are at high risk, for first-time parents, and for those who request a conference. The prenatal visit should include anticipatory guidance, pertinent medical history, and a discussion of benefits of breastfeeding and planned method of feeding per AAP statement "The Prenatal Visit" (1996).
2. Every infant should have a newborn evaluation after birth. Breastfeeding should be encouraged and instruction and support offered. Every breastfeeding infant should have an evaluation 48-72 hours after discharge from the hospital to include weight, formal breastfeeding evaluation, encouragement, and instruction as recommended in the AAP statement "Breastfeeding and the Use of Human Milk" (1997).
3. For newborns discharged in less than 48 hours after delivery per AAP statement "Hospital Stay for Healthy Term Newborns" (1995).
4. Developmental, psychosocial, and chronic disease issues for children and adolescents may require frequent counseling and treatment visits separate from preventive care visits.
5. If a child comes under care for the first time at any point on the schedule, or if any items are not accomplished at the suggested age, the schedule should be brought up to date at the earliest possible time.
6. If the patient is uncooperative, rescreen within 6 months.
7. All newborns should be screened per the AAP Task Force on Newborn and Infant Hearing statement, "Newborn and Infant Hearing Loss: Detection and Intervention" (1999).
8. By history and appropriate physical examination; if suspicious, by specific objective developmental testing. Parenting skills should be fostered at every visit.

9. At each visit, a complete physical examination is essential, with infant totally unclothed, older child undressed and suitably draped.
10. These may be modified, depending upon entry point into schedule and individual need.
11. Metabolic screening (eg, thyroid, hemoglobinopathies, PKU, galactosemia) should be done according to state law.
12. Schedule(s) per the Committee on Infectious Diseases, published annually in the January edition of Pediatrics. Every visit should be an opportunity to update and complete a child's immunizations.
13. See AAP Pediatric Nutrition Handbook (1998) for a discussion of universal and selective screening options. Consider earlier screening for high-risk infants (eg, premature infants and low birth weight infants). See also "Recommendations to Prevent and Control Iron Deficiency in the United States." MMWR. 1998;47 (RR-3):1-29.
14. All menstruating adolescents should be screened annually.
15. Conduct dipstick urinalysis for leukocytes annually for sexually active male and female adolescents.
16. For children at risk of lead exposure consult the AAP statement "Screening for Elevated Blood Levels" (1998). Additionally, screening should be done in accordance with state law where applicable.
17. TB testing per recommendations of the Committee on Infectious Diseases, published in the current edition of Red Book: Report of the Committee on Infectious Diseases. Testing should be done upon recognition of high-risk factors.

Key:
● = to be performed
S = subjective, by history
◄ • ► = the range during which a service may be provided, with the dot indicating the preferred age.
★ = to be performed for patients at risk
O = objective, by a standard testing method

These guidelines represent a consensus by the Committee on Practice and Ambulatory Medicine in consultation with national committees and sections of the American Academy of Pediatrics. The Committee emphasizes the great importance of **continuity of care** in comprehensive health supervision and the need to avoid **fragmentation of care.**

MIDDLE CHILDHOOD⁴				ADOLESCENCE⁴										
5y	6y	8y	10y	11y	12y	13y	14y	15y	16y	17y	18y	19y	20y	21y
•	•	•	•	•	•	•	•	•	•	•	•	•	•	•
•	•	•	•	•	•	•	•	•	•	•	•	•	•	•
•	•	•	•	•	•	•	•	•	•	•	•	•	•	•
O O	O O	O O	O O	S S	O O	S S	S S	O O	S S	S S	O O	S S	S S	S S
•	•	•	•	•	•	•	•	•	•	•	•	•	•	•
•	•	•	•	•	•	•	•	•	•	•	•	•	•	•
•	•	•	•	•	•	•¹⁴	•	•	•	•	•	•	•	•
•						•¹⁵								
★ ★	★ ★	★ ★	★ ★	★ ★	★ ★	★ ★	★ ★	★ ★	★ ★	★ ★	★ ★	★ ★	★ ★	★ ★
				★	★	★	★	★	★	★	★	★²⁰	★	★
• • •	• • •	• • •	• • •	• • •	• • •	• • •	• • •	• • •	• • •	• • •	• • •	• • •	• • •	• • •
•	•	•	•	•	•	•	•	•	•	•	•	•	•	•

18. Cholesterol screening for high-risk patients per AAP statement "Cholesterol in Childhood" (1998). If family history cannot be ascertained and other risk factors are present, screening should be at the discretion of the physician.
19. All sexually active patients should be screened for sexually transmitted diseases (STDs).
20. All sexually active females should have a pelvic examination. A pelvic examination and routine pap smear should be offered as part of preventive health maintenance between the ages of 18 and 21 years.
21. Age-appropriate discussion and counseling should be an integral part of each visit for care per the AAP *Guidelines for Health Supervision III* (1998).
22. From birth to age 12, refer to the AAP injury prevention program (TIPP®) as described in *A Guide to Safety Counseling in Office Practice* (1994).
23. Violence prevention and management for all patients per AAP statement "The Role of the Pediatrician in Youth Violence Prevention in Clinical Practice and at the Community Level" (1999).
24. Parents and caregivers should be advised to place healthy infants on their backs when putting them to sleep. Side positioning is a reasonable alternative but carries a slightly higher risk of SIDS. Consult the AAP statement "Changing Concepts of Sudden Infant Death Syndrome: Implications for Infant Sleeping Environment and Sleep Position" (2000).
25. Age-appropriate nutrition counseling should be an integral part of each visit per the AAP *Handbook of Nutrition* (1998).
26. Earlier initial dental examinations may be appropriate for some children. Subsequent examinations as prescribed by dentist.

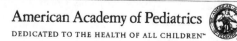

American Academy of Pediatrics
DEDICATED TO THE HEALTH OF ALL CHILDREN™

- How are visits for acute illnesses handled? Can you make an appointment on short notice if your child needs to see the pediatrician because of a sore throat or an infection, for example?

- Does the doctor communicate clearly, using straightforward language (not medical jargon) to explain illnesses and treatments, and does the doctor make an effort to ensure that all your questions are answered?

- What are the doctor's usual fees for sick visits, routine examinations, and immunizations? What is the office policy regarding the processing of insurance forms?

- In what managed care programs does the doctor participate?

- Does the pediatrician's office serve as its patients' "medical home"? If your child should ever develop a complex illness that necessitates the care of one or more specialists, will your pediatrician coordinate care among all the specialists providing treatment?

Managed Care

Many Americans receive their healthcare in managed care plans. These plans, typically offered by employers and state Medicaid programs, provide services through health maintenance organizations (HMOs) or preferred provider organizations (PPOs). The plans have their own networks of pediatricians and other physicians, and if you or your employer change from one managed care plan to another, you may find that the pediatrician you have had a relationship with is not part of the new network. Once you have a pediatrician you like, ask what plans she is in, and see if you can join one of them if there's a need to switch from one HMO or PPO to another.

Managed care plans attempt to reduce their costs by having doctors control patient access to certain healthcare services. Your pediatrician may act as a "gatekeeper," needing to give approval before your child can be seen by a pediatric medical subspecialist or surgical specialist. Without this approval, you'll have to pay for part or all of these services out of pocket.

To help you maneuver effectively through your managed care plan, here are some points to keep in mind:

- To determine what care is provided in your managed care plan, carefully read the materials provided by the plan (often called a certificate of coverage). If you have questions, talk to a plan representative or your employer's

Keeping Medical Records

Because you might change pediatricians from time to time, it's useful to keep accurate medical records of your child's health. Your records should include the following information:

- **Physicians.** Include the name and address of your child's previous pediatrician.

- **Hospitalizations.** List dates, illnesses, and treatments.

- **Immunizations.** Include the dates on which they were administered.

- **Your child's height and weight.** Height and weight are measured at each well-child visit with the pediatrician.

- **Special care.** If your child has received treatment for particular diseases or conditions, note these, the age at which they began, and what therapies were used.

- **Screening tests.** Include the results of tests done to evaluate your child's vision, hearing, lead levels, and other aspects of health.

- **Family history.** List health conditions that run in your extended family—including allergies, asthma, diabetes, heart disease, and high blood pressure—that might be important for your pediatrician to know about.

benefits manager. All plans limit some services (e.g., mental health services, home health services), so find out what's covered and what's not.

- When you are part of a managed care plan, primary and preventative care visits usually will be covered, including well-child checkups, treatment for illnesses or injuries, and immunizations. In many plans, you will have a co-payment—a fixed charge that you pay—for each primary care visit.

- Once you've chosen a pediatrician, it's best to stay with her. But if you feel the need to switch, all plans allow you to select another doctor from among those who are part of their network. The plan administrator can give you information on how to make this change. Some plans allow you to switch only during certain periods, called open enrollment.

■ If you feel that your child needs to see a pediatric subspecialist, work with your pediatrician to find one who is part of your plan, and obtain approval to schedule an appointment with her. Check your plan contract for details about whether your insurer will pay at least a portion of these costs. Also, if hospital care is needed, seek your pediatrician's guidance in selecting a hospital in your plan that specializes in the care of children. Most hospital procedures and surgeries require prior approval.

■ Know in advance what emergency services are covered, since you won't always have time to contact your pediatrician. Most managed care plans will pay for emergency room care in a true emergency, so in a life-threatening situation, go immediately to the nearest hospital. In general, follow-up care (e.g., removing stitches) should be done in your pediatrician's office.

■ To file a complaint—for example, if coverage of certain procedures is denied—start by expressing your concern to your pediatrician. If she is unable to resolve the problem, contact your plan's member service representative or your employer's employee benefits manager about filing a com-

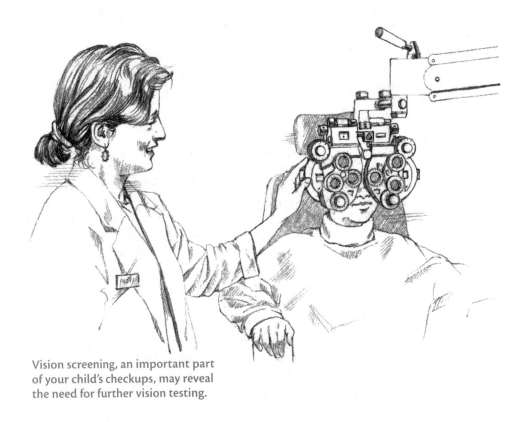

Vision screening, an important part of your child's checkups, may reveal the need for further vision testing.

plaint. If a claim has been denied, you typically have fifteen to thirty days to file an appeal, and you could receive a decision about the appeal within thirty to ninety days of the request. If you still are dissatisfied, you may decide to seek help from the office of your state insurance commissioner, or you can take legal action.

Resolving Problems

Your child can continue to be treated by a pediatrician through adolescence. However, no matter how carefully you have made your choice of a pediatrician, sometimes the chemistry between doctor and patient or between doctor and parent may become less than ideal. After several office visits you may decide that your expectations are not being met. In these instances, make an effort to discuss the problem with the pediatrician. Most difficulties can be smoothed out and resolved. On occasion, you might make a decision to switch physicians if the relationship continues to be unsatisfactory.

When to See Your Pediatrician

The American Academy of Pediatrics recommends that your middle-years child have a routine well-child examination every year. During these doctor's visits, your physician will conduct a number of evaluations, such as measurement of height, weight, and blood pressure, a check of vital functions, a vision and hearing screening, and a complete physical examination. The doctor will ensure that your child's immunizations are up to date, and ask about your child's diet, exercise habits, and sleep patterns. He or she can also refer you to other health professionals; for example, children should receive regular dental checkups twice a year, and if a pediatrician detects eye problems during routine screening, he or she may refer your child to an ophthalmologist for further evaluation and care.

YOUR PEDIATRICIAN IS interested not only in your child's physical health but also in his or her mental and emotional well-being. It is appropriate to discuss such concerns as your child's school experiences, relationships with peers, family transitions or difficulties, and daily stresses.

Health Maintenance

There are many preventative measures that your family can take to reduce your child's risk of illness and injury. As always, encourage your child to use good per-

Yearly Well-Child Visit with Your Pediatrician
(ALSO KNOWN AS HEALTH SUPERVISION VISIT)

Children ages 5–7 years: Annual visits to the pediatrician allow the doctor to monitor prepubertal growth, ensure vaccines are up to date, and assess social and school acclimation.

Children ages 8–10 years: Children this age need annual visits with their doctor. Girls may be showing early signs of puberty. Vaccines prevent infections and disease, and a child's emotional and social development is discussed.

Children ages 11–12 years: These are particularly exciting years for school-age children. At this age kids should see their pediatrician every year. Schools will likely require physical forms and sports forms, and your pediatrician will recommend disease-preventing vaccines based on age and assess your child's growth as she approaches or begins puberty.

sonal hygiene habits: bathing regularly, routinely washing hands before eating and after going to the bathroom to prevent the spread of infectious diseases, brushing teeth at least twice a day, and flossing once a day.

Immunizations

The success of modern vaccines is one of the truly extraordinary accomplishments of medical science. Immunizations are the greatest public health advancement of the twentieth century. In earlier generations many school-age children contracted communicable diseases such as polio and whooping cough (pertussis), frequently with devastating consequences. Some children died; others were left with permanent impairments, perhaps dependent on a wheelchair. But the development of vaccines has made many of these childhood illnesses relatively rare and has thus improved the lifetime health and well-being of millions of people. These immunizations help children build their own defenses against infectious diseases by forming infection-fighting substances called antibodies, which kill the invading bacteria or viruses.

Unfortunately, some parents have become complacent about their children's immunizations. They have erroneously presumed that these serious diseases have disappeared or have been eradicated. Some parents are concerned by reports of possible side effects associated with certain vaccines. Despite the accessibility of information on the internet, parents need to be able to distinguish quality health information from inaccurate claims that are not backed by scientific investigation. Anecdotes circling on social media platforms do not trump scientific research findings.

The risks of not receiving immunizations are immense. As a responsible parent, *you need to ensure that your child receives all of the currently recommended vaccines*. Today's vaccines are extensively tested and safe, and they generally produce only mild side effects (such as fever or localized redness at the injection site). Severe adverse reactions are extremely rare. See the vaccine schedule on page 634 for more information.

For maximum effectiveness, immunizations should be administered at specific times to protect those particular ages. Based on recommendations from the Centers for Disease Control and Prevention and the American Academy of Pediatrics, your pediatrician can advise you as to when your child should receive immunizations.

Many of the recommended immunizations are given in the infant and toddler years, prior to starting school. On or after the fourth birthday, prior to entering school, children should receive booster doses of diphtheria, tetanus, and pertussis (DTaP); polio; measles, mumps, and rubella (MMR); and varicella (chicken pox) vaccines. If your school-age child has not received these booster immunizations, they should be given promptly. An additional Tdap (tetanus, diphtheria, and pertussis) booster is recommended at age 10, and then every ten years. At age 11 years, the meningococcal and human papilloma virus (HPV) vaccine series are recommended, with a meningococcal booster at 16 or 17 years.

Because scientific research continues to develop new and improved ways to protect children from serious diseases, immunization guidelines will continue to evolve. Talk with your pediatrician about her recommendations for your child. Here are some of the current recommendations for middle childhood:

- **MMR booster.** Every child should have an initial measles, mumps, and rubella vaccine at 12 months of age, with a second booster dose given at 4 to 6 years of age. In recent years, physicians have become particularly concerned about outbreaks of measles. Measles is the most infectious of the vaccine-preventable diseases, and outbreaks of measles are an unfortunate result of a decrease in immunization rates in a community, putting children, especially infants too young to receive certain vaccines and those who medically cannot receive vaccines (such as a child receiving chemotherapy or who has undergone organ transplantation), at risk.

- **Pneumococcal vaccine.** This vaccine can prevent meningitis and pneumonia caused by *Streptococcus pneumoniae* bacteria. Previously healthy children can develop a serious illness from these bacteria. Thanks to the success of this vaccine, research has shown that *Streptococcus pneumoniae* is no longer the most common cause of ear infections and pneumonia. All babies, toddlers, and young children should receive multiple doses of the pneumococcal vaccine that covers thirteen different serotypes (PCV13). Children above the age of 2 years with certain conditions or diseases are more vulnerable and thus should be vaccinated with pneumococcal polysaccharide (PPSV23). These high-risk children include those with chronic lung disease or sickle cell disease, or those who have had their spleens removed (either because of an accident or as part of the treatment for certain illnesses). This pneumococcal inoculation also is advised for children whose immune system is suppressed, either because of cancer treatments or because of medications that have weakened their immunity.

- **Influenza vaccination.** An annual flu shot each fall is recommended for all children above the age of 6 months. Influenza can cause serious illness or even death in previously healthy children. The flu vaccine is especially recommended for those whom an infection by the influenza virus would be particularly severe, including those with heart disease, an impaired immune system, chronic lung disease (including asthma and cystic fibrosis), and abnormalities of hemoglobin, the substance that carries oxygen in the blood. The siblings and parents of these children also should be vaccinated.

- **Chicken pox (varicella) vaccination.** A vaccine to protect against chicken pox is recommended for all healthy children between 12 and 18 months of age who have never had the disease, with a booster dose after the fourth birthday. Certain children are at a higher risk of developing severe problems from varicella infection, including children who are under one year of age, have weak immune systems, have eczema and other skin conditions, or are adolescents. Children over age 13 who have not had varicella (chicken pox) should receive two doses of the vaccine, one month apart.

- **Hepatitis B vaccine.** A vaccine series to prevent hepatitis B is recommended to be given to children during their first year of life. Hepatitis B is a viral illness that affects the liver. Infected children can have no symptoms or a mild illness; however, hepatitis B, especially if long-standing, can progress to severe liver disease and can lead to the development of liver cancer. The virus can be passed from mother to infant at the time of birth or from one household member to another via saliva. It can be spread through contact with infected blood from contaminated needles or contaminated surgical or dental instruments. Teenagers can also contract this disease through sexual intercourse.

Most children in their middle years will have received hepatitis B immunization during infancy. Children who have not been vaccinated may begin the three-dose series during any childhood visit to their pediatrician. Because adolescence is a time of increased risk of contracting hepatitis B, it is important that children are completely immunized by age 13. The second dose is ordinarily given at least one month after the first, and the third dose is administered at least four months after the first dose and at least two months after the second.

■ **Human papilloma virus (HPV) vaccine.** HPV is a virus that can cause genital and oral warts in both males and females, and can lead to cervical, oropharyngeal (mouth and pharynx), and other cancers. Many parents wonder why an 11-year-old requires a vaccine that protects against an infection spread by sexual contact; parents should know that research studies have shown that the HPV vaccine gives a much stronger immune boost when given to 11- and 12-year-olds, rather than waiting until after 15 or 16 years of age. Rates of HPV nationally have declined significantly thanks to the success of the vaccine. If this vaccine is given starting at 11 years of age, two doses spaced six months apart are needed. A third dose is needed if the child is over the age of 15 years.

■ **Meningococcal vaccine.** An initial dose is recommended at 11 years with a booster at 16 years. This vaccine helps prevent meningitis, an infection of

WHERE WE STAND

The American Academy of Pediatrics believes that the benefits of immunizations far outweigh the risks incurred by childhood diseases, as well as any risks from the vaccines themselves. The AAP believes that immunizations are the safest and most cost-effective way of preventing disease, disability, and death, and it urges parents to ensure that their children are immunized against dangerous childhood diseases in a timely fashion.

The middle school years provide an opportunity to protect against certain infections that can impact the rest of your child's life—for example, the human papilloma virus. Scheduling regular health maintenance visits with your pediatrician ensures that you will learn about the most up-to-date, recommended immunizations to keep your child healthy for decades to come.

the fluid surrounding the brain and spinal cord. Meningococcal disease can be devastating, resulting in permanent disability or death.

- **Hepatitis A vaccine.** Children above the age of 12 months should receive two doses of hepatitis A vaccine spaced six months apart. Hepatitis A is a liver virus that is spread via the fecal-oral route—in other words, by eating contaminated food. Domestic outbreaks can occur with fruit or other produce, and international travelers are strongly recommended to receive this vaccine.

- **Tetanus, diphtheria, and acellular pertussis vaccine (Tdap).** Infants and toddlers receive a different version of this vaccine, and children 10 years and older should receive a dose every ten years. Tetanus causes infection by contaminated soil, most commonly with puncture wounds, and can cause debilitating illness.

Your Child's Teeth

Good oral hygiene is very important. A child in the middle years who ignores the day-to-day care of his teeth—including brushing them at least twice a day and flossing once a day—runs the risk of tooth decay, toothaches, and lost teeth.

Your child may need some help brushing until he is between ages 7 and 10. Even if his intentions are good, he may not have the dexterity to clean his teeth well. You might consider an electric toothbrush for additional motion and keeping a child's interest. Ideally, the teeth should be brushed within five to ten minutes after eating. Also, for long-term dental health, your child needs to care for his gums as well; he should be taught to floss regularly, preferably once a day, in order to help prevent periodontal (gum) disease in adulthood.

A tartar-control toothpaste can help keep plaque from adhering to your child's teeth. Also, fluoride in the toothpaste can strengthen the exposed outer enamel of the child's teeth and help prevent cavities. Fluoride also has been added to the water supply in most cities. If your own tap water has less than the recommended levels of this nutrient, or if your home uses well water, your pediatrician may suggest that you add fluoride to your child's diet beginning at age 6 months, often as part of a vitamin supplement.

Your dentist may also suggest placing sealants on your child's molars. Sealants may need to be reapplied during adolescence. With a combination of sealants and fluoride treatment, the incidence of cavities can be reduced by 90 percent.

Diet can also play a role in healthy teeth. In particular, minimize your child's contact with high-sugar and sticky sweets and other carbohydrates. Gummy-type

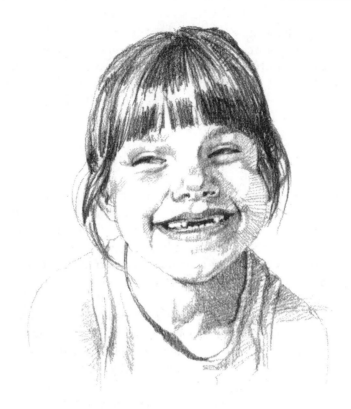

fruit snacks, or even gummy vitamins, can get stuck in teeth and contribute to dental decay. Cut back on snacking on sweets between meals, when these foods are more likely to linger in the mouth without brushing.

Make sure your child has dental checkups twice a year for cleaning, as well as for X-rays as recommended by your dentist. Parents may choose to utilize a pediatric dentist, a dentist with special interest and expertise in children's dentistry. Regular preventive appointments will significantly decrease your child's chances of having to undergo major dental treatment. Also, contact your dentist whenever your child complains of a toothache. This pain could be a sign of a decayed tooth. Until the dentist can see your child, treat the pain with acetaminophen by mouth.

Erupting permanent teeth cause the roots of baby teeth to be reabsorbed so that by the time they are loose there is little holding them in place besides a small amount of tissue. Baby teeth ordinarily are shed first at about age 6 when the incisors, the middle teeth in front, become loose. Molars, in the back, are usually shed between ages 10 and 12, and are replaced with permanent teeth by about age 13. Children usually wiggle their teeth loose with their tongues or fingers, eager to hide them under their pillow for the Tooth Fairy. If your child wants you to pull out the already-loose tooth, grasp it firmly with a piece of tissue or gauze and remove it with a quick twist. Occasionally, if a primary tooth is not loosening sufficiently on its own, your child's dentist may suggest extracting it.

Around the time of puberty, parents begin to worry about whether their child has an adequate bite and whether his teeth are symmetrical. Your dentist is an excellent source of information about whether a consultation with an orthodontist is advisable.

Children ages 5–7 years: Ensure that children brush their teeth morning and evening, ideally after meals. Kids this age brush better when dental care is fun—a reluctant brusher may benefit from an electric toothbrush meant for kids that lights up for the length of time needed to brush. Dental visits every six months are an important aspect of good oral care. Cavities of baby teeth *can* impact later dental health.

Children ages 8–10 years: While more independent, children between 8 and 10 still require parental monitoring and guidance. Ensure your kids have developed a flossing habit; kids' flossers, plastic single-use flossing devices, help small hands maintain this healthy habit.

Children ages 11–12 years: Kids in this age group may require orthodontia, which makes proper oral care all the more important. Your dental and orthodontic teams will have special instructions on how to properly clean orthodontic work. Twice-a-year visits to the dentist continue to be important.

~ 2 ~

Nutrition

PROPER NUTRITION IS one of the most important influences on your child's well-being. A varied, balanced diet—containing vitamins, minerals, protein, carbohydrates, and healthy fats—promotes growth, energy, and overall health. Food preferences are developed early in life, mostly during early and middle childhood. The earlier you encourage healthful food choices for your child, the better his lifelong eating habits will be.

From early on, your child learns from your example and watches you for clues to proper food choices. She will copy many of your habits, likes, and dislikes. During the middle years, the model you provide at home will be extremely important in both guiding and reinforcing good eating habits. However, as children begin to spend many hours a day away from home, in school and with friends, a variety of social and other factors influence what and when children eat. As they hurry to catch the school bus in the morning, they may speed through breakfast. For lunch at school—despite schools' efforts to offer healthy choices—your child might choose high-fat or sugar-laden foods that do not contribute to a balanced diet, or pack processed, simple carbohydrate-rich foods from home. If available, they may choose soft drinks rather than milk, or a candy bar instead of fresh fruit.

The most important step a family can take in order to eat healthfully is to prepare simple meals together at home. Cooking at home is well worth the time investment of planning, buying groceries, and actual meal preparation. Families who cook together pass along healthy eating habits to their children. Food cooked at home often has less fat and salt than food from a fast-food drive-through lane or a restaurant. Kids reinforce their math and science lessons from school by cooking, and learn important life skills of meal preparation. By 10, 11, and 12 years of age, children should have more independence in the kitchen and be able to prepare a simple meal or sandwich for themselves.

Monitoring Nutritional Needs

In general, it is the parents' job to determine *what* and *when* the child eats, and the child is in the best position to decide *how much* to eat. Normally, healthy and active children's bodies do a good job of "asking" for just the right amount of food, although their minds may lead them astray when choosing which foods to eat. You can easily overestimate the amount of food your child actually needs, especially during the younger years of middle childhood. Children this age typically do not need adult-size servings of food. It is best to avoid making mealtimes a battleground, as well as avoid any rules about "cleaning" one's dinner plate by eating everything on it. Mealtime should be a pleasant and social time to not only nourish the body but also nurture communication and relationships within the family to reconnect after a busy day of school, work, and activities.

Regular checkups with your pediatrician are one way for you to monitor your child's nutrition. There is rarely a reason for you to count calories for your children, since they tend to control their intake quite well. As the middle years progress, children's total energy needs will increase and thus their food intake will rise, especially as they approach puberty. Between ages 7 and 10, both boys and girls consume about 1,600 to 2,400 calories per day, although caloric needs obviously vary considerably even under normal circumstances. Most girls experience a significant increase in their growth rate between ages 10 and 12 and will take in about 200 calories more each day, while boys go through their growth spurt about two years later and increase their food intake by nearly 500 calories a day. During this time of rapid growth, they will probably require more total calories and nutrients than at any other period in their lives—from calcium (to encourage bone growth) to protein (to build body tissue).

Appetites can vary, even from day to day, depending on factors such as that day's activity level. Every child's caloric needs are different. A child also may go through what some call "food jags" where one day she eats more protein and another day is focused on fruits, for example. One meal or one day may not be nutritionally complete, but the week as a whole may still have good representation from a variety of food groups. Sweets and higher-fat choices should not be forbidden; rather, they should be a special "once-in-a-while" treat, served in moderation using appropriate portion sizes.

Picky Eaters

Some children simply do not eat as much as their peers. Their appetite may not be as large, or they may be selective or "finicky" eaters, unwilling to even taste certain types of foods. Appetites may fluctuate as your child grows. Even within the same family, brothers and sisters may vary considerably in the amounts and types of food they desire. Generally, children increase their food consumption considerably as they enter the growth spurts associated with puberty; until then, however, a child's appetite may be unpredictable.

Some children are less open to trying new foods than others. Most important is exposing your children to a variety of tastes and flavors from a young age. If the family is having a certain meal for dinner, that should serve as the main meal. Avoid the temptation to be a short-order cook and prepare a separate meal for your selective eater, as this perpetuates the picky eater cycle. Try introducing new foods as part of familiar foods that your child already enjoys. Look at cookbooks together, grocery shop together, and involve your child in the meal preparation process. Many kids end up nibbling on vegetables as they are being prepped for the main meal. Children who participate in the cooking process in an age-appropriate way are more likely to try new foods. By letting kids work in the kitchen, smelling and tasting new foods, you can help kids feel more comfortable trying new foods, which can help build healthy habits and teach them to make healthier food choices too.

Avoid rewards or strong, coercive encouragement for trying something new. If you introduce foods in a confrontational way, you and your child may become caught up in a battle, and your child will likely resist these foods even more as a way of asserting her independence. Offering rewards for particular foods may give your child the impression that the food would otherwise be undesirable.

As frustrating as your child's picky eating habits may be, keep in mind that you, too, may have foods you like and dislike. It is important for parents to remain calm at mealtimes, as drama at the dinner table will only perpetuate the problem. A daily multivitamin may put some of your fears to rest and help you relax and enjoy mealtimes more, which will help your child feel comfortable experimenting with new foods.

Healthy Food Choices
Variety and Portions

Your child should consume a variety of fruits and vegetables, grains, proteins, and dairy. Each food group supplies important nutrients, including vitamins and minerals. The USDA has replaced the former "food pyramid" format with the Choose My Plate format (ChooseMyPlate.gov; see graphic below), which visually shows the ideal distribution and portions of foods for a typical meal, representing all five food groups. Half of the plate should consist of fruits and vegetables, a quarter should be protein, a quarter should be grains (preferably whole grains), and a side of dairy rounds out the meal.

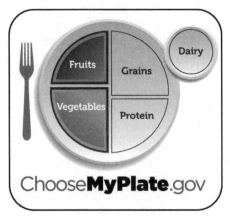

Teach your child the importance of eating a variety of foods from the five major food groups, in appropriate portion sizes.

- **Vegetables:** 3–5 servings per day. A serving may consist of 1 cup of raw leafy vegetables or ½ cup of other vegetables, raw or cooked.

- **Fruits:** 2–4 servings per day. A serving may consist of ½ cup of sliced fruit or a medium-size whole fruit, such as an apple, banana, or pear.

- **Bread, cereal, or pasta:** 2–3 servings per day. Aim for whole grains whenever possible for the added fiber. Each serving should equal 1 slice of bread, ½ cup of rice or pasta, or 1 ounce of cereal.

- **Proteins:** 2–3 servings of 2–3 ounces of cooked lean meat, poultry, or fish per day. A serving in this group may also consist of ½ cup of cooked beans or 1 egg.

- **Dairy products:** 2–3 servings per day of 1 cup of low-fat milk or yogurt, or 1½ ounces of cheese.

- **Water:** Proper hydration is important! Often thirst can mimic the feeling of hunger. Ensure kids are drinking plenty of water throughout the day, regardless of the season or activity levels. School-age kids should bring re-fillable water bottles to school and sip throughout the day. Many schools have installed automatic water bottle fillers similar to those found in airports.

Fiber

Fiber is a carbohydrate component of plant foods that is usually indigestible. It is found in foods like fruits, vegetables, whole-grain breads, cereals, brown rice, beans, seeds, and nuts. A diet high in fiber has been linked with a reduction of chronic gastrointestinal problems, including colon cancer, irritable bowel syndrome, and diverticulitis. Fiber also helps ease constipation—providing bulk that can promote regular frequency of bowel movements, soften the stools, and decrease the time it takes food to travel through the intestines.

Protein

Your child requires protein for the proper growth and functioning of his body, including building new tissues and producing antibodies that help battle infections. Without essential amino acids (the building blocks of protein), children would be much more susceptible to serious diseases. Protein-rich plants—such as dried beans and peas (legumes), grains, seeds, and nuts—can be used as valuable sources of protein. Other protein-rich foods include meat, fish, milk, yogurt, cheese, and eggs. These animal products contain high-quality protein and a full array of amino acids.

Bear in mind, however, that red meat and shellfish not only are rich in protein and an important source of iron but are higher in fat and cholesterol as well. Thus, your child should consume them only in moderate amounts. Select lean cuts of meat and trim the fat before cooking. Likewise, remove skin from poultry and excess fat from fish before serving.

Healthy Fats

Dietary fats are a concentrated source of energy, providing essential fatty acids that are necessary for a variety of bodily processes such as metabolism, blood clotting, and vitamin absorption. However, high fat intake—particularly a diet

Healthy Family Eating Habits

Family eating habits determine what your child will learn to eat and enjoy.

- Keep fresh fruits and vegetables readily available. Parents can maintain a stocked fruit bowl in the kitchen with apples, bananas, and oranges in sight as a visual reminder, ready for snacking. Clementines are easy for school-age kids to peel independently. Grapes, washed and ready to eat, are another example of a healthy grab-and-go snack. Kids can enjoy fruit and vegetable snacks freely through the day without limitations.

- Serve whole-grain bread and cereals.

- Skim or 1 percent milk is preferable to 2 percent or whole milk.

- Limit high-calorie toppings that do not provide additional nutritive value, including butter, sour cream, and gravy.

- Serve lean meats, such as chicken, turkey, fish, lean beef cuts (lean hamburger, top loin, top round, eye of round), and lean pork cuts (tenderloin, loin, chops, ham). Cut away visible fat and remove the skin from poultry.

- Choose frozen fruit bars, angel food cake, or frozen yogurt instead of richer, creamier desserts.

- When cooking, use nonstick vegetable sprays to cut down on added fat.

- Baking, broiling, poaching, grilling, and steaming are good methods of preparing meat, fish, and poultry. Limit the use of extra butter and oils when preparing or serving vegetables.

- Serve vegetable-based and broth-based soups. Choose low-fat milk when making cream soups.

high in *saturated* fats—can cause problems. Saturated fats are usually solid at room temperature and are found in fatty meats (such as beef, pork, ham, veal, and lamb) and many dairy products (whole milk, cheese, and ice cream). They can contribute to the buildup of atherosclerotic plaques in blood vessels and lead to coronary artery disease later in life. A diet rich in saturated fats also can increase blood cholesterol, particularly in people who have inherited a tendency toward high cholesterol levels.

As a general guideline, fats should make up less than 30 percent of the calories in your child's diet, with no more than about one-third of those fat calories coming from saturated fat and the remainder from unsaturated (that is, polyunsaturated or monounsaturated) fats. Oils and fats derived from animal origin are saturated. Avocados and almonds are a good source of heart-healthy monounsaturated fats.

Sugar

Sugar serves an important function for our bodies as the fuel to provide energy for our bodily processes and daily activities. Sugar includes not only the simple table sugars that most of us think of when we hear the word "sugar," but also honey, molasses, and high fructose corn syrup. Sugar naturally occurs in produce, most notably in fruit and berries (where it accounts for the sweet taste) but also in vegetables and milk. Most of us, kids included, prefer the sweet taste of sugar, and modern diets arguably contain too much sugar. Unfortunately, many processed foods, including snack bars and convenience packets of instant oatmeal, include a surprising amount of sugar.

The problem with excessive daily sugar intake is that the excess of calories from sugar can contribute to weight gain, obesity, and a pre-diabetic state (a beginning stage of diabetes; for more on type 2 diabetes, see page 589). Often a diet with excessive sugar is also lacking in other nutrients such as whole grains. How to limit daily sugar intake? A simple step is to avoid juice and soft drinks on a regular basis by limiting their availability to special occasions. Portion control is also smart: when having an ice cream treat, for example, prepare smaller serving sizes by using smaller bowls. Often we are surprised when reading a product's nutrition label by what is considered a true "single serving" amount.

Salt

Researchers have found a relationship between dietary salt and high blood pressure in some individuals and population groups. High blood pressure can contribute to heart attacks and strokes in older adults. The habit of using extra salt is an acquired one. As much as possible, serve your child foods low in salt. In the kitchen, minimize the amount of salt you add to food during its preparation, using herbs, spices, or lemon juice instead. Also, take the salt shaker off the dinner table, or at least limit its use by your family.

Because of the preservative properties of salt, processed foods and fast foods often contain large amounts of it. Salt-rich foods may include processed cheese, instant puddings, canned vegetables, canned soups, hot dogs, cottage cheese, salad dressings, pickles, certain breakfast cereals and snack bars, potato chips, and other snacks.

Vitamin Supplements

Vitamins and minerals are important elements of your child's nutritional requirements. Because the human body itself is unable to produce adequate amounts of many vitamins, they must be obtained from the diet. The body needs these vitamins in only tiny amounts, and in a balanced diet they are usually present in sufficient quantities in the foods your child eats. For these reasons, supplements are rarely needed in middle childhood.

For some children, however, pediatricians may recommend a daily supplement. If your child has a poor appetite or erratic eating habits, or if she consumes a selective diet such as a vegan diet containing no dairy products, a vitamin supplement should be considered. Chewable tablets are available for children who have difficulty swallowing pills. Gummy vitamins can contribute to tooth decay; if these are used, make sure your child brushes her teeth afterward. A daily multivitamin can also help parents feel more relaxed at mealtimes, which will in turn help kids feel more comfortable about trying new foods.

Over-the-counter supplements are generally safe; nonetheless, they are drugs. If

WHERE WE STAND

The American Academy of Pediatrics believes that healthy children receiving a normal, well-balanced diet do not need vitamin supplementation over and above the recommended dietary allowances. Megadoses of vitamins—for example, large amounts of vitamins A, C, or D—can produce toxic symptoms, ranging from nausea and rashes to headaches, and sometimes to even more severe adverse effects. Talk with your pediatrician before giving vitamin supplements to your child.

taken in excessive amounts (in tablets, capsules, or combined with other supplements), some supplements—particularly the fat-soluble vitamins (A, D, E, and K)—can be toxic. Always consult your pediatrician before giving your child supplements. And don't leave a bottle of vitamins on the table as though they were a condiment like salt or pepper; taking vitamins should be done with careful consideration.

Vitamins and minerals found in actual food are more bioavailable to your child's body than those found in a supplement, meaning that it is easier for the body to utilize them. As much as possible, maximize the vitamins your child receives in her regular meals.

Vitamin A promotes normal growth, healthy skin, and tissue repair, and aids in night and color vision. Rich sources include yellow vegetables, dairy products, and liver.

B vitamins promote red blood cell formation and assist in a variety of metabolic activities. They are found in meat, poultry, fish, soybeans, milk, eggs, whole grains, and enriched breads and cereals.

Vitamin C strengthens connective tissue, muscles, and skin, hastens the healing of wounds and bones, and increases resistance to infection. Vitamin C is found in citrus fruits, strawberries, tomatoes, potatoes, Brussels sprouts, spinach, and broccoli.

Vitamin D promotes tooth and bone formation and regulates the absorption of minerals like calcium. Sources include fortified dairy products, fortified orange juice, fish oils, and egg yolks. Sunlight also contributes to dietary sources of vitamin D, stimulating the conversion of a naturally occurring compound in the skin to an active form of the vitamin; however, the risks of sunlight exposure leading to skin cancer outweigh the benefits, so obtaining vitamin D from the diet or vitamin supplementation is the best course of action.

Especially during periods of rapid growth, **iron** is essential for the production of blood and the building of muscles. When iron levels are low, your child may demonstrate symptoms such as irritability, listlessness, depression, and an increased susceptibility to infection. However, a deficiency of iron is much more common in adolescence than in middle childhood. Once girls begin menstruation, they need much more iron than boys do. The best sources of iron include beef, turkey, pork, and liver. Beans and prunes also contain modest amounts of iron. Some cereals and flour are enriched with iron.

As your child matures, **calcium** is necessary for healthy bone development. An inadequate calcium intake during childhood can not only affect present growth but could also contribute to the development of weakened and porous bones (osteoporosis) later in life. Low-fat milk, cheese, yogurt, and sardines are excellent sources of calcium. Some vegetables, such as broccoli, also contain modest amounts of calcium.

Age-Appropriate Kitchen Tasks

There is no better way to get your kids involved in family mealtimes than including them in food preparation. Research shows that kids who regularly eat meals with their family develop good communication skills, are less likely to abuse alcohol and illicit drugs, get better grades in school, and are less likely to be obese. Increased involvement in kitchen preparation is all about baby steps; Rome wasn't built in a day, and kids need to develop cooking skills with smaller tasks at younger ages. In the short term, involving children in meal preparation may seem like *more* work, to clean up the inevitable spills and messes. Teach your kids to clean as they go, though, and over the years their skills will develop and will be more than worth the investment of initiating cooking skills from an early age.

When it comes to kids and kitchen skills, every child is different. While some kids may be able to progress more quickly, consider your individual child's development and maturity to determine the most appropriate tasks and steps.

Children ages 5–7 years: Can you say salad? Kids in this age range can help tear lettuce for salads, mix salad dressing, toss the salad, and set the table. Children in early elementary school grades can wash fruits and vegetables, pick herb leaves off stems, use a salad spinner, and use a citrus juicer for lemons, oranges, and limes. Whisking, stirring, kneading, mashing, rolling with a rolling pin, and spreading glaze with a pastry brush are all fun for kids this age. Kids can sprinkle salt, use a pepper grinder, and break eggs with adult help. Kids this age generally are not ready for true knife usage; some families allow kids this age to use a plastic knife instead, which can get the job done safely.

Children ages 8–10 years: Most children in this age group can perform the above tasks in addition to new tasks, such as measuring ingredients with measuring spoons and cups, and can learn the difference between measuring wet and dry ingredients. With close adult supervision, kids can learn beginner knife skills to slice bread, chop vegetables, and slice fruits, as well as grate and peel produce. A rolling pizza cutter is a great idea to help younger kids learn easy cutting; if you have multiple kids, consider buying more than one for simultaneous use. Kids can help pound chicken layered in plastic wrap. Kids this age should learn the importance of keeping raw meats and poultry separated from produce (e.g., using separate cutting boards) as a way of minimizing bacterial risks and food poisoning. Kids this age can slice and scoop avocado, grate cheese, form patties and evenly sized cookies, use a can opener (a no-sharp-edges can opener is much safer), and scoop batter into muffin tins.

Children ages 11–12 years: Older children can and should have increased responsibilities in the kitchen, including all the above tasks as well as mastering new tasks. The goal for this age group is to advance kitchen skills to the point of working independently (with an adult present nearby who can assist in case of emergency). Good beginner stovetop preparation skills include making simple dishes such as grilled cheese sandwiches and scrambled eggs. Before increasing a child's independence, ensure your child has good stovetop and oven safety techniques (e.g., turns pot handles toward the back of the stovetop to avoid spills), has appropriate knife safety skills, and unplugs electrical appliances when not in use. One of the final kitchen tasks to learn is how to drain a pot of cooked pasta in the sink, being mindful of the burn risks of steam; this step should be modeled and assisted for quite some time before independence.

Reading Food Labels

When grocery shopping, shopping the perimeter of the store is a way to eat healthfully. The perimeter or outside edges of the store is where fresh produce, meats, and dairy are kept; the center aisles are reserved for the prepackaged, processed foods. The best foods to eat—for example, fresh apples—do not require a label with nutritional information on them.

Read product labels to learn the amounts of fat, cholesterol, sodium, vitamins, and minerals, and the percentage of calories from fat. Pay close attention to portion sizes, which can sometimes cause confusion. For example, breakfast cereal packages often provide the nutritional content of the cereal when combined with half a cup of milk; thus, the serving may seem nutritious due to the addition of milk, even though the cereal itself provides little nutritional value. Keep in mind that because these listed portion sizes are arbitrary, they may not be equivalent to the portions actually consumed by your own family. When comparing different products, make sure the portion sizes on the labels are equal, or do some quick refiguring of your own.

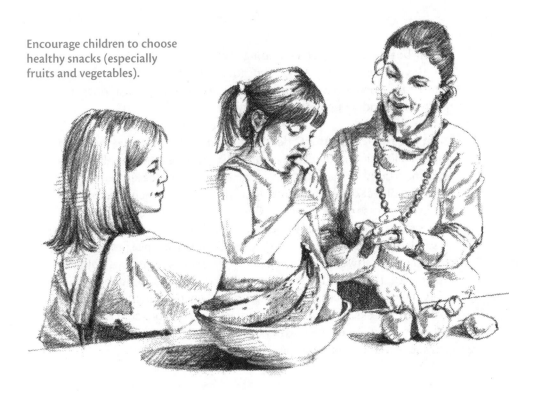

Encourage children to choose healthy snacks (especially fruits and vegetables).

Choosing Healthy Snacks

Many children arrive home from school and head straight to the refrigerator for a snack. Thirst can often feel similar to hunger, so a glass of water is a great first step when returning home after school or activities; drinking water will help curb an excessive appetite. Healthy snacks round out kids' nutritional requirements and provide as much as one-fourth of their calories. In general, occasional snacks will not ruin appetites for regular meals, as long as the snack is not eaten shortly before they sit down to lunch or dinner. Snacks are another opportunity for parents to provide healthy food choices to their children while reinforcing good eating habits—learning to get hungry, rather than eating to feel full all the time.

"Snacks" should not mean only processed, packaged foods; think of them as mini meals with similar nutrient portions as a regular meal. Remember that what is brought home from the grocery store is what will get eaten; if you feel your child excessively prefers a particular processed snack, leave it off your shopping list for a while. There is a difference between special once-in-a-while foods and routine healthy snack options. When snacking, children often reach for the closest

Healthy Snacks for Any Mood

Your child's snacking moods may vary, but he can still consistently maintain healthy snacking habits. Encourage plenty of water throughout the day. For instance, if his snacking mood is:

Thirsty: Water! All of us, kids and adults alike, should drink more water. Other good hydration choices include cold skim or low-fat milk, or water with lemon.

Smooth: Yogurt, banana, papaya, mango, cottage cheese, or a fruit smoothie. For an easy fruit smoothie, blend 1 cup of skim milk, three ice cubes, your favorite fresh fruit, and a dash of vanilla or honey, cinnamon, and nutmeg in a blender.

Crunchy: Raw vegetables (asparagus, bell pepper, broccoli, cabbage, carrots, cauliflower, celery, zucchini), apples, corn on the cob, unbuttered popcorn, puffed-rice cakes, or wheat crackers.

Juicy: Fresh fruit (berries, cantaloupe, grapes, grapefruit, kiwi, nectarine, orange, peach, plum, watermelon, tomato, pear) or frozen juice pops.

Fun: Fruit, frozen grapes, frozen bananas, fruit kabobs.

Really hungry: Hard-boiled eggs, granola, oatmeal, sandwich, cereal with milk, bran muffin, peanut butter or soy nut butter on crackers or bread, nuts, cheese.

convenient food at hand. If your cupboard has cookies in it, that is probably what your child will eat. However, if there are healthier items in the refrigerator or on the kitchen table, your child will become accustomed to snacking on these foods instead. The healthiest and simplest choices are fruits and raw vegetables that require little if any preparation. Encourage your child to make healthy snacks a habit by keeping fruit and cut vegetables (carrots, cucumbers, celery, peppers, broccoli) washed, prepped, and handy. Kids enjoy helping with these preparation steps; for more information on this, see the box above.

Children in the older range of the middle years (10, 11, 12 years) also can learn some simple cooking techniques. As they prepare snacks for themselves, you can teach them to differentiate between more and less healthy choices. However, be sure they learn appropriate safety precautions for the use of a stove, oven, microwave, or other cooking appliance. For more on age-appropriate kitchen tasks, see the box on pages 28–29.

Cooking with Your Children

One of the best ways to familiarize your child with good food choices is to encourage her to cook with you. Let her get involved in the entire process, from planning the menus to shopping for ingredients to the actual food preparation and its serving.

Particularly in her first few efforts at helping in the kitchen, let her select recipes that she and other family members have enjoyed in the past, so she can see what's involved in preparing them. For more on age-appropriate kitchen tasks, see the box on pages 28–29.

In assigning tasks to your child, keep in mind that they need to be age-appropriate. For instance, you wouldn't give a 6-year-old a sharp knife to chop vegetables, although she can certainly wash the lettuce. Nor would you let her remove a hot, heavy casserole pot from the oven, although she can carefully open the oven door for you. Here are some other guidelines to keep in mind:

- Make certain that you or another adult is in the kitchen at all times when your child is helping out.

- When your child pares vegetables, show her how to point sharp edges away from her to avoid accidents.

- Explain how she should weigh and measure ingredients.

- When cooking on the stovetop, make sure that pot handles are turned inward so children can't accidentally knock them off the stove.

- Teach your child the importance of using oven mitts or potholders when touching hot saucepans and other items.

- Shut off the oven and stovetop burners when you're finished cooking.

Cooking at Home Compared to Eating Out

Between work, school, activities, and more, families are busy and cannot always cook at home. Unfortunately, traditional, fast-casual, and fast-food restaurant meals tend to be relatively high in calories, salt, and total fat. Meals prepared at home are typically the healthier option.

Families can use time-saving strategies to prepare meals at home despite a hectic family schedule. Batch meal prep on the weekend is one idea: prepare more than one meal so that it is ready for the hectic weekday. Slow cookers are a useful tool: put ingredients together in the morning and have a prepared meal ready later in the evening. Adding fresh ingredients at the end of the cooking process can liven up a slow cooker meal. Alternatively, pressure cookers can cook meals in a fraction of the time of traditional cooking methods. Use the internet or cookbooks from your public library for new meal ideas to add into your family rotation, and share the cookbooks with your kids for additional inspiration and suggestions.

Children learn most from watching the adults in their world and how they lead by example. Parents should model and encourage healthy eating habits that a child can maintain for decades to come. Practice balance, variety, and moderation in your own and your family's diet, and your children are likely to follow suit.

~ 3 ~

Healthy Nutrition and Specific Considerations

Childhood Obesity: An Epidemic

Studies show that today's children tend to be heavier than their counterparts were a generation ago, and that over 15 percent of America's school-age children are now overweight. Obesity can contribute to physical problems such as high blood pressure and diabetes, limit a child's athletic abilities, and impair self-esteem.

The Body Mass Index (BMI) is a helpful tool to monitor your child's weight at annual visits with the pediatrician. It is a number calculated using the child's weight and height. HealthyChildren.org, the parenting website of the American Academy of Pediatrics, has a BMI calculator available for parents. Growth charts and BMI tell only part of the story because neither method directly measures a child's body fat. That said, subtle shifts and increases in the BMI over the childhood years can indicate that adjustments need to be made in both a child's level of daily activity and her diet. A healthy BMI varies by age; in general, if your child's BMI is less than the 5th percentile or greater than the 85th percentile, your pediatrician will want to discuss this with your family. Generally speaking, a BMI above the 85th percentile means the child is overweight. At times, however, some children who are athletic or muscular may have a higher BMI without having excess fat. Most children with a BMI above the 95th percentile have an excess amount of body fat, however.

What is a reasonable approach to maintain a healthy weight and BMI, or tackle a rising BMI? First, you need to determine if your child is overweight. Talk with your pediatrician, who will consult growth charts to determine the most appropriate target weight range for your child. This ideal range will depend on a number of factors, including your child's sex, age, height, and body build.

Children tend to gain weight at a fairly steady rate through the middle years, with an increase in weight gain and growth during and just prior to puberty. Parents and their children should not become alarmed by this increase in weight. Usually the goal is not necessarily to *lose* weight; rather, it is to *maintain* weight as the child's height increases.

Various factors can influence the likelihood of a child's becoming overweight. A child who is physically inactive is more likely to have a weight problem. Too much screen time (videogames, time spent online social networking, television, etc.) means more time the child is sedentary and less time he is running, playing, and moving muscles (for more information on media use, see page 315). Family genetics play a role as well, and if your family's meals tend to emphasize high-calorie foods, that can cause excess weight gain. Although certain metabolic and

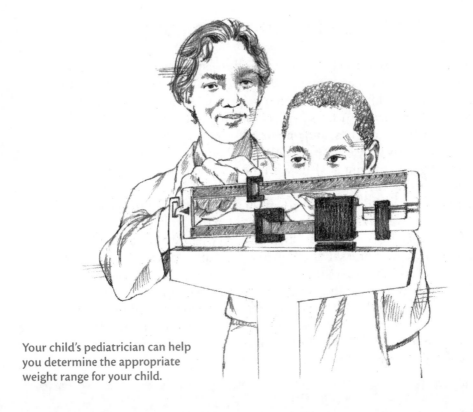

Your child's pediatrician can help you determine the appropriate weight range for your child.

endocrine disorders may contribute to obesity, they are the cause in only about 5 percent of obese children.

Stress can also play a role in some overweight problems. Children often have little control over their lives, and thus have fewer options with which to respond to emotional peaks and valleys. They may be prone to changing the way they eat as their moods and behavior change—for instance, when they are bored, anxious, or depressed.

If your child's BMI is increasing each year, do not ignore the problem. A sedentary lifetime of poor eating habits can increase your child's chances of developing serious diseases that could shorten his life span. Together, you and your child should set realistic goals. In middle childhood, actual weight loss may not be an appropriate objective for many overweight children. The goals you agree upon should not be principally about weight, but rather about *healthy living*—eating appropriate amounts and kinds of food, exercising, and dealing with personal and social factors that encourage poor lifestyle habits. Working together as a family is a great idea. A team approach to more physical movement and improved food choices, as well as agreeing to limit the availability of juice, soda, and other "treat" foods, helps all family members improve their health. Kids always learn best by having a good example set for them.

As part of a comprehensive program, your pediatrician may suggest the *maintenance* of current weight, keeping your child's weight at its present level while he continues to grow in height, thus causing him to slim down. However, for children who are more than 40 percent overweight for their age, sex, and height, your doctor may recommend a comprehensive plan, including dietary changes aimed at small increments of weight loss. Obese children should avoid fad diets and instead consume a variety of foods relatively low in calories but high in nutritional value. Foods like vegetables, fruits, fish, and poultry fit this description. While you can limit portion sizes, do not severely restrict your child's caloric intake or you may run the risk of impeding normal growth.

Support your child by modeling your own good eating habits. Ensure that the foods brought home from the grocery store are healthy options. Cook low-calorie meals for the entire family. You cannot expect your child to successfully change his eating and exercise habits on his own, particularly if others in the household are not setting good examples. Your goal should be to help him learn and adopt healthier *lifetime* eating habits that can keep his weight permanently under control.

A key step in maintaining a healthy BMI is for your child and entire family to become more physically active. The best step of all is to increase time spent simply playing outdoors. Regular exercise can play an important role in the maintenance of a healthy weight over the long term. You can become a good role model for physical activity, even involving your child in your own exercise program, perhaps bicycling, swimming, or brisk walking as a family. Encourage your child to exercise, knowing that as he becomes more physically fit, his overall sense of well-being and his feelings of self-worth are likely to improve.

Physical activity and movement should be *fun* for school-age kids. Formal youth sports programs can be a great source of exercise; however, for most kids, more free time playing outdoors will do the trick. Do not feel the need to invest financially in sports teams; family walks after meals, limiting screen time (no screen time until all homework is completed and time spent playing outside), and setting a timer on screens, television, or other media use are good strategies families should employ.

Families can even make increasing daily movement a friendly competition; there are many low-cost pedometers available, and family members can "compete" to see who can track the most activity each day. Keeping activity *fun* is a key step to nurturing physical fitness as a lifetime healthy habit, not just a temporary measure.

What About a Formal Weight Loss Program?

Many community hospitals and specialized clinics offer formal weight loss programs for children. For some obese children, these programs may be worth considering. The best candidates are children who are at least 30 to 40 percent overweight and who are in basically good health, without any significant physical or psychological problems. Families must be willing to provide support and help their offspring implement and follow through on the eating and exercise plans that are recommended.

When you're evaluating a particular weight loss program, keep in mind that the most effective ones tend to be those that help children adopt long-term, lifestyle-based behavioral strategies. Doing so in a group setting not only provides support but helps your child develop her social skills too. These programs also should help a child increase her physical activity.

As children enter a program, they should be assessed by a variety of health professionals. The best weight loss programs include one or more registered dietitians or qualified nutritionists, exercise physiologists, pediatricians or family physicians, and psychiatrists or psychologists. A pediatrician should document that the child has sufficient excess weight to warrant her participation and to confirm that she has no significant underlying health problems. A nutritionist or registered dietitian should determine what the child's nutritional habits are and create a personalized eating plan. A psychologist or other mental health professional should evaluate your child to identify any existing psychological difficulties, as well as to determine whether family problems may be interfering with the child's efforts at weight control.

Once your child begins participation in a formal weight loss program, her success will require you to make certain aspects of the program part of your family's day-to-day life—from making sensible food choices to encouraging the entire family to become more physically active together. Also, with guidance from the program's staff, encourage your child to set reasonable, short-term (week-by-week) goals that she has a high likelihood of achieving. Changes in eating and exercising—and the accompanying improvements in weight—should be slow and gradual.

Rewards (ideally not money or material items, but rather experiences) should

Elements of a Weight Control Program

Here are some sensible guidelines for healthy weight management:

- Have your child participate in daily vigorous physical activity, sufficient to increase his heart rate and make him sweat. Free time spent playing outdoors is best. It does not need to be a specific amount of continuous time; ten-minute bursts sprinkled through the day can actually be an easier goal to set and maintain. He can try fast walking, jogging, bicycling, and skating. Team sports are fun, but not all team sports are vigorous enough to be sufficient alone for weight management.

- Monitor your child's diet by writing down what he eats and drinks. Review this record together each day, and find foods that he could eliminate by substituting healthier choices. Add more vegetables and fiber to his diet, and use fruits as desserts rather than cake, pie, cookies, pudding, and ice cream. Watch the portion size of each serving, and avoid second helpings.

- Support your child's efforts by eliminating undesirable foods from the household. "Cleaning up" the food environment is critical. Keeping high-calorie foods in the house for special occasions or for other family members is cruel and will undermine the child's efforts.

- As a parent, positive praise goes a lot further than negative reinforcement. You are not the "food police," and thus you should not remind, nag, or scold your child. If you yourself practice healthier habits and keep undesirable foods out of the house, it will make it easier for the entire family to do together.

be given immediately upon achieving the goals rather than setting them off in the distance (such as a visit to the amusement park next month, or a trip next summer). The best rewards are those that provide the child with additional, enjoyable times with the family, such as outings and sports activities.

High Blood Cholesterol Levels

Atherosclerosis (fatty plaque formation and hardening of the arteries) has initial stages in childhood that progress as a child grows into adulthood. The physiological processes that cause plaques to form on the walls of the arteries, clogging the arteries and thus interfering with blood flow, begin in childhood. Blood cholesterol levels may be one indicator of this ongoing disease process.

High levels of total cholesterol and of low-density lipoprotein (LDL or "bad") cholesterol are associated with a higher risk of atherosclerosis. *Low* levels of high-density lipoprotein (HDL or "good") cholesterol are also associated with developing atherosclerosis, while having increased amounts of this HDL cholesterol is protective. Though high blood levels of LDLs promote the deposit of cholesterol and other fatty substances in the walls of the arteries, HDLs act as scavengers in the bloodstream, removing the cholesterol that could damage the arteries.

WHERE WE STAND

The American Academy of Pediatrics recommends that all children between 9 and 11 years old be screened for high blood cholesterol levels. Other children may also need cholesterol testing during the school years:

- Children whose parents have had a heart attack by their 50s

- Children whose families have high cholesterol

- Children whose family history is not known

- Children who show signs of heart disease such as obesity or high blood pressure

Cholesterol Levels in Children and Adolescents		
Classification	Total Cholesterol[a]	Low-Density Lipoprotein[a]
Acceptable	< 170	< 110
Borderline	170–199	110–129
High	> 200	> 130
[a] Milligrams per 100 ml of blood		

The treatment of high cholesterol depends on if it is inherited from the family or is due to lifestyle patterns such as diet and exercise. Detecting cholesterol issues early is important to begin treatment and minimize the chances of long-term problems.

Food Allergies

For information about living with food allergies, see page 484.

Vegetarians and Vegans

In recent years, vegetarianism has grown in popularity for both nutritional and ethical reasons. Vegetarian diets tend to be high in fiber and polyunsaturated fat, and low in cholesterol and calories. If your family or child is following a vegetarian diet, you need to guard against nutritional deficiencies. There are various degrees of vegetarianism, and the strictness of the diet will determine whether your child is vulnerable to nutritional shortcomings.

Following are the common categories of vegetarians. Although none eat meat, poultry, or fish, there are other areas in which they vary:

- **Lacto-ovo-vegetarians** consume eggs, dairy products, and plant foods.

- **Lacto-vegetarians** eat dairy products and plant foods but not eggs.

- **Vegans** eat only plant foods, no eggs or dairy products.

Children can be well nourished on all three types of vegetarian diet, but nutritional balance is difficult to achieve if dairy products and eggs are completely eliminated. Vegetarians sometimes consume insufficient amounts of calcium and vitamin D if they remove milk products from their diet. Because of the lack of meat products, vegetarians sometimes have an inadequate iron intake. They may also consume insufficient amounts of vitamin B_{12}, zinc, and other minerals. If their caloric intake is also extremely low, this could cause a delay in normal growth and weight gain.

Vegetarians may also lack adequate protein sources. As a result, you need to ensure that your child receives a good balance of essential amino acids. As a general guideline, his protein intake should come from more than one source, combining cereal products (wheat, rice) with legumes (dry beans, soybeans, peas), for example; when eaten together, they provide a higher quality mixture of amino acids than if either is consumed alone.

Other planning may be necessary. To ensure adequate levels of vitamin B_{12}, you might serve your child commercially prepared foods fortified with this vitamin. While calcium is present in some vegetables, your child may still need a calcium supplement if he does not consume milk and other dairy products. Alternative sources of vitamin D might also be advisable if there is no milk in the diet. Your pediatrician may recommend iron supplements, too, although your child can improve his absorption of the iron in vegetables by drinking citrus juice at mealtime.

Nutrition and Sports

Even in middle childhood some kids who participate in competitive sports are looking for an edge that might make them run a little faster or throw a little harder. Often they will turn to nutrition for help. However, there is no magical food or supplement that can transform an average athlete into a superstar. No matter what age your child is, optimal performance depends more on a balanced diet, sufficient nutrients to meet the demands of physical activity, and adequate rest. Sports activities may require increases in:

- **Caloric (energy) intake.** Without adequate calories your child may feel weak and fatigued, and her athletic performance may suffer. To raise caloric consumption, your child should rely primarily upon carbohydrates (potatoes, rice, pasta, beans, bread), which are excellent sources of energy during exercise.

- **Protein intake.** The protein needs of an athlete may be only a little higher than those of a more sedentary individual. Even so, some evidence suggests that a small increase in protein, in conjunction with exercise, may be important when trying to increase muscle mass and lean tissue. Often, simply by increasing caloric intake in a well-balanced diet, a child will obtain any additional protein she may require. In general, protein supplementation is discouraged for children, as it may burden a growing child's kidneys.

■ **Fluid intake.** During exercise, you perspire and can lose fluid that must be replaced to prevent dehydration and overheating. Children should drink plenty of water before exercising, and then drink again every ten to twenty minutes during exercise itself, even if they are not thirsty. This is particularly important when exercising in hot weather.

Fluid intake needs can vary widely from child to child, based on his or her body size, level of physical activity, and the weather. These requirements generally range from 1½ to 3 quarts per day of fluid; your child should drink an extra 8 to 12 ounces of water for every half hour of strenuous physical activity.

Thanks to persuasive advertising, many children and coaches believe that commercially prepared electrolyte or sports drinks have some advantages over water. These drinks do provide some replacement for the salts and sugars that are lost with vigorous exercise. However, they may be high in sugar, which can sometimes cause cramps, nausea, and diarrhea. Water is usually the best choice.

If your child is involved in a sport where his weight is important—perhaps wrestling or gymnastics—he might be drawn to unhealthy weight management strategies, perhaps adopting a crash diet, taking laxatives, or consuming special supplements. Wrestlers, for example, in an attempt to "make weight," may be tempted to fast, which is potentially harmful. You might choose to consult your child's pediatrician or a registered dietitian to evaluate the adequacy of your child's diet. The doctor will probably advise against rapid reduction in body weight.

~ 4 ~

Physical Fitness and Sports

DAILY PHYSICAL ACTIVITY is a habit that kids should develop from a young age. Children who exercise daily are more likely to maintain this healthy lifestyle for many decades. Physical fitness is a stress reliever, helps kids stay focused, develops both large and small muscle groups, enhances coordination, and is just plain fun! The benefits of fitness and daily activity extend beyond the physical; research indicates daily activity helps kids' ability to concentrate and focus on academic pursuits. Engaging in physical activity with your child is an excellent way to connect and establish a healthy habit for the whole family. Younger kids benefit most from simple free play outdoors. Older kids may benefit from organized sports or school programs. Schools should protect children's structured recess time during the school day. Just as adults can refresh and rejuvenate with a simple walk outdoors, the same holds true for kids.

Physical Activity as a Way of Life

Kids benefit from more time spent in unstructured play, ideally outdoors, and less time spent sedentary (sitting on the couch watching television, playing videogames, or engaging in other types of screen time). The family goal should be increased movement, and there is no better movement than kids engaging in free play outdoors. When the activity is fun and kid-directed, this can be the best exercise of all.

Physical activity should be as routine a part of children's lives as eating and sleeping. Physical activities such as cycling (always with a helmet), swimming, basketball, walking briskly, dancing, and soccer are fun and promote health. Some sports, like baseball, that require only sporadic activity are beneficial in a number of ways, but have different levels of sustained physical exertion.

Every day, children should be exerting themselves a minimum of thirty to sixty minutes a day. These minutes do not need to be continuous; shorter, intense bursts do provide the health benefits of a sustained longer burst of physical activity. More formal exercise ideally should be preceded and followed by a gradual warm-up and cool-down period, allowing muscles, joints, and the cardiovascular system to ease into and out of vigorous activity, thus helping to guarantee a safe workout. This can be accomplished by a general warm-up for a few minutes before and stretching after exercise.

Physical activity can be healthful in the following ways:

Increase cardiovascular endurance. Regular physical activity can help protect against heart disease later in life. Exercise can improve your child's fitness, make him feel better, and strengthen his cardiovascular system. Exercise also releases the body's natural endorphins for an emotional boost and mood lifter; see "Reduce Stress" opposite.

Aerobic activity can make the heart pump more efficiently, thus reducing the incidence of high blood pressure. It can also raise blood levels of HDL (high-density lipoprotein) cholesterol, the "good" form of cholesterol that removes excess fats from the bloodstream. Even though most cardiovascular diseases are thought to be illnesses of adulthood, fatty deposits have been detected in the arteries of children as young as age 3, and high blood pressure exists in about 3 to 5 percent of children.

Improve core muscle strength, large muscle strength, and endurance. As your child's muscles become stronger, he will be able to exercise for longer periods of time, as well as protect himself from injuries—strong muscles provide better support for the joints. Kid-friendly yoga and Pilates are both excellent boosts for flexibility and core body strength. Modified sit-ups (knees bent, feet on the ground) can build up abdominal muscles, increase lung capacity, and protect against back injuries. For upper body strength, he can perform modified pull-ups (keeping the arms flexed while hanging from a horizontal bar) and modified push-ups (positioning the knees on the ground while extending the arms at the elbow).

Increase flexibility. For complete physical fitness, children need to be able to twist and bend their bodies through the full range of normal motions without overexerting themselves or causing injury. Flexibility encourages agility.

In most stretching exercises, your child should stretch to a position where he begins to feel tightness but not pain, then hold steady for twenty to thirty seconds before relaxing. He should not bounce as he stretches, since this can cause injury to the muscles or tendons. Yoga and Pilates both help with flexibility.

Maintain proper weight. Approximately 15 percent of children in the pre-puberty years are overweight, with a higher percentage in Hispanic and black populations. Oftentimes, few of these kids are physically active. Time spent in the fresh air outdoors playing not only strengthens muscles and boosts the cardiovascular system but also is time that the child is not sedentary and bored, reaching for a sweet treat to pass the time. Exercise can effectively burn calories and fat.

Ask your pediatrician to help you determine whether your child has a healthy percentage of body fat for his age and sex. (For a more complete discussion of weight problems, see page 35.)

Reduce stress. Unmanaged stress can cause muscle tightness, which can contribute to headaches, stomachaches, and other types of discomfort. Your child needs to learn not only to recognize stress in his body but also to defuse it effectively. Exercise is one of the best ways to control stress. Physical activity releases the body's natural endorphins, which is a natural mood-lifter. A physically active child is less likely to experience stress-related symptoms than his more sedentary peers. (For more information, see "Stress and Your Child" on page 565.)

Enhance the brain's ability to focus. Research studies indicate that children who engage in regular daily activity have an improved ability to focus and concentrate in an academic setting. Schools with regular outdoor recess help kids maximize the time spent in academic pursuits. Simply an hour a day spent in group physical activity was shown to enhance cognitive performance and brain function during tasks requiring greater executive control. Physical exercise boosts brain health as well as benefiting the body.

Recreational League, Park District, and Formal Club Sport Programs

Organized sports can contribute to physical fitness and develop basic motor skills. Participation in a sports activity suited to your child's capabilities can also boost self-confidence, enhance social development, teach the importance of teamwork and sportsmanship, develop leadership skills, and help her deal with both success and failure. By participating in sports and general play activities, children often find exercise enjoyable and are more likely to establish lifelong habits of healthful exercise. There are many ways for children to be fit and become active without participating in a team sport. Individual sports such as competitive swimming and cross-country are excellent choices, as the child can compete with herself to achieve her personal best effort and performance.

The goals of participating in any youth athletic program should be to have fun, socialize, and improve overall fitness. Before your child enters a youth sports program, evaluate his objectives as well as your own. If either you or your child places winning at or near the top of your list of goals—and if you put pressure on your child to win a tournament or kick a goal—your priorities need reevaluation. Winning certainly adds to the fun and excitement of sports, but it should *not* be a primary goal.

Choosing a Sports Program

Once your child has decided that she wants to become involved in a sports activity, she will have to decide which one to select. Of course, she should choose one that *she* will enjoy; even though your first love may be baseball or softball, let her choose soccer if that is what appeals to her.

Some children prefer individual sports rather than team sports. These individual activities—such as swimming, running, tennis, martial arts, and cycling—can become lifetime sports, offering enjoyment and health advantages throughout adulthood. Many of these same activities (running and swimming, for example) provide an aerobic workout too. Competitive swimming is a fantastic individual sport in which the child "competes" with her own best times at meets. Swimmers

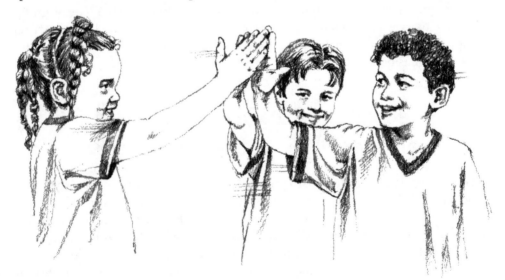

Participation in sports can boost your child's self-confidence and help develop friendships.

also have the camaraderie of group relay events with which to experience the team dynamic. Another option at the junior high level is cross-country running, in which the goal is to improve one's own PR, or personal record. Many elementary schools have running clubs intended for younger children, with just as much emphasis on fun as on physical fitness.

If your child selects a team activity, investigate the programs available in your community. There are both contact and noncontact sports (see table on page 51), and you and your child should evaluate which are more appropriate for his or her size, interests, and abilities. Many team sports (basketball, soccer) involve at least some contact, although others (T-ball, swimming, tennis) are purely noncontact activities. The nature of how some sports are played changes with a child's age. For example, soccer for younger children is played without much contact and rarely results in collisions.

Participation in Sports at Different Ages

Children ages 5–7 years: Children of this age should not participate in tackle or contact sports. The focus at these younger ages should be to try a variety of different sports to see what appeals to the individual child and her interests and abilities. Many park districts offer courses specifically intended to introduce children this age to a variety of sports.

Children ages 8–10 years: At this age, children may have their first experiences with contact sports (e.g., ice hockey); ensure appropriate safety gear is utilized.

Children ages 11–12 years: Older children may feel pressure to "specialize" in a single sport. Experts caution against early specialization, as this can lead to overuse injuries, joint problems, and stress fractures. Kids this age who participate in different sports develop diverse muscle groups and agility.

As you might expect, there is a greater chance of injury in contact and collision sports, but many children still enjoy these activities, particularly if the coach emphasizes participation, not winning. Also, take into account your child's physical maturity. His ability to compete with his peers—particularly in the collision sports—

depends more on body size and weight than on age. A late-maturing junior high school student, for instance, may have fewer skills and be much more susceptible to injury in contact or collision sports than his more physically mature teammates and opponents. Do not pressure your child to participate in a sport for which he may lack the proper physical maturity level. You, your child, and your pediatrician should discuss the most appropriate activities or sports for your child, and whether the advantages of a contact or collision sport outweigh the potential risks.

Also important to consider are financial and time commitments, including travel times. Depending on how many children you have, you may need to make choices to provide opportunities for your kids. See what resources your commu-

What Is Your Child's Physical Maturity Level?

Throughout middle childhood, children grow at varying rates and at different times. At first glance you might think that the early maturers would have clear physical advantages over their later-maturing peers. However, both groups of children face certain difficulties.

Kids who mature early are more likely to experience athletic success during the elementary and junior high years. Yet, with time, their peers will catch up with them, eliminating any advantages the early maturers once had and, often, deflating their self-esteem in the process. Formerly a star athlete, the early maturer has to adjust to being just one of the gang.

If your children fall into this category, you can help ease them through the adjustment process by encouraging them to participate in athletic activities with children who are also early maturers. Their maturity level is a more important factor than age. Also, urge your kids to develop other interests in addition to sports—areas in which they can excel and activities they can enjoy even when their maturity status no longer gives them an advantage over their classmates.

Late-maturing children face different types of challenges. These children, smaller than most kids their age, tend to lag behind in their strength level and motor skills. Regardless of their size, these children should be encouraged to participate in athletic activities, choosing those where maturity level and size are not as important—perhaps tennis, gymnastics, or certain track events. Later, when they catch up with their earlier-maturing peers, they can participate in sports where size plays a more significant role.

Classification of Sports by Contact		
Contact/Collision	**Limited Contact**	**Noncontact**
Basketball	Baseball	Archery
Boxing*	Bicycling	Badminton
Diving	Cheerleading	Bowling
Field hockey	Canoeing/kayaking	Canoeing/kayaking
Football	(whitewater)	(flat water)
Flag	Fencing	Crew/rowing
Tackle	Field	Curling
Ice hockey	High jump	Dancing
Lacrosse	Pole vault	Field
Martial arts	Floor hockey	Discus
Rodeo	Gymnastics	Javelin
Rugby	Handball	Shot put
Ski jumping	Horseback riding	Golf
Soccer	Racquetball	Rope jumping
Team handball	Skating	Running
Water polo	Ice	Sailing
Wrestling	Inline	Scuba diving
	Roller	Swimming
	Skiing	Table tennis
	Cross-country	Tennis
	Downhill	Track
	Water	Yoga
	Softball	
	Squash	
	Ultimate Frisbee	
	Volleyball	
	Windsurfing/surfing	

*Participation is not recommended.

nity has to offer; if you live five minutes from the nearest aquatic center but thirty minutes from the nearest ice arena, this is an important factor to consider when selecting sports for participation. Consider the cost of needed gear, equipment, and team fees as well.

What Else Should You Consider?

Before making a final decision on the right sports for your child, investigate the philosophy of the program under consideration. Here are some questions to ask:

- Do all team members get equal playing time? (Studies show that children would prefer to play regularly on a losing team rather than be relegated to the bench of a winning one.)

- Does the program emphasize mastery of the sport rather than winning? Is each child encouraged to reach his or her own potential in terms of skills development?

- Are kids given unconditional approval, with good efforts praised and mistakes met with gentle encouragement and constructive correction?

- Is the teaching of good sportsmanship emphasized?

- Are the needs of the children taken into consideration? For example, are practices at a convenient time and place, and are they limited to a reasonable length of time? Will the time demands prevent the children from participating in other activities and assuming other responsibilities?

- Are safety rules adhered to during practices and games? Is appropriate equipment available? Are children matched with others of the same size and strength? (This is particularly important in contact sports.)

- What expenses are involved, including the costs of equipment and travel?

- What are the expectations and demands on the parents' time?

Also, investigate the coach or coaches for whom your child will be playing. They can serve as important role models for your children. They should enjoy being with children and communicate well with them. They should respect each member of the team as an individual, not showing favoritism toward the best athletes on the team. They should be knowledgeable about the game they are coaching, not only in order to help children learn the sport properly but also to minimize the chance of injury. Their practices should be instructive, safe, and enjoyable, and games should emphasize participation, learning, and fun—not winning. Even when their players do not perform up to expectations, the coaches should provide support rather than react angrily.

Evaluate your children's athletic needs and expectations, investigate the sports that are available and which ones are most appropriate for them, estimate the quality of your child's experience, and decide whether a particular activity lends itself to a lifelong habit of exercise. Sports are one aspect of your child's life in which being an active advocate can have big payoffs.

Strength Training

Age and developmental stage are big factors in the decision of when to introduce the concept of strength training to young athletes. Keep in mind that not all strength training means the use of free weights. Many strength training maneuvers use one's own body weight as resistance, such as leg lifts and chair step-ups. For young age groups before puberty, lighter weights with more repetitions are the rule, with supervision by a trained professional or coach who can monitor technique and encourage proper form to prevent injury.

To perform strength training effectively, athletes must have correct form and be able to move the weight in a safe and efficient manner. Balance, control, posture, and coordination start to mature to adult levels by around 7 to 8 years of age. Strength training should not be the main focus at early ages; rather, in early childhood it is important to be involved in activities or programs that work on general foundational skills, like running, jumping, hopping, kicking, and throwing. This can provide a base to build on for future physical activity and strength training programs. An increased attention span, ability to stay focused, and maturity are necessary developmental milestones.

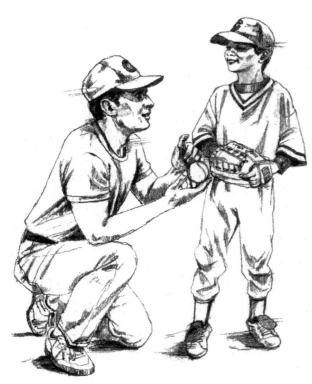

Coaches can serve as important role models for your child.

Commonly Asked Sports Questions

SHOULD I ALLOW MY CHILD TO QUIT A TEAM?

Sometimes a child's interest in a sport will fade. Or her participation may become a negative experience, perhaps because of a volatile coach, frustration about not playing as much as she would like, or a mismatch between her own physical size and that of the players against whom she competes.

In cases like this, find out the exact reasons why your child wants to quit. Listen to her and discuss her concerns. Working together, decide on the best course of action. Although it may not be wise for your child to make a habit of avoiding difficult situations, dropping out of a program may be the most sensible option in some instances. Your child is learning lifelong lessons in the world of athletics; rather than abruptly quitting in midseason, it is strongly encouraged that your child finish up the season you signed up for, and then refrain from signing up for the following season. This situation presents an excellent opportunity to teach the greater lesson of completing what you started.

IF MY CHILD IS HAVING TROUBLE KEEPING HER GRADES UP, SHOULD SHE STILL BE PERMITTED TO PARTICIPATE IN SPORTS?

In most cases, the answer is yes. All children need physical activity as part of their day. Without this physical outlet, many have difficulty concentrating on their academic work. If practices and other sports-related demands are excessive, however, talk to the coach about your child's need to devote adequate time to studies.

There is another important factor to consider: sometimes children who have difficulty with schoolwork can use a boost in self-esteem, which sports often can provide. As they feel a sense of accomplishment in athletics, this renewed self-confidence can often carry over to other areas of their lives, including academics. In fact, many research studies show a strong correlation between athletics and classroom success, suggesting that physical stimulation also stimulates the brain. Physical activity is also a great release for children with attention deficit hyperactivity disorder, allowing them to concentrate better in the classroom.

MY CHILD IS FINDING HER SPORTS PARTICIPATION TOO STRESSFUL. HOW CAN I ALLEVIATE HER ANXIETY?

Sports can be stressful, but so can other childhood activities, such as school exams and band solos. However, you should try to minimize the stress in your child's athletic endeavors in the following ways:

- Emphasize that sports participation is fun; do not let a "win at all cost" attitude interfere with your child's enjoyment of the game.

- Let your child know that she is not being judged by her success (or lack of it) on the athletic field. When she strikes out or misses a free throw, be supportive and praise her for trying her best.

- Help your child improve her athletic skills, which will reduce her stress levels during competition; if necessary, ask for some outside instruction from a cooperative coach.

- Stay away from coaches who are abusive toward your child.

- Speak with other parents to see if there is a common problem that needs to be addressed.

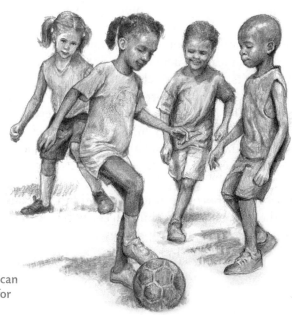

Playing any sport can be a great outlet for fun and exercise.

If Your Child Has a Chronic Condition

Exercise is a way for children to keep fit, have fun, build self-esteem, and relate to other children. Kids with a chronic illness can and should enjoy the benefits of participating in safe and appropriate physical activity.

Talk with your pediatrician about whether restrictions are necessary for your child with a chronic illness. She should not be in an athletic environment where her limitations place her in danger or significantly limit her opportunity to have some success. Nearly every child can find an appropriate level of activity in which she can participate successfully and without frustration, while developing muscle strength and coordination. Every child should be encouraged to become as active as possible.

Most chronic health issues require few, if any, restrictions. Children with asthma, for example, can and should participate in sports; they may have to follow their doctor's guidelines for medication administration before exercising. Regular physical exercise is a fantastic way to boost a child's lung capacity, especially during this significant growth phase of childhood.

Children with well-controlled seizure disorders can enjoy nearly all sports, from baseball to basketball to soccer—although if a child has occasional seizures, it is probably sensible to avoid activities such as rope climbing, high diving, and workouts on parallel bars, where a fall could cause a serious injury. While swimming, these children should be supervised by an adult who is in the water with them.

Children with heart disease or high blood pressure can participate in most sports, although your child's cardiologist may have specific recommendations about how strenuous an activity should be. Children with musculoskeletal problems like scoliosis can also lead an active life, as can most children with rheumatoid arthritis; swimming is an excellent choice in both these situations.

Some children have impaired, uncorrectable vision in one eye. In these cases, talk to an ophthalmologist about protecting the good eye from injury. Special protective eyewear may be suggested. Children who participate in sports where eyes are frequently injured, such as baseball, racquetball, and handball, are also advised to use protective eyewear.

The Special Olympics program offers unique, exciting experiences for disabled children, providing opportunities for physical fitness, competition, and enjoyment. Through their participation, children can enhance their self-esteem, and parents can connect with a valuable support system.

Sports Injuries

Improvements in the quality of protective equipment—such as padding and helmets—have made sports participation safer than ever before. Even so, children's bodies are still vulnerable to injury. As children move through middle childhood—becoming bigger, stronger, faster, and more aggressive—the incidence of injuries rises. Children between 5 and 14 years old account for approximately 40 percent of sports-related injuries for all age groups.

Injury prevention should be a paramount concern. Your child should be wearing a well-fitted helmet, mouthpiece, face guard, padding, eye gear, protective cup, or other equipment appropriate for the sport.

The majority of sports-related injuries involve the body's soft tissues rather

The ICE Treatment

As soon as an injury occurs, use the three-step "ICE" first-aid treatment to minimize swelling:

1. **Ice:** Apply an ice bag or a plastic bag of ice over the injured area. (Caution: overuse of ice can cause skin damage. Never apply ice for longer than twenty minutes, or more often than every two hours.) A frozen bag of peas from the freezer works well; it's convenient and melds to the shape of the body part nicely.

2. **Compression:** After removing any part of the child's clothing that covers the injured region, wrap an elastic bandage around the skin. The last section of the bandage should be wrapped firmly around the ice bag. Maintain compression even after ice is removed.

3. **Elevation:** Raise the injured leg or arm higher than the level of the heart, keeping it elevated as much as possible until the pain or swelling subsides.

This is the only treatment you should apply on your own until a doctor has diagnosed the injury. Do not tape or splint an injured arm or leg. Do not administer any drugs that have not been prescribed by a doctor. When helping your child leave the field of play, keep her from using or putting weight on the injured part.

than the bones. About two-thirds of all injuries are strains (overstretching or over-extension of the muscles) and sprains (wrenching of a joint with partial tear of the ligaments).

Many injuries are caused by overuse of or repetitive stress on the affected body part. When a child overdoes it or trains inappropriately—for example, pitching too many innings or throwing improperly—the stress placed on the joints, tendons, and muscles can cause damage.

Overuse injuries can often be prevented by advising your child to stop exercising at the first sign of discomfort. "No pain, no gain" may be a catchy phrase, but it is bad advice. "Slow but sure" makes a lot more sense. Overuse injuries make up about 50 percent of sports injuries, and the large majority of them are preventable.

Once an injury occurs, it needs to be properly diagnosed and treated. Even children with injuries that appear to be quite minor may benefit from being examined by a pediatrician. In addition to recommending specific types of treatment, the doctor may suggest that your child reduce the level of athletic participation for a while and do rehabilitation exercises, allowing the injury to heal while maintaining some use of the injured body part. Improperly treated and incompletely healed sports injuries can set the stage for future injuries. Because children in middle childhood are unable to fully contemplate the future, parents have to be firm to ensure that medical guidelines are followed.

It is also important to identify the cause of the injury before returning to the sport. Was the playing field in bad shape? Was the safety equipment not being used? Was training or fitness not adequate? Was the coaching poor? If parents neglect these factors, injuries are likely to recur.

Children in contact sports are much more vulnerable to serious injury, with the knees bearing the brunt of more injuries than any other part of the body. The ankles, shoulders, and elbows are also particularly susceptible to injuries that can put young children on the disabled list during the healing process.

Concussion

A concussion happens when a hit to the head results in brain function alteration. Concussions can occur in any sport, but they happen more frequently in contact sports (see table on page 51). A collision with another player, colliding with the ground or a pole, or getting hit in the head with a moving ball can all cause a concussion.

Concussion symptoms may be noted immediately after the injury, or may take hours or days to become apparent. In most concussions, the athlete does *not* lose consciousness. There may only be one symptom, such as headache, or there may be a collection of multiple symptoms. Symptoms can include headache, vomiting, dizziness, balance problems, vision changes, sensitivity to light or noise, difficulty concentrating, memory problems, irritability, or drowsiness. If a concussion is suspected, the athlete should stop the activity and seek medical attention. The physician will confirm the concussion, determine if further testing is needed, and create a plan for return to play. It is important to let the physician know if there have been prior concussions.

Most kids who have had a concussion need a plan of modified physical and mental activities. Screen time should be limited during the recovery process, and stopped altogether if it makes any symptoms worse. School attendance and participation, including physical education and recess, may need to be modified in addition to athletic participation. If symptoms are worsening over time instead of improving, the family should notify the physician.

Recovery from a concussion can vary based on the individual child, the severity of the concussion, and any history of prior concussions. Typically, the child should have complete resolution of symptoms at rest before reintroducing physical and mental activities in a stepwise fashion. Your child will most likely need a doctor's note to be able to return to full activity.

ACL Tears

The anterior cruciate ligament (ACL) is the ligament connecting the femur (thigh bone) and tibia (shin bone) inside the knee joint. The ACL provides stability in the knee joint, especially when a child pivots, jumps, and lands. ACL tears, unfortunately, can occur with sports participation, and can result in sudden knee pain, most commonly from a twisting, knock-kneed, or overextension injury, at times with a "pop" sensation. Swelling and weakness can follow.

ACL tears occur in all sports, but jumping, cutting, and pivoting sports such as basketball, soccer, and volleyball present the highest risk, and girls are affected more often than boys. Instruction in good running, jumping, landing, and squatting technique can reduce the chances of tearing the ACL.

Be a Good Role Model

If physical activity is fun, it will be a lifelong habit. The best way to get children to enjoy exercise is to make it a family affair, with parents setting a good example and encouraging their children to join them. The entire family can participate together in many physical activities, from swimming to cycling to hiking. Not only will everyone's fitness improve, but the unity of the family can be strengthened too.

If you can get your child interested in fitness at a young age, you will improve the chances that physical activity will become a lifetime habit. Long-term health will be the ultimate result.

PART II

Promoting Health and Development

~ 5 ~

Physical Development

AS A CHILD grows from an infant into a school-age child, time seems to fly by. Wasn't it only yesterday that you sang lullabies over your child's crib, watched her crawl for the first time, or cheered as she took her first steps? Now she is bigger, more coordinated, more independent, forming social relationships outside of the family—and moving toward the much more dramatic changes of puberty that lie ahead.

The steady physical development that occurred during the preschool years will continue during middle childhood, although it will not proceed nearly as rapidly as the growth that will follow in adolescence. The present changes tend to be more gradual and steady, all part of the evolution toward adulthood.

Your child should visit the pediatrician every year for a well-child check. Even if your school does not require new forms or vaccines, the annual checkup is a great opportunity to monitor your child's physical and mental health, and discuss any concerns with your physician.

Your Child's Growth

On average, the steady growth of middle childhood results in an increase in height of a little over 2 inches a year. Weight gain should

2 to 20 years: Boys
Stature-for-age and Weight-for-age percentiles

NAME _____

RECORD # _____

Mother's Stature _____ Father's Stature _____

Date	Age	Weight	Stature	BMI*

*To Calculate BMI: Weight (kg) ÷ Stature (cm) ÷ Stature (cm) x 10,000
or Weight (lb) ÷ Stature (in) ÷ Stature (in) x 703

AGE (YEARS)

STATURE

WEIGHT

Published May 30, 2000 (modified 11/21/00).
SOURCE: Developed by the National Center for Health Statistics in collaboration with
the National Center for Chronic Disease Prevention and Health Promotion (2000).
http://www.cdc.gov/growthcharts

CDC

SAFER · HEALTHIER · PEOPLE™

2 to 20 years: Boys
Body mass index-for-age percentiles

NAME _____

RECORD # _____

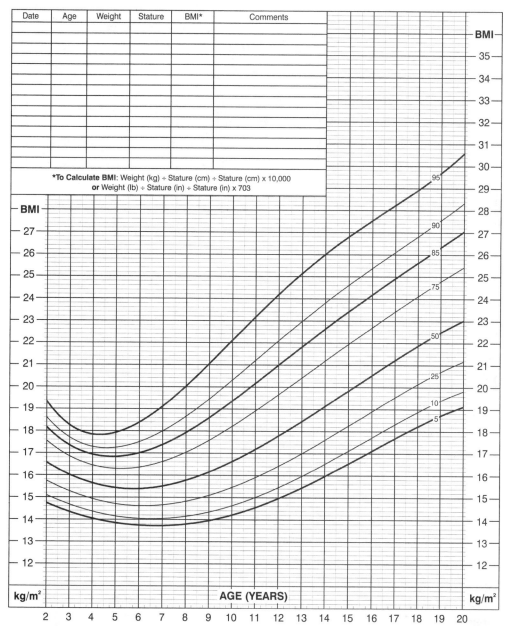

Date	Age	Weight	Stature	BMI*	Comments

*To Calculate BMI: Weight (kg) ÷ Stature (cm) ÷ Stature (cm) x 10,000
or Weight (lb) ÷ Stature (in) ÷ Stature (in) x 703

AGE (YEARS)

kg/m²

BMI

Published May 30, 2000 (modified 10/16/00).

SOURCE: Developed by the National Center for Health Statistics in collaboration with
the National Center for Chronic Disease Prevention and Health Promotion (2000).
http://www.cdc.gov/growthcharts

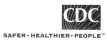

SAFER · HEALTHIER · PEOPLE™

2 to 20 years: Girls
Stature-for-age and Weight-for-age percentiles

NAME _____

RECORD # _____

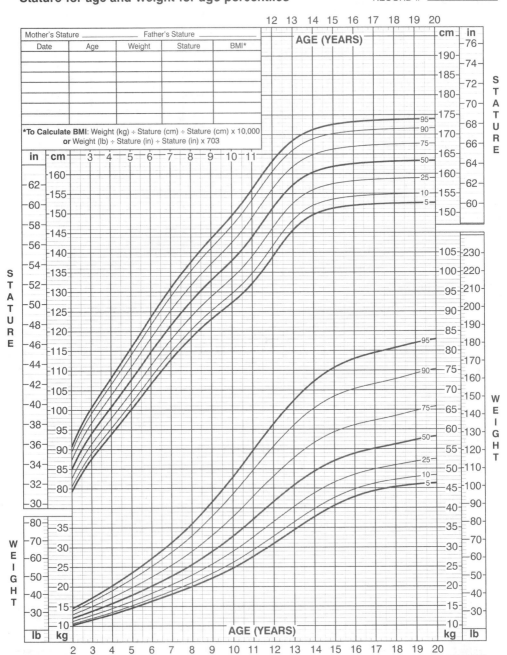

*To Calculate BMI: Weight (kg) ÷ Stature (cm) ÷ Stature (cm) x 10,000
or Weight (lb) ÷ Stature (in) ÷ Stature (in) x 703

Published May 30, 2000 (modified 11/21/00).
SOURCE: Developed by the National Center for Health Statistics in collaboration with
the National Center for Chronic Disease Prevention and Health Promotion (2000).
http://www.cdc.gov/growthcharts

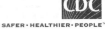

SAFER · HEALTHIER · PEOPLE™

2 to 20 years: Girls
Body mass index-for-age percentiles

NAME _____

RECORD # _____

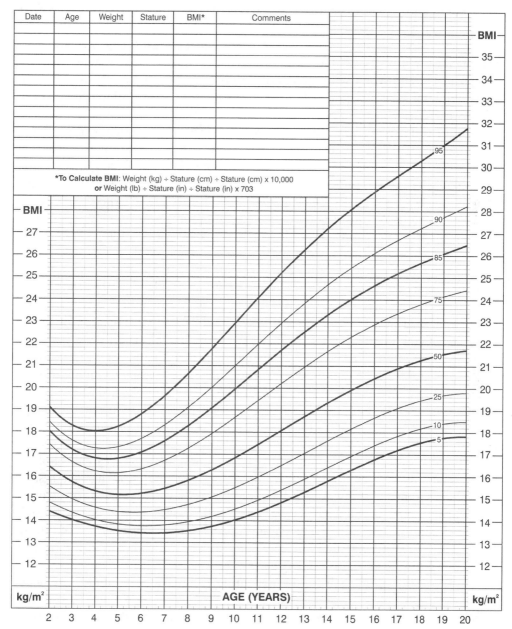

Date	Age	Weight	Stature	BMI*	Comments

*To Calculate BMI: Weight (kg) ÷ Stature (cm) ÷ Stature (cm) x 10,000
or Weight (lb) ÷ Stature (in) ÷ Stature (in) x 703

AGE (YEARS)

kg/m²

Published May 30, 2000 (modified 10/16/00).
SOURCE: Developed by the National Center for Health Statistics in collaboration with
the National Center for Chronic Disease Prevention and Health Promotion (2000).
http://www.cdc.gov/growthcharts

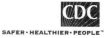

SAFER · HEALTHIER · PEOPLE™

average about 6 ½ pounds a year. However, these are only averages. A number of factors, including how close the child is to puberty, will determine when and how much your child grows. In general, there tends to be a period of slightly increased growth rate between ages 6 and 8 years.

Perhaps more than any other factor, your child's pattern of growth and ultimate height will be influenced by family genetics and heredity. While there are exceptions, tall parents usually have tall children, and short parents usually have short children. Genetics play a large role in the growth of children during the school years.

If your child seems *unusually* short or tall relative to her friends of the same age, talk with your pediatrician. The doctor may recommend an X-ray of the wrist, called a "bone age" X-ray, to determine your child's skeletal growth stage. Examining the growth plates can help your physician determine if your child's growth matches his chronological age, is more advanced than expected, or is delayed, which could indicate potential future catch-up growth. If there are concerns, your pediatrician may consult with a pediatric endocrinologist (a growth and hormone specialist).

Just as height can vary from child to child, so can the timing of a child's growth. Despite the averages mentioned above, many middle school children often experience clear growth spurts, followed by periods in which they grow very little. Some children grow as much as three times faster during a particular season of the year, compared with their "slow" seasons. These individual variations in timing—along with hereditary factors—are largely responsible for the wide variations in size among children of the same age. Height differences among children in a typical elementary school classroom range from 4 to 5 inches. In addition, parents should keep in mind that a particular school grade level's students have birthdays that range over twelve months' time; a difference of ten months in age, for example, can result in a big difference in growth stages.

A number of other factors, such as environmental influences, can affect physical development as well. Nutrition is important to normal growth processes, so your child should consume a well-balanced diet. Your child's need for calories rises during times of rapid growth, gradually increasing as she moves through middle childhood into puberty. However, if the calories consumed exceed those expended, your child may develop a weight problem, which could lead to health problems (for more on obesity, see page 35).

Some parents worry their child is not eating as much as he "should." Remember that parents decide what and when to serve meals, but the child decides the amount that is ingested. Often adults overestimate what a child truly needs. Even with what seems to be relatively low food intake, children can grow at normal rates. If your school-age child is a picky eater, you do not usually have to worry that this frustrating behavior is impairing his growth. During these picky-eater phases, do not make mealtimes a battleground that will lead to further power struggles. Do not fall into the trap of feeling that he will starve if you don't give in to his desire for junk food or cook a second, smaller meal just for him. His fluctuating eating habits may be due to normal slow-growth periods, or he may simply have personal, unpredictable preferences or distastes for certain foods. Continue to serve a wide array of nutritious foods, and limit treat or junk foods to special occasions. In general, children outgrow these food preferences without any harm to their physical well-being. As long as your child is gaining weight appropriately and is eating a variety of healthy foods, you can feel comfortable that his nutritional needs are being met. A daily multivitamin may provide peace of mind for some parents and reduce dinner table battles (for more information on nutrition, see Chapter 2, "Nutrition").

In our relatively affluent society, severe malnutrition is uncommon. Nevertheless, when a child's caloric intake is severely restricted—for example, due to an eating disorder or during a chronic illness—then her development and overall health can be seriously impacted. If your child is losing weight, discuss this situation with your doctor. (For more information about eating disorders, see page 553.) Your pediatrician can help you assess whether more assessment or intervention is required.

Maturation of Strength, Coordination, and Fine Motor Skills

Children ages 5–7 years: Five-year-olds can skip, walk on tiptoes, and broad-jump. Kids this age should tie their own shoes, cut and paste, and draw a person with a head, body, arms, and legs. By age 6, a child can bounce a ball four to six times, skate, ride a bicycle, skip with both feet, and dress herself completely without help.

Children ages 8–10 years: Kids in this age group can master new skills. A 9-year-old can build a model or learn to sew. A 10-year-old can probably catch a fly ball.

Children ages 11–12 years: Older children can perform many tasks, notably in the kitchen (for more information, see "Age-Appropriate Kitchen Tasks" on page 28). Kids this age have mastered electronic devices; parents should realize this mastery also means they can operate simple household appliances to help with chores such as the laundry.

Your child also needs to have daily movement and exercise to ensure appropriate physical development. Children who spend their free time playing videogames, watching TV, using other electronic devices ("screen time"), or engaging in other sedentary activities, rather than participating in time spent playing outdoors, may have impaired bone strength and an increased risk for obesity. Encourage your kids to be active during recess and at home, and make sure they have opportunities for exercise in their daily schedules.

During middle childhood, you will probably notice a number of prepubertal changes. Your child will become stronger as her muscle mass increases. Her motor skills—in both strength and coordination—will improve as well, which will be reflected in gradual improvements in tasks ranging from tying her shoes to throwing a ball accurately.

The Onset of Puberty

Puberty is typically made up of a clear sequence of stages, affecting the skeletal, muscular, reproductive, and other body systems (see the chart on page 73 for more information on the progression of puberty). Puberty often begins earlier than parents think.

Breast budding in girls—their first sign of puberty—starts at age 10 on average, with some girls starting as early as 8 and others not starting until 13. The peak growth period (in height, weight, and muscle mass) in girls occurs about one year after puberty has begun. Menstruation usually starts about two years after the onset of puberty; on average, the first menses occurs at about 12½ years of age.

Boys enter puberty about one or two years later than girls. The first sign is enlargement of the testes and a thinning, reddening, or darkening of the scrotum, which happens at an average age of 11 but may occur anytime between 9 and 14 years. For boys, the peak growth period occurs about two years after the beginning of puberty.

Although boys and girls are generally of similar height during middle childhood, that changes with the beginning of puberty. Particularly in middle school, girls are often taller than their male classmates, but within a year or two, boys catch up and usually surpass their female classmates. About 25 percent of human growth in height occurs during puberty.

There are many opportunities during this time of life for you to talk to your child about what she is experiencing. Your child needs to understand the physical changes that will occur in her body during puberty. You should emphasize that these changes are part of the natural process of growing into adulthood, stimulated by hormones (chemicals that are produced within the body). Discussing puberty with your child is not a single conversation; rather, you should discuss

A Series of Conversations About Body Changes

Discussions with your child about body growth and changes will evolve over the years. Your children will naturally have questions; answer these questions in a calm, nonjudgmental manner. Reassurance and matter-of-fact explanations help kids understand that our bodies and the changes of puberty are normal.

Children ages 5–7 years: Body discussions inevitably arise during bath time or when changing clothes. Use proper names (such as "penis" and "vagina") for body parts; avoid the use of nicknames for defining anatomy, as this can be confusing for kids and can send a message that the body is something to be embarrassed about. Kids this age may ask why their bodies look different from those of adults; simple explanations should suffice for most children.

Children ages 8–10 years: Kids this age are ready to learn more. They often have an increased awareness of the concept of privacy when changing clothes and bathing. This is a good age to begin discussing that just as we brush our teeth and comb our hair, we also need to care for our body by bathing, showering, and using deodorant. Outline body changes that will occur. Open-ended questions are a good conversation starter; you can ask your child, "What do you know so far?" Often kids this age have already chatted with their peers and likely have questions you can answer, or misconceptions that you can correct.

Children ages 11–12 years: Older children will often have had some form of formal puberty discussion at school; parents should remember that they are still the most significant source of health information for their kids. This period is a great opportunity to share your family's values with your child. Remember that our role as adults is not to perform a one-sided lecture; rather, these should be conversations, a two-way exchange, in which you ask your child what they already know, what they think, or what they may need clarification on. Let your child know he can come to you with questions or concerns at any time, and follow through on this promise.

Stages of Puberty

As children approach and move through adolescence, they proceed through the following five stages of puberty:

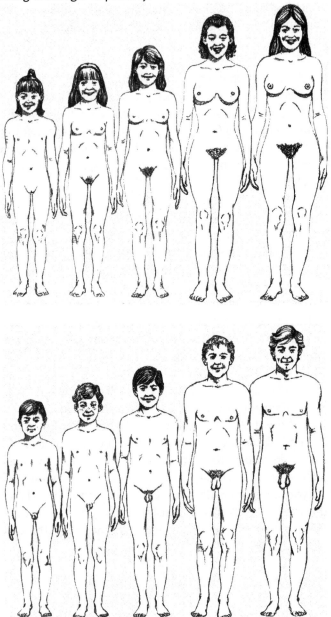

Stages of Puberty

	Boys	Girls
Stage one	Prepubertal No sexual development	Prepubertal No sexual development
Stage two	Testes enlarge Body odor	Breast budding First pubic hair Body odor Height spurt
Stage three	Penis enlarges Pubic hair starts growing Ejaculation (wet dreams)	Breasts enlarge Pubic hair darkens, becomes curlier Vaginal discharge
Stage four	Continued enlargement of testes and penis Penis and scrotal sac deepen in color Pubic hair curlier and coarser Height spurt Male breast development	Onset of menstruation Nipple is distinct from areola
Stage five	Fully mature adult Pubic hair extends to inner thighs Increases in height slow, then stop	Fully mature adult Pubic hair extends to inner thighs Increases in height slow, then stop

body changes with your child in a series of mini-conversations, keeping the discussion age-appropriate. A 5-year-old naturally has questions; a conversation about body changes at 5 years of age will be different from what you will discuss with your child when she is 10 or 11 years of age.

While fully respecting his desire for privacy, keep track of your child's bodily changes. As the age ranges above indicate, there are wide variations of "normal" in regard to the time when puberty begins; remind your child that while he and his friends will grow at different rates, they will eventually catch up with one another.

On occasion, children start puberty either early or late. Girls should be checked by their physician if they begin pubertal changes before age 8, while boys should be evaluated if they enter puberty before age 9. Likewise, see a doctor if there are no pubertal changes in a girl by age 13 or a boy by age 14.

Also, contact your physician if your child's pubertal development does not follow the expected pattern on the preceding chart—for example, if your daughter begins menstruation before she experiences breast development. Your child should continue to visit her pediatrician for yearly well-child visits throughout these times of dramatic physical changes and adolescence.

Puberty Changes in Girls

Menstruation. Many concerns about puberty center on menstruation. Spend time helping your daughter prepare for her first period. There is no reason for a girl to be surprised by her menarche, not knowing what is happening or why.

Remember, menstruation may begin sooner than you expect. Certainly, once your daughter's breast development has started, the two of you should fully discuss this topic. If you do not have adequate knowledge, ask your pediatrician to refer you to some informational sources. Some pediatricians schedule special educational visits at the time of puberty. Age-appropriate books intended for young girls on the subject of body and puberty changes can be a great resource for your child and can open the door of communication between child and parent as additional questions arise. As a parent, lend a supportive, understanding ear; avoid judgment or inappropriate joking, despite any qualms you may have about discussing this momentous change with your child; and let your child know that she can come to you with concerns or questions at any time.

Discuss the biology of menstruation, describing it as a normal bodily process. Mention that her periods may be irregular, particularly in the beginning as her body adapts to rapid physiological changes. Also, let her know that several months before her first period, fluid may be secreted by glands within her vagina. This substance may be clear or white in color, and watery to thick in consistency. Tell her not to worry, and that this physiologic leukorrhea (a type of vaginal discharge) is normal.

In addition, discuss hygiene related to menstrual cycles. Be certain your daughter has the supplies she will need for her first period. Since she may be away from home when the first period begins, discuss how to use pads or tampons, and let her know her school nurse will also have these supplies on hand in case this happens during the school day and she is caught off guard. She should understand the need to change pads or tampons several times a day. Of course, girls can shower or bathe while menstruating. Explain that she may experience some cramping before or during her periods, and options for managing it.

Many girls will ask if they can participate in activities such as sports, including swimming, or physical education classes. Reassure your daughter that she can take part in normal activities while menstruating. Physical exercise is a good way to ease the cramps associated with periods.

Breast Development. It is not uncommon for girls to have anxieties about breast development. For example, one breast usually begins to develop before the other. Explain to your daughter that as her breasts develop, it is quite normal for one to be somewhat larger than the other, and that breast size is seldom completely symmetrical. Also, when a girl first notices the lump beneath one nipple, she may worry that this is cancer; reassure her that one breast is beginning to develop before the other. If questions persist, consult your doctor.

If a girl's breasts start to develop relatively early, she may feel embarrassed and self-conscious. To help your daughter feel more comfortable in a situation like this, a sports or athletic bra is a simple way to provide some coverage and comfort.

Puberty Changes in Boys

As with girls and puberty, your son will have questions about his body changes. Speak with your pediatrician regarding these transitions. Age-appropriate books geared toward growing boys can help your son to learn more, as well as open the door of communication for additional questions and discussions.

Voice Changes. As the larynx (or voice box) enlarges and the muscles or vocal cords grow, boys' voices may "crack" as they speak before their voice gets lower. While this can be embarrassing, it is a normal part of the growth process.

Wet Dreams. Boys may awaken in the morning with damp pajamas and sheets. These "wet dreams," or nocturnal emissions, are caused by an ejaculation, not urination, that occurs during sleep; they are not an indication that the boy was having a sexual dream. Explain this phenomenon to your son, and reassure him that you understand that he cannot prevent it from happening. Wet dreams are just part of growing up.

Involuntary Erections. During puberty, boys get erections spontaneously, without touching their penis and without having sexual thoughts. These unexpected erections can be quite embarrassing, especially if they occur in public—at school, for example. Inform your son that these unexpected erections are normal and are a sign that his body is maturing. Explain that they happen to all boys during puberty, and that with the passage of time they will become less frequent.

Temporary Breast Enlargement. Many boys experience swelling of the breasts during the early years of puberty. Most often, your son may feel a flat, button-like bump under one or both nipples. His breasts may also feel tender or even painful. After a few months—sometimes longer—the swelling will disappear; these boys will not develop true breasts. If questions persist, talk to his pediatrician.

One Testicle Lower Than the Other. Uneven testicles are both normal and common.

Considerations as Kids Begin Puberty

Privacy

As your child approaches and enters puberty, be sensitive to his need for privacy. Preteens will tend to become more modest while they bathe, for example, or change their clothes. Respect this desire for privacy, not only as it relates to their bodies but in other aspects of life as well, such as not reading their mail and remembering to knock before entering their rooms. Online activity, however, should continue to be supervised by parents; find more on this subject on page 315.

Body Image

Children also become more sensitive about their body image during this time. Their interest in grooming increases, and they are more likely to be self-conscious about their appearance, largely due to the influence of their peers and the media. Watch for signs of a child who has a distorted body image, which can contribute to mental health issues such as eating disorders (see page 553) or anxiety disorders.

Avoid even good-natured teasing of your child about her pubertal development. Because most children feel self-conscious during this time, they will become embarrassed if they are kidded about the changing shape of their bodies or their deepening voices. Help your child feel comfortable raising questions with you about the pubertal process; an open door of communication will serve both of you well as your child matures into adolescence.

Gender Identity

The changes that accompany puberty can be stressful for all children, but this can be a particularly difficult time for children who are transgender. Transgender children are children who have a gender identity that is different from what would be expected based on their sex assigned at birth. For example, a child who was identified as a female at birth (based on having a vagina) may identify as a boy as the years pass. Exploring gender identity is normal for all children, and transgender gender identity is a normal variation of the spectrum of gender. As a transgender child's body starts to change in puberty, this can be a time of particular stress, as the body may be changing in a way that does not align with the child's gender identity. Consider a child who identifies as a boy and starts to experience breast development or have menstrual periods, or a child who identifies as a girl whose voice starts to change to a lower pitch. For transgender children, puberty can be a time of increased risk of depression, anxiety, and even self-harm related to these stresses of their changing body. If your child is expressing concerns related to gender identity, your pediatrician can assist you in finding resources in your area to help you best support your child.

~ 6 ~

Safety: Prevention of Injuries and Substance Use

WITH INCREASED INDEPENDENCE comes a need for an increased awareness of safety and injury prevention. Between the ages of 5 and 12, unintentional injury is the leading cause of death, far outnumbering deaths by any other cause. Each year children are involved in automobile crashes as passengers or pedestrians. Others drown, suffer severe burns, or are victims of gunfire or other injuries—most of which are preventable. While some of these injuries result in death, many more leave children with lifelong impairments. Bicycle safety, fire prevention, and protection from firearms are all important considerations. Awareness and education regarding the use of substances such as alcohol, tobacco, and marijuana are also important to keep a child safe.

Injury Prevention

Car Safety

In middle childhood, automobile crashes are responsible for more deaths than any other cause. In 2015, 1,361 U.S. children younger than 15 years were killed and 191,662 were injured as occupants in motor vehicles.

Most fatalities and injuries can be avoided with the use of car safety seats, booster seats, and seat belts. As a driver, before even starting the engine of your car, check to make certain that all children in your vehicle are buckled in place, and then buckle your own belt. Follow this simple rule consistently: the car does not move unless all occupants are properly buckled, no excuses. Children must be appropriately restrained, even if the distance traveled is just a block; the majority of crashes occur within a five-mile radius of home.

Proper car safety habits should be established as early in life as possible, using car safety seats, booster seats, and seat belts. It is important to teach your children to take personal responsibility for buckling their own belts, whether riding with you or another adult. Remember, children learn by example, so to reinforce seat belt use, set a good example and buckle your own belt whenever you are in the car, whether you are the driver or a passenger.

Booster Seats

Booster seats are for school-age kids who have outgrown their forward-facing car safety seats. All children whose weight or height exceeds the forward-facing limit for their car safety seat should use a belt-positioning booster seat until the vehicle seat belt fits properly. Typically that happens when children have reached 4 feet 9 inches in height and are 8 through 12 years of age. Most children will not fit in most vehicle seat belts without a booster until 10 to 11 years of age. All children younger than age 13 should ride in the back seat.

Instructions that come with the car safety seat will tell you the height and weight limits for the seat. As a guideline, you know that your child has outgrown a forward-facing car safety seat when he reaches the top weight or height allowed for his seat with a harness, his shoulders are above the top harness slots, or the tops of his ears have reached the top of the seat.

Booster seats are available in both high-back and backless models. Many high-back booster seats come with harness straps that can be used until the child reaches the manufacturer's forward-facing weight or height limit, and are then removed for an older child to use the seat as a booster. Booster seats are used with lap and shoulder seat belts in your vehicle, the same way an adult rides. They are designed to raise a child up so that lap and shoulder seat belts fit properly over the chest and breastbone (sternum), which are the strongest parts of the child's body that will provide support in the case of a crash. Most booster seats are not secured to the vehicle seat with the seat belt or lower anchor and tether, but simply rest on the vehicle seat and are held in place once the seat belt is fastened over a child. However, some models of booster seats can be secured to the vehicle seat and kept in place using the lower anchors or top tether.

When using a booster seat, always read the vehicle owner's manual and the car safety seat instruction manual before installing the seat. Booster seats often have

Types of Car Safety Seats

While this chart can be used as a guideline, it is also important to continue your research to learn about each car safety seat your child will use, as safety guidelines are continually being updated.

Age Group	Type of Seat	General Guidelines
Infants and toddlers	Rear-facing only Rear-facing convertible	All infants and toddlers should ride in a rear-facing seat until they are at least 2 years of age or reach the highest weight or height allowed by their car safety seat manufacturer
Toddlers and preschoolers	Forward-facing convertible Forward-facing with harness	Children who have outgrown the rear-facing weight or height limit for their convertible seat should use a forward-facing seat with a harness for as long as possible, up to the highest weight or height allowed by their car safety seat manufacturer.
School-aged children	Booster	All children whose weight or height exceeds the forward-facing limit for their car safety seat should use a belt-positioning booster seat until the vehicle seat belt fits properly, typically when they have reached 4 feet 9 inches in height and are 8 through 12 years of age. All children younger than 13 should ride in the back seat.
Older children	Seat belts	When children are old enough and large enough for the vehicle seat belt to fit them correctly, they should always use lap and shoulder seat belts for the best protection. All children younger than 13 years of age should ride in the back seat.

a plastic clip or guide to correctly position vehicle lap and shoulder belts. When using a booster seat, make sure the lap belt lies low and snug across your child's upper thighs, and the shoulder belt crosses the middle of your child's chest and shoulder and is off the neck. Older lap-only belts should not be used with a booster seat; lap *and* shoulder belts are always needed.

When purchasing a booster seat, make sure it has not been recalled. You can find out by calling the manufacturer or contacting the National Highway Traffic Safety Administration (NHTSA) Vehicle Safety Hotline at 888-327-4236. You can also visit the NHTSA website at SaferCar.gov. Do not use a booster seat that is too old, has visible cracks, has an unknown history (meaning you do not know if it was involved in a prior crash), does not have a label with the manufacture date and model number, or does not come with instructions. Any booster seat that has been involved in any crash, even a minor one, must be replaced.

If you have questions or need help installing your booster seat, find a certified child passenger safety technician (CPST). Lists of certified CPSTs and child seat-fitting stations are available at the National Highway Traffic Safety Administration's Parents Central website safercar.gov/parents/index.htm, or the National Child Passenger Safety Certification website at cert.safekids.org and click on "Find a Tech" or call (877-366-8154). The NCPSCT website also includes a list of CPSTs fluent in Spanish and other languages, as well as technicians who have extra training in transportation of children with special needs.

Seat Belts for Older Children and Adults

A car's seat belts are made for adults. Children should stay in a booster seat until adult seat belts fit correctly, typically when children reach about 4 feet 9 inches in height and are 8 through 12 years of age. Most children will not fit in a seat belt alone until 10 to 11 years of age. When children are old enough and large enough to use the vehicle seat belt alone, they should always use lap and shoulder seat belts for the best protection. All children younger than 13 should ride in the back seat.

An adult seat belt fits correctly when the shoulder belt lies across the middle of the chest and shoulder, not the neck or throat. The lap belt should be positioned low and snug across the upper thighs, not the belly. Your child should be tall enough to sit against the vehicle seat back with her knees bent over the edge of the seat without slouching, and can comfortably stay in this position throughout the trip. Make sure your child does not tuck the shoulder belt under her arm or behind her back. This leaves the upper body unprotected and adds extra slack to the seat belt system, putting your child at risk of severe injury in a crash or with sudden braking. Never allow anyone to "share" seat belts. All passengers must have their own car seats or seat belts.

Car Safety Reminders

Parents, as kids' greatest role models, should set a good example for their children by always buckling up themselves. Avoid distracted driving, including driving while holding a handheld phone or texting while driving, and absolutely never drive after using alcohol or other substances. Be consistent with car safety seat and lap/shoulder belt usage so that all family members are on the same page and know what to expect. Kids should not be alone in or around cars due to the dangers of elevated heat inside a parked car, the strangulation risk of power windows, or being backed over by a driver who does not realize a child is nearby.

About Airbags

Front airbags are installed in all new cars. When used with seat belts, airbags work well to protect teenagers and adults; however, airbags can be very dangerous to children, particularly those riding in rear-facing seats, and to preschool- and young school-age children who are not properly restrained. Vehicles with no back seat or a back seat that is not made for passengers are not the best choice for traveling with small children; however, the airbag can be turned off in some of these vehicles if the front seat is needed for a child passenger. See your vehicle owner's manual for more information.

Side airbags are available in most new cars. Side airbags improve safety for adults in side-impact crashes. Read your vehicle owner's manual for more information about the airbags in your vehicle. Read your car safety seat instructions and the vehicle owner's manual for guidance on placing the seat next to a side airbag.

Important Car Safety Tips

■ Head and all limbs should stay inside the car window.

■ Keep all doors locked while the car is in motion.

■ Pick up and drop off children at the curb or driveway.

■ Use power window locks if they are available on your car.

- Equip each car with a fire extinguisher and first-aid kit.

- Loose objects—particularly heavy ones, such as luggage or bicycles—should be placed in the car trunk or on the roof rack rather than inside the car. Not only can these unsecured items obstruct the driver's view, but they can be tossed about the car in a crash—as can an unbuckled driver or passenger—striking and injuring the occupants.

- Never leave young children alone in the car.

- Lock your car when it is parked, even in your garage or driveway, so children cannot get in unsupervised.

As your children become more involved in extracurricular activities, you'll be driving them back and forth more, and carpooling will probably make sense. Not only does carpooling save time, it is also a valuable opportunity to learn more about your child's friends and observe the group dynamic. When you drive children in a carpool, you must be as responsible for every child in the car as you are for your own. Be clear about your expectations of your child riders: everyone must buckle up and safety rules must be obeyed. Children in groups can get unruly, so pull over if any child gets out of control; don't drive if you are distracted by misbehavior. And never transport more children than your car can safely accommodate.

WHERE WE STAND

Many children and adolescents are injured or killed each year while riding in the back of pickup trucks. These young people are often ejected from the back of the truck during a collision or a rollover. Their deaths or injuries, however, could have been prevented.

The American Academy of Pediatrics believes that passengers should be prohibited from riding in truck beds or in any other area of a vehicle that does not have a seat and a seat belt. Only a few states presently have such bans. We also urge you to educate your children about the dangers of riding in open truck beds, and never allow them to do so.

Other Motorized Vehicles

Although school-age children cannot drive automobiles, some of them (usually with their parents' blessings) are still being allowed into the driver's seat of other types of motorized vehicles. While children in this age group are physically able to turn the steering wheel and reach the gas pedal of these motorized vehicles, they lack the coordination, the reflexes, and the judgment to avoid crashes. For that reason, children should *not* be allowed to drive them. This includes tractors, lawn-mowers, personal watercraft, mopeds, minibikes, trail bikes, all-terrain vehicles (ATVs), and snowmobiles. Even if some of these vehicles are marketed as designed to be used by school-age children, they are not safe.

These motorized vehicles achieve high speeds but provide no protective covering. Therefore, when a crash does occur, there is a high risk of serious injury. Minibikes (two-wheeled vehicles that resemble small motorcycles) have a much higher crash rate than bicycles, with most injuries occurring from falls or collisions.

ATVs have received considerable attention in recent years—much of it negative because of their high crash rates. These off-road vehicles can achieve speeds as high as 30 to 50 miles per hour. ATVs are prone to overturning on hills and slopes. Many children have died, often after suffering serious head injuries. Head injuries also are responsible for deaths on snowmobiles, which can achieve high rates of speed and are prone to rollovers. Tractors, riding mowers, and personal watercraft also tend to roll over, causing serious injuries. None of these vehicles are appropriate for children to drive.

Bicycle Safety

Mastering the art of riding a two-wheel bicycle gives most children a feeling of pride and newfound independence. Overnight they acquire a new means of transportation to school or the playground. Learning to ride a bicycle is similar to learning other motor skills—some children are ready earlier than others. Starting with training wheels is helpful but not always necessary to learn to coordinate watching, listening, pedaling, steering, and balancing. Younger children may depend on training wheels until they are 5 or 6, and sometimes older. Use a bicycle helmet from the *very first* time your child climbs on a bicycle or tricycle. With this new skill comes responsibility, as riding a bicycle does pose a risk of injury.

The majority of bicycle-related deaths involve collisions between a bicycle and an automobile, often when the child darts out of a driveway or alley and strikes, or is struck by, a car. Or the bicyclist may be riding on the street *against* rather than *with* the flow of traffic. Most of these collisions are preventable if both parents and children learn the rules of the road, wear helmets, and avoid riding at night.

Many more injuries happen when a child falls off a bicycle, which can cause everything from serious contusions to a broken arm to a severe head injury. These events often occur when children ride too fast and lose control of the bike, ride on a rough surface, or are double riding or stunt riding. Some injuries are caused when the child's clothes become entangled in the bicycle mechanism.

Do not let your child ride on the street or in traffic until she can ride confidently and adhere to the basic rules of the road. Make sure she understands and abides by these safety guidelines:

- **Wear a bicycle helmet *at all times*.** This first point is particularly important. Buy a helmet at the same time you purchase your child's first bicycle, ensuring that it is a proper fit for your child. Also encourage your child to use the same helmet for other types of play like roller-skating and skateboarding. The helmet should adhere to the safety standards of the Consumer Product Safety Commission. (Look for a sticker affixed to the helmet and a label on the package indicating that the helmet meets the CPSC standard.) These helmets can help absorb the impact of a crash, thus protecting the head from serious injury; studies show that helmets can reduce the risk of brain injury by up to 85 percent. Adjust the straps so the helmet fits snugly over the top of the head and forehead and does not move when pushed or pulled, and keep the chin strap fastened at all times. Make helmet use a firm rule; your child should not be riding a bike without using a helmet. Model safe behavior by always wearing a properly fitted helmet yourself.

- Stop at all points where a driveway, sidewalk, alley, or side street intersects with a street. Look both ways before proceeding.

- Obey all traffic lights and signs. They are there for bicycles as well as automobiles.

- When cycling with friends, ride in single file instead of riding abreast of one another and perhaps extending out into traffic. Use bicycle paths if at all possible.

- Avoid all trick and double riding, such as a second child riding on the handlebars.

- Do not ride at dusk or after dark.

- Ride in the same direction as traffic.

- Do not wear loose-fitting pants or other clothing that could become caught in the bicycle chain or other mechanism. Wear shoes and tie the laces.

- Do not wear earphones while riding. Listening to music muffles the traffic sounds that help you ride safely.

- If objects need to be carried, they should be placed in a backpack or a basket, allowing both hands to remain on the handlebars at all times. The backpack should not be so heavy that it affects the balance of the rider.

Choose your child's bicycle carefully. If her bike is the wrong size for her, she is more likely to lose control and be injured. Although some parents tend to buy a bike that their child can "grow into," an oversized bike is dangerous.

When shopping for a bike with your child, first have her sit on the seat; while gripping the handlebars she should be able to put the balls of both feet on the ground. Make sure that she can place both of her feet flat on the ground when straddling the center bar, with about a one-inch clearance between the bar and her crotch. Although coaster brakes are more appropriate for a younger child, an older child who prefers hand brakes should try them out, making sure she can grasp them comfortably and apply enough pressure to bring the bike to a halt.

Teach your child to keep her bicycle in good condition. Have her check the seat and handlebar height, the brakes, and the tire inflation regularly.

Water Safety

Drownings rank behind only motor vehicle crashes as the leading cause of death among children in middle childhood. Most often, these tragedies occur when children swim without adequate adult supervision. In most cases, these children (and their parents) have overestimated their swimming ability and their knowledge of water survival skills.

- Never allow your child to swim alone or play by or in water away from the watchful eye of an adult. Ideally, this adult should be trained in cardiopulmonary resuscitation (CPR). Also, teach your child to use the buddy system even when swimming with large groups of friends.

- Make sure your child learns how to swim from an experienced and qualified instructor. Check for available lessons at local recreation centers, YMCAs, school and park districts, and summer camps. Keep in mind that even strong swimmers can drown, and swim lessons do not provide "drown-proofing" for swimmers of any age.

- Do not allow your child to engage in horseplay that might result in injury.

- Prohibit your child from diving unless someone has already determined the depth of the water and checked for underwater hazards.

- Do not allow your child to swim in areas where there are boats or people fishing. Nor should he swim at beaches where there are large waves, a powerful undertow, or no lifeguards. Make sure he understands that swimming in one body of water (e.g., a backyard pool) may be different from swimming in another (a river or ocean).

- While riding in a boat, you and your child should always wear a life jacket.

- Do not permit your child to rely on an air mattress, inner tube, or inflatable toy as a substitute for a life jacket. If these devices deflate, or your child slips off them, he could be in serious trouble.

- Your child should never be permitted to swim during a lightning storm.

- If you have a backyard swimming pool, it should be enclosed with high and locked fences on all four sides. The fence should completely separate the pool from the house and the rest of the yard.

- When your child is old enough he should learn lifesaving skills such as CPR, taught in most cities through community agencies or the American Red Cross. Many local fire departments offer babysitting courses that include

WHERE WE STAND

The American Academy of Pediatrics feels strongly that parents should never—even for a moment—leave children alone near open bodies of water, such as lakes or swimming pools, nor near water in homes (bathtubs, spas). For backyard pools, rigid, motorized pool covers are not a substitute for four-sided fencing, since pool covers are not likely to be used appropriately and consistently. Parents should learn CPR and keep a telephone and emergency equipment (such as life preservers and shepherd's hooks) ready poolside.

CPR training and are approved for kids as young as 11 years of age. Kids who learn CPR at a younger age should continue to freshen their skills with recertification courses.

Fire and Burn Prevention

Your family's best protection against fire-related injuries is to equip your home with smoke alarms and ensure regular maintenance of these alarms. Thousands of lives could be saved every year if smoke alarms were in place, awakening families in time to allow them to escape their burning homes. Install the alarms throughout the house, mounting them on the ceiling or on the wall 6 to 12 inches below the ceiling. They should be placed inside each bedroom, in halls adjacent to the bedrooms, and in the living room, garage, and other parts of the home where they can awaken the family if a fire has broken out. Every level of the house should have at least one alarm, and every alarm should be tested monthly. It is best to use smoke alarms that use long-life batteries, but if yours have traditional batteries, change the batteries at least once a year.

Home fire extinguishers are also a good idea. Keep extinguishers in the parts of the house where a fire is most likely to start (the kitchen and the workroom, for example). However, use the extinguisher only for a small fire; if the fire is large, everyone should leave the dwelling *immediately*, and you should call the fire department from a cellphone or a neighbor's home. If children are home alone, instruct them to evacuate the house at once in case of a fire, even if it is a small one. Your child should learn to call 911, but he should understand that his own safety comes first, and he should make the call once he is safely outside the home.

Hold regular fire drills with everyone in the family participating. During these drills, plan and rehearse all possible escape routes for fires occurring in various parts of the house, as well as a place for family members to meet once they are outside. Since many fires—including most fatal ones—occur at night, conduct some of your drills after dark. A flashlight should be available at the bedside of every family member. Also, teach your children to "stop, drop, and roll" if their clothing should catch fire. Reassure your younger children that while a fire is unlikely, by performing these drills everyone will know what to do in case of an emergency. Kids ages 5–12 years are accustomed to fire drills, natural disaster drills, and lockdown drills in the school setting; similar preparedness is a smart idea for the household.

Educate your children never to play with matches, lighted candles, cigarette lighters, or other flammable devices. Also, keep in mind that most fatal home fires are caused by adults and their cigarettes; typically, a cigarette or its ashes fall on a bed or a couch, smolder for several hours, and then burst into flames, often after the family is asleep. Do not smoke in your house. Portable heaters also are responsible for many home fires and burns, and if their use is necessary, they should be used only with great caution.

Many burns are *not* related to fires. Most often, these are scalds from hot liquids—for example, when a child turns over a cooking pot upon himself, or turns the knobs on a bathtub faucet so hot water flows on him. Children also sometimes suffer burns by taking hot foods out of the microwave or by touching a hot iron, a coil on an electric stove, a curling iron, a hot barbecue grill, or fireworks.

To avoid scald burns, reduce the temperature of your water heater so the water at the tap is never hotter than 120 degrees Fahrenheit. Keep hot irons out of children's reach and use caution around the stovetop when food is cooking. Keep portable heaters away from children and from flammable materials, such as curtains. Use a cool mist humidifier instead of a hot steam vaporizer. Teach your child not to play with matches.

On average, between 10,000 and 12,000 people are treated each year in hospital emergency departments for fireworks-related injuries; around half are children. Every type of legally available firework has caused serious injury or death. Even sparklers burn at 1,200 degrees Fahrenheit and can cause significant burns. Fireworks should never be used by children or other family members. Rather than risk your child's health and safety, families should attend public fireworks displays conducted by professionals.

Skateboard Safety

Young skateboarders have a high center of gravity and may not be successful at safely breaking their falls. Additionally, newer products such as longboards, battery-powered hoverboards, and powered scooters may be more difficult to control than traditional skateboards. As a result, these products continue to cause many injuries, most often to the arms, legs, head, face, and neck. Falling on an outstretched arm is one of the most common ways kids get a bone fracture.

If your child rides a skateboard or similar product, she should wear a helmet, knee pads, elbow pads, and wrist guards to minimize the chances of injury. Also, she should never ride the skateboard in or near traffic. Many communities have designated skate parks, often located adjacent to public playgrounds, that are much safer for kids to develop skills on without the risk of oncoming traffic. Skate parks designed for younger kids are a safer bet than a homemade ramp in a driveway that leads onto a (possibly busy) street.

Roller Skates and In-Line Skating

Traditional roller skates and in-line skates provide an opportunity to skate outdoors in warm temperatures. This low-impact sport can provide good aerobic exercise. Skates differ widely in price and construction. Children's feet should feel comfortable in the boot, and their ankles should be well supported by a snugly buckled or strapped top. In general, children should be able to properly put on and remove their skates.

Skate wheels vary in size and hardness. Smaller wheels provide a lower center of gravity that may help beginning skaters feel more stable. Large wheels are faster and last longer. Softer wheels absorb bumps from small irregularities better than hard wheels, and provide better traction on smooth surfaces. In-line skates also come with a brake that drags along the ground when the child shifts weight.

Safe in-line skating takes both practice and precaution. Helmets, knee and elbow pads, and wrist guards should be standard equipment for skaters. Wrist guards are particularly important, as falling onto an outstretched hand is the cause of one of the most common fractures in children. Children should learn to skate on flat, open paved surfaces free from traffic. Basic technique should be learned and practiced slowly; speed and technique should progress together. Consider an empty parking lot for initial practice that is flat and devoid of cars and traffic. Parents should set clear rules for when and where skating is permissible.

Here are some safety guidelines for your middle-years child:

- Always wear protective gear.

- Skate under control and leave plenty of room to stop.

- Always skate on the right side of paths and sidewalks, and pass on the left.

- Avoid uneven pavement and areas with heavy traffic.

- Observe traffic regulations, and yield to pedestrians.

- Kids should not skate while exercising a pet on a leash; entanglement easily leads to injuries.

Too often, children venture into streets and try out stunts before they are fully able to control their skating.

Staying Safe While Home Alone

Every child is different, but until about the age of 11 or 12, most children are not able to handle stressful or emergency situations that require mature decision making on their own. Therefore, it is best for parents to arrange for an adult or a responsible older adolescent to be at home when they are not present, or for some other structured supervision.

However, your child may be an exception and be sufficiently mature at the age of 10 years to be home alone after school or for other short periods of time. Before her first time on her own, however, you need to make sure she feels safe and secure, and that she is prepared for dealing with knocks on the door, emergencies, and injuries. Some communities and local fire departments offer courses in babysitting that can also serve as good preparation for self-care. Nevertheless, your child should not be home alone until she is comfortable with that arrangement. Here are some issues that you should discuss with her:

- Does she know her full name, address, and phone number? Does she know your full name as well, your cellphone number, and the address and phone number of your workplace, or other ways to reach you at work? You might call every day, text message, or even use face-to-face video chat to be sure your child has arrived home safely and that nothing at home is out of the ordinary; children appreciate the sense of security this form of supervision provides.

- Does she have an established routine to follow so she knows what she is supposed to do and where she is supposed to be?

- Can your child use the telephone correctly, particularly when calling you, a neighbor, or emergency services (911)? Any number that might be needed in an emergency should be written down or stored in your child's phone contacts list.

- When she returns home from school every day, does your child know how to lock the door behind her? Can she remember to call you or a neighbor as soon as she arrives home, and then check in again at designated times?

- Have you instructed your child never to enter your home if a door is ajar, or if a window is open or broken?

- Have you talked about what to do if someone knocks at the front door while she is home alone? She should not open the door under any circum-

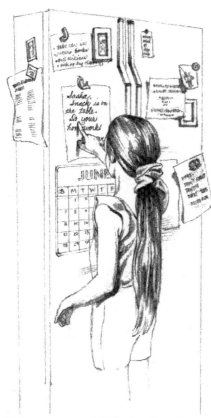

Make sure your child feels safe and secure and is well prepared to deal with emergencies if she will be home alone after school.

stances, nor give any impression she is home alone.

■ Have you and your child discussed how she should exit your home quickly in case of a fire? Does she know which exits are safest, depending on the location of the fire? Does she know what to do in case of an emergency or a natural disaster such as thunderstorm, tornado, or earthquake, and is she familiar with basic first aid (e.g., applying pressure to a cut)?

Gun Safety

Firearm violence is a public health crisis in the United States. Guns are widely available in our society and are kept in millions of American homes. In a study of gun-owning Americans with children under 18 years of age, 21.7 percent stored a gun loaded, 31.5 percent stored a gun unlocked, and 8.3 percent stored at least one gun unlocked and loaded. Many children are either unaware of or ignore the possible consequences of handling these lethal weapons. Their mere presence poses a very real danger to children.

School-age children are curious about and often attracted to guns. They sometimes see guns as symbols of power. So do many adolescents and adults. Parents often mistakenly believe that their children do not know where the gun is stored or how to access it. They may think they can teach their child not to handle a gun; however, several studies show that gun-avoidance teaching does not prevent children from handling guns and may actually increase it instead. No amount of teaching can overcome a child's natural curiosity.

The availability of handguns in settings where children live and play has led to a devastating toll in human lives, reflected in some sobering and almost unthinkable statistics: every two hours, a child is killed with a gun, either in a homicide, in a suicide, or as a result of an unintentional injury. In addition, an unknown but large number of children are seriously injured—often irreversibly disabled—by guns but survive.

Parents should realize that a gun in the home is much more likely to be used to kill a friend or family member than a burglar or other criminal. To compound this problem, depressed preteenagers and teenagers die by suicide with guns more frequently than by any other means. Suicide by firearm is much more likely to be fatal than other methods, with approximately a 90 percent mortality rate. Those who survive a suicide attempt usually do not die of a subsequent attempt, but there is no second chance with a gun. Keeping guns out of the hands of children and adolescents is important to reducing the risk of suicide.

The best preventive measure against firearm injuries and deaths is not to own a gun. However, if you have firearms in your home, adhere to these rules for gun safety:

- Never allow your child access to your gun(s). No matter how much instruction you may give him or her, a child in the middle years is not mature and responsible enough to handle a potentially lethal weapon and cannot be trusted not to handle a gun if it is found.

- Never keep a loaded gun in the house or the car.

- Guns and ammunition should be locked away safely in separate locations in the house; make sure children don't have access to the keys.

- Guns should be equipped with trigger locks.

- When using a gun for hunting or target practice, learn how to operate it before ever loading it. Never point the gun at another person, and keep the safety catch in place until you are ready to fire it. Before setting the gun down, always unload it. Do not use alcohol or drugs while you are shooting.

WHERE WE STAND

The American Academy of Pediatrics strongly supports gun control legislation. We support the strongest possible legislative and regulatory approaches to prevent firearm injuries and deaths.

Even if you don't have guns in your own home, that won't eliminate your child's risks. Half of the homes in the United States contain firearms, and many unintentional shootings of children take place in the homes of their friends, neighbors, or relatives. It is your responsibility as a parent to ask if guns are present in the homes where your child visits, and if so, whether they are stored safely, locked up and unloaded with the ammunition locked in a separate place.

Here is some important information you need to communicate to your child:

- Let them know that risks of gun injuries may exist in places they visit and play.

- Tell them that if they see or encounter a gun in a friend's home or elsewhere, they must steer clear of it, and tell you about it.

- Talk with the parents of your child's friends, and find out if they have firearms in their home. If they do, insist that they keep them unloaded, locked up, and inaccessible to children. This may be an uncomfortable conversation for you to initiate, but other parents are often thankful to have the issue raised; the more often this conversation happens, the safer our society as a whole will be.

- Make sure your children understand that violence on TV, in the movies, and in videogames is not real. They need to be told—and probably reminded again and again—that in real life, people are killed and hurt badly by guns. Although the popular media often romanticizes gun use, children must learn that these weapons are extremely dangerous.

Substance Use

Substance Use Prevention

Drugs, including alcohol, tobacco, and other substances, are unfortunately available even to school-age children. As a parent, you have a significant role in your child's decision not to use substances. Children as young as grade school should hear parents' values and learn about the dangers of substance use, before they are readily available or being offered to your child. Parents begin these difficult conversations, which are then supported by school programs on substance use prevention. Talk with, and listen to, your child. Support your child's good choices and friends, and teach your child how to speak up for herself and say no when necessary.

Parents serve as kids' greatest role models; children watch how the adults in their world use alcohol and other substances at home and in their social life. Model good habits by drinking only in moderation and never driving after drinking. Speak honestly with your child about healthy choices and risky behaviors.

Learn the facts about the harmful effects of substance use, and share these with your child. Talk with your child about the negative effects alcohol and drugs would have on their brains and bodies and their ability to learn or play sports.

It does not matter what choices other families at school or in the community make; your family determines its own set of values. Correct any misperceptions your child has about substance use. Use TV commercials for alcohol as a teaching opportunity to share your values with your child. Eating together as a family is a good time to talk and learn about what's going on in their lives at the moment. Let your kids know you care about them, and talk with them about being safe.

Help your child make good choices and friendships. A good sense of self-worth and knowing what is right and wrong will help your child say no to substances and other risky behaviors. Check to see that the friends your child spends time with are safe and have values similar to yours. Find ways to get your child involved in sports, hobbies, school clubs, and other activities that develop character and lead to good peer relationships. Look for activities that you and your child or the entire family can do together. Help your child learn the importance of being a responsible individual and what it means to be a real friend. Children need to learn that real friends do not ask friends to do risky things like use alcohol, tobacco, or drugs, or reject friends when they don't want to do something that they know is wrong.

Teach your child how to respond to someone offering drugs. It is much easier to say no when prepared ahead of time. Role-playing and practicing for this situation helps your child feel natural when the time comes to say no, say why not, suggest something else to do, or leave the situation entirely.

Efforts aimed at the prevention of substance use must begin *before* the teen years, during the middle years of childhood. Prevention, including raising awareness of risks, the communication of values, and providing the example of desirable behavior, must occur in all arenas of the child's life—home, school, and community. The degree and effectiveness of this education can influence what behavior will occur during adolescence.

The use of alcohol, tobacco, or other substances begins with experimentation and casual usage. The use of these substances starts in a social setting, usually under strong peer pressure. But what begins as a social event may turn into drug dependency. The longer one of these substances is utilized, the more habitual its use becomes, and the greater the risk of both psychological and physiological addiction.

When a young person starts experimenting with drugs, he often has the illusion that he can control its use, denying that the substance is potentially addictive. Also, children are notoriously unable to see the connection between present behavior and future consequences, and they feel immune to bad outcomes. Nevertheless, as habitual use gradually becomes established and dependence upon the substance grows, the child increasingly loses control of the drug use.

Researchers believe that an individual's use of drugs progresses along what is called a *substance use hierarchy*. The entrance or "gateway" drug for many young people is tobacco, but they then move on to alcohol. They then may experiment with marijuana, cocaine, and other types of substances. Across the country, heroin use has become a growing concern. Many youths do not realize that their first time trying a substance could be their last; the first use of heroin can result in death. However, it is known that adolescents who engage in one type of risky behavior, like smoking, are more likely to be involved in others, such as drug use and sexual activity. They are also more likely to have academic problems.

How susceptible is your own child to the temptations of substance use? Many factors contribute to his potential vulnerability: his self-esteem, his emotional needs, existing behavioral problems, and the values of the family and community. Your own attitude toward substance use is probably *the* major factor determining whether your child will use drugs. If you smoke, that is the example you are setting for your child; kids often do what they see. It will be harder for you to persuade him not to use cigarettes when he sees you smoking. And when you bring

Secondhand Smoke and Children

If you smoke and are having difficulty motivating yourself to stop, bear in mind that the research is conclusive: parental smoking is a serious health hazard for both you and your children. Children who live in the same households as smokers inhale cigarette smoke. As a result, they run a higher risk of developing asthma, bronchitis, pneumonia, and middle-ear disease. These children also have more difficulty getting over colds. Of the more than 4,000 chemicals that have been identified in tobacco smoke, at least 40 are known to cause cancer.

The American Academy of Pediatrics suggests:

- If you would like to quit smoking but have been unable to, contact your physician; there are many low-cost programs available to help.

- If your spouse or another member of your household is a smoker, provide him or her with support to quit.

- If you or other members of your household are not able to give up cigarettes, do not smoke inside the house. And by no means should anyone smoke in an automobile in which children ride.

cigarettes into the home or leave incompletely smoked cigarettes in ashtrays, they become too easily available if your child or his friends decide they want to try one.

If you want to help your child avoid the added health risks caused by smoking, you must first start by stopping smoking yourself. Children whose parents smoke are more likely to use cigarettes than are the children of nonsmokers. In the same way, if either parent is a heavy alcohol or substance user, a child is much more likely to become involved in their use, due to both exposure and availability.

The media play another influential role in substance abuse. Celebrities who appear in the media with a drink in their hand or a cigarette in their mouth can influence children. Advertisers are targeting children and adolescents in efforts to encourage future use of tobacco products and alcohol. Advertising attempts to "normalize" the use of alcohol and tobacco—conveying the impression that "everyone is doing it."

All children and adolescents desire the approval of peers as they become increasingly independent of their families and develop their own identities. If your child's friends have substances available, he will be encouraged to try them. Children and teens who report feeling connected to their family or school report fewer high-risk behaviors, such as substance use, and greater numbers of prosocial behaviors, such as sports, arts, music, or extracurricular activities.

Some children are much more vulnerable to these peer influences than others. Children with a poor self-concept or a strong need for acceptance will tend to try harder to win approval from their peers and will more readily conform to their friends' behavior. These same children may have conduct problems, depression, anxiety, or family stresses, and they may also find a numbing relief and excitement in the use of illicit and self-destructive substances. Substance use also may give them a sense of pleasure, freedom, and independence, and a chance to rebel and assert themselves in a world that otherwise seems to give them little control or autonomy.

How to Help Your Child Be Substance-Free

A child with healthy self-esteem has much less need to use substances. A number of factors can contribute to a child's feeling good about himself, many of which come from positive interactions within the family and from his successful performance at school and in other social settings. The section "Self-Esteem," on page 139, discusses this topic more thoroughly, but here are a few ways you can strengthen your child's self-concept.

- Raise your child to feel that he is important in your life and to believe that his feelings and thoughts really matter. Be respectful of his wishes, and try to understand his perspective and instill in him a sense of self-worth. Show an interest in his schoolwork.

- Participate in his hobbies and other activities. Spend time reading books together or playing games of his choice.

- Be honest with your child in all aspects of your relationship with him. Parents who lie or break promises give their child reasons to distrust them and give the impression that it is somehow okay to be deceitful and hide substance use.

- Acknowledge and celebrate your child's successes and achievements, which can help him build a sense of personal confidence and power in the world. Cheer his successes in school and with peers, and when he demonstrates responsibility at home.

- Clearly articulate your own attitudes about substance use. At the same time, examine your own use of substances and what kind of model you are presenting to him.

WHERE WE STAND

Alcohol is the substance most often abused by the largest number of children and adolescents. The American Academy of Pediatrics is strongly opposed to the use of alcohol by children and adolescents and supports a ban on alcohol advertising and promotion.

Alcohol use can result in impaired judgment, poor coordination, drowsiness, vomiting, or depression. Long-term use can result in blackouts, vitamin deficiencies, hepatitis or cirrhosis, heart disease, or stroke.

While driving under the influence is an obvious hazard of alcohol usage, impaired judgment can put even younger kids in danger of a difficult situation of being taken advantage of physically or sexually.

Parents should discuss alcohol use with their kids, and model appropriate behaviors. Share your values about the use of alcohol and other substances with your children, even if you have used them yourself in the past.

An important part of this educational process is to educate your child about the health hazards associated with tobacco use. Cigarettes cause lung cancer and heart disease, and are the most common cause of lung diseases like chronic bronchitis and emphysema. Even though these are chronic diseases that may take many years—even decades—to develop, let your child know that the earlier he starts smoking, the greater his chance of becoming addicted and eventually developing these conditions.

Children are not particularly motivated by long-term consequences, so remind your child of the more immediate drawbacks to smoking. Young people may believe that kids who smoke are "cool" and sophisticated. Cigarette advertising, for example, stresses the social desirability of smoking. But in fact, smoking stains teeth. It causes bad breath and a hacking cough, plus it leaves a strong tobacco odor on clothes. The habit costs quite a lot. And for children who like sports, the use of cigarettes can keep them from running or swimming as well as they could if they didn't smoke.

What About Chewing Tobacco or E-Cigarettes?

A growing number of young people are using chewing (smokeless) tobacco or e-cigarettes as an alternative to cigarettes.

The potential for chewing tobacco use is particularly high among young boys who imitate some adult professional athletes. The nicotine in smokeless tobacco is as addicting as the nicotine in cigarettes. Smokeless tobacco can cause sores and white patches in the mouth and throat, and cracking and bleeding of the lips and gums. It can interfere with a child's sense of taste and smell, and can lead ultimately to the development of cancer of the throat, mouth, and gums.

E-cigarettes, also called electronic nicotine delivery systems (ENDS), are becoming more popular among adolescents and adults. ENDS, e-cigarettes, vape pens, "juuling," e-cigars, or vaping devices heat a mixture of nicotine and flavored liquid that is then inhaled by the user. Unfortunately, they are not yet regulated by the U.S. Food and Drug Administration. The AAP supports actions to prevent kids from using or being exposed to ENDS vapors. The solution in these devices can contain harmful chemicals and carcinogens (cancer-causing agents). The nicotine is addictive and can harm the still-developing brain. Some of these devices have exploded, causing burns. The long-term effect of users and that of secondhand smoke are still not known.

You should discourage your child's use of these products as strongly as you resist his use of traditional cigarettes.

What to Do if Your Child Is Using Substances

Many children involved in using substances are not receiving adequate parental supervision of their activities. If you discover your school-age child experimenting with cigarettes or alcohol, take this opportunity to communicate your own attitudes about smoking and drinking. At the same time, learn from your child why she has smoked or used alcohol. Discuss the peer pressure she may be experiencing, and together consider how to deal with it effectively. Talk about how the values of her friends and their families may conflict with your own. Be clear about what you believe is right and wrong, healthy and unhealthy, safe and unsafe. Teach your child to use her conscience as a guide; this will encourage her to be responsible for herself, and it will demonstrate that you trust her to show good judgment and make good choices.

When children in the middle years use tobacco, alcohol, or other substances repeatedly, it is no longer experimentation, it is a problem. Children who engage in this type of risky behavior are more likely to engage in other high-risk activities. You need to consider what might be motivating your child to jeopardize her health in this way. Look at this substance use in the context of what else is happening in her life. It signals a serious problem, including her association with peers who are supplying her with the illicit substance.

In the middle childhood years, it is not too late to help your child nurture good friends who are good influences. Discuss with her what she values in a friendship, and how to meet and make friends with children whose values are similar to hers

WHERE WE STAND

The American Academy of Pediatrics opposes the use of tobacco in any form. Smoking should be prohibited in all public places, and children should not be exposed to tobacco smoke at home or school. We also support a complete ban on tobacco advertising, the use of harsher warning labels on cigarette packages, and an increase in the cigarette excise tax.

Currently 43 percent of children ages 2 months to 11 years live in a home with at least one smoker. If you smoke, quit. If you can't quit, don't smoke around children (especially indoors or in the car). Children of parents who smoke have more respiratory infections, bronchitis, pneumonia, and reduced pulmonary function than children of nonsmokers.

and those of your family. Set limits on her association with children who appear to lead her away from your own values, thus protecting her and teaching her to make good judgments.

Your pediatrician can recommend evaluation by a child psychiatrist or psychologist, or participation in an alcohol- or drug-use program, which are critical before the pressures of adolescence begin.

~ 7 ~

Emergency Preparedness

NATURAL AND MAN-MADE disasters can affect anyone. Planning for a disaster may feel overwhelming; however, taking a few simple steps can help protect your family, ensure that your children feel safe, and make it easier to recover after a disaster. As kids approach middle school age, knowing what to do in an emergency situation is an important life skill.

Based on where you live, you may be at risk for natural disasters such as forest fires, floods, tornadoes, winter weather, hurricanes, or earthquakes. Human-caused disasters, such as terrorism or hazardous material spills, can also affect you and your community. Basic preparation will help you in any type of disaster.

A disaster plan should include all the needs of each family member. True family readiness is achieved when a family has prepared and planned together. Include children in family preparedness discussions and decisions in an age-appropriate way to empower them.

Emergency Supply Kit

Keep a supply kit of things you may need in case of an emergency. Flashlights and extra batteries will be necessary if you do not have power, and bottled water is a good idea. Keep a supply kit in your car also in case your car breaks down. Check your kits at least once every six months. Items may need to be replaced or updated. For example, replace expired food or clothing children have outgrown. Visit online resources such as Ready.gov, RedCross.org, and HealthyChildren.org for more information about what to include in a supply kit.

In addition to preparing a kit, update personal and medical records. If you have copies of important documents at home, make sure to give a copy to a trusted person in another region, and save any details that you can on your phone or in a web- or cloud-based system.

If you have a child with special healthcare needs, you may want to make him a "go bag." It may be a bag your child takes to school each day. You can keep the special bag with your family kit, but it should be easy to carry.

Make a Plan

An emergency plan must include communication, transportation, and reunification. You should consider steps to take if you need to leave your home quickly or if you need to shelter for an extended time.

Communications Plan

Talk with your kids! Discuss how to prepare for disasters that could happen in your area. Teach them what the different danger or warning signals sound like (for example, a fire alarm and a tornado siren). Show them where you keep a list of contacts, such as family members, emergency contacts, doctors' and veterinary offices, and pharmacies. Children should know their parents' names, phone numbers, and addresses. Consider using a child ID card (either homemade or a version included with your child's yearly school portraits), and place a copy of this card in your child's kit or backpack. Your child should understand 911 usage and when to call this number. Choose an out-of-state family "check-in" member and make sure everyone in the family knows how to contact that person. If you fear you may become separated from your younger child, then write your phone number on her forearm with permanent marker (or provide him with an emergency bracelet). Do this even if your child knows your phone number; when younger kids are stressed or hurt they may not be able to recall a phone number. Decide on local and out-of-state meeting places if you become separated from your family. During a disaster, cell communications may not work. Make sure all family members know how to text, or make a plan to inform members through an agreed-upon social media platform.

Transportation Plan

Let child care or school staff know who can pick your child up if you are not able to do so, and let your kids know about this backup plan. Know your evacuation routes as well as alternative routes. If possible, find a friend's or relative's place that is far away (hundreds of miles) where you and your family could stay. Print directions to this location and keep these in your car and in your disaster kit. Identify the shelters in your area. Find out which shelters can suit your needs, such as medical, family, or pets. Use the Red Cross Shelter App to find a shelter near you.

Reunification Plan

Create a family password or safe phrase to prevent your children from going with a stranger. Identify a family meeting place outside the home (for example, a neighbor's house). Take and store photos on your phone of all forms of identification cards for your family, and consider having a hard copy on you at all times, in case you misplace your phone.

Be Informed

As part of your plans, consider working with others to create networks of neighbors, relatives, friends, and coworkers who will help each other in an emergency. Talk with your neighbors and learn who has special skills such as doctors, nurses, and firefighters. Find out who has special needs and may need extra help such as elderly or disabled persons. Buy a battery-operated or weather radio, such as a National Oceanic and Atmospheric Administration (NOAA) radio, for your home. Talk with your kids about the difference between a weather watch and warning so they understand the different messages the radio will provide. Download the American Red Cross Emergency App to your phone, and for older kids who have their own phones, download it to their phones also. The app is free and will send text alerts when there is a watch or warning for your area. You also can use it to see what emergency shelters have been set up after a disaster. Show your kids where the smoke alarms and carbon monoxide alarms are located in your home, and review with them what they need to do for each alarm if they go off. Learn about environmental risks in your area and plan for each risk. Risks may include tornadoes, floods, hurricanes, or earthquakes. Check with your child's school or child care program to find out what plans are in place to help kids stay safe.

Get Involved

Have your kids help you when you test the smoke alarms in your home. Check your alarms at least every six months when reviewing your kit; this gives your kids a chance to hear what the alarms sound like. Smoke alarm batteries should be changed once a year; some families do this on the same day each year, such as January 1, to help them remember. Show your kids where the fire extinguisher is and how to use it. Talk with your kids' teachers and school to find out what the school disaster plans are and how often they drill them. Check with your local fire department to see if they offer Community Emergency Response Team training. Take a Red Cross first-aid and CPR class; many local fire departments offer these classes for children 11 years and older as part of a babysitting certification course.

While it can be daunting to think of a natural or man-made disaster, emergency preparedness can help families feel more secure knowing that if the unexpected strikes, they will be ready. These preparation steps also help kids learn important life skills.

~ 8 ~

Your Growing Child and Sex Education

AS CHILDREN GROW through the school years, they learn about sex from the world around them. The behaviors and attitudes modeled by adults (including their parents), the media and popular culture, and certainly peers all play a role in their education. Parents in particular hold a significant role in a child's sex education, and should guide their children to accurate, age-appropriate information. Even if you feel uncomfortable talking to your child about sex, remember that she will learn about it from the world around her, and it is best that *you* are also a part of that conversation.

Children in their middle years have great curiosity about sex. Five-year-olds will ask questions about body parts during bath time. A 7-year-old will wonder why grown men look different from grown women. A relative will announce a pregnancy, leading to questions regarding how babies are made. A fifth-grader may hear a joke about sex at the playground at recess. An 11-year-old searching on the internet stumbles upon inappropriate sexual content. It is not a matter of *if* your child will have questions, but *when*.

The process of learning about sex and sexuality begins in early childhood, as soon as children are able to observe, listen to, and sense the world around them. Initially, most of their learning took place at home, but now, as they move through middle childhood, many messages about sexuality come from the outside environment—not only from their peers but also from the media, including the internet, social networks, movies, television, advertisements, and other media.

Talking to Your Child About Sex

Parents of prior generations had "the talk" with their children—a single, onetime discussion of the "birds and bees." The notion of a single conversation is outdated. Rather, parents should have a series of mini-conversations with children about various sexual topics over time, in an age-appropriate manner. At all stages, these smaller talks should be modified for that child's age and developmental stage, and these chats will often be quite brief and to the point for younger children.

When younger children ask inevitable questions about body parts or a relative's growing pregnancy, use the situation as a teaching opportunity to define terms and convey information in a calm, matter-of-fact manner. Often a younger child's innocent questions cause panic in a parent, but remember that brief explanations are best; a topic this significant should not be covered in a single discussion. Try not to think about sex as a taboo or anxiety-producing topic—it is normal human behavior, and should be taught in a way that is comfortable and natural. The biggest barrier to ensuring successful sex education is parental hesitation.

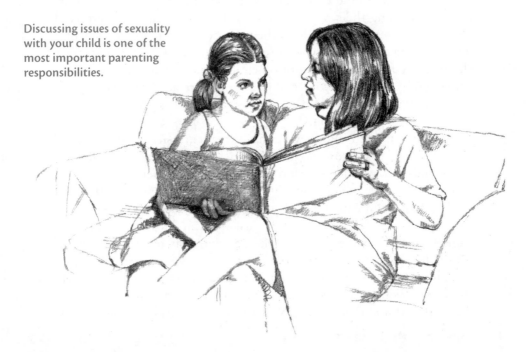

Discussing issues of sexuality with your child is one of the most important parenting responsibilities.

Everyday opportunities—"teachable moments"—often provide the best time to discuss sexuality-related topics.

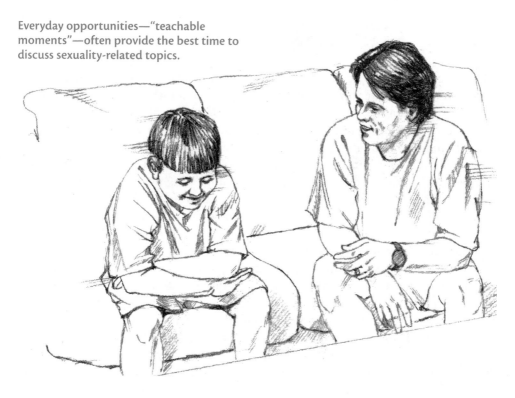

While many school systems offer sexuality education in middle school, there is no better place for children to learn about sexuality than from their parents. Of key importance is that you have an important opportunity to discuss with your child the *values* you associate with sex. In a one-on-one conversation, you can personalize the issues with your child, discuss your child's fears and worries, and make sure sexuality education, as well as your family's values, are offered well ahead of the time that pressures for sexual behavior increase.

Children learn about sexuality not only from what parents say but also from parents' behavior, observing the interactions of those they love. Keep in mind that for a child, sexual interest is not synonymous with sexual activity. When kids in middle childhood pose questions about sex, they are not interested in engaging in physical acts themselves, but may be fascinated with the subject because they sense that it is taboo or secret. The physical changes your child will experience at puberty will trigger a lot of questions (for more on puberty, see page 70). While these questions should be answered directly, proper education about sexuality also encompasses topics such as sexual roles, sexual orientation, the concept of consent and ownership over one's own body, avoiding substance use in order to make appropriate choices and stay safe, and establishing relationships in the future. (For more on gender issues and sexual orientation, see page 148. For more on substance use, see page 95.)

How Do I Start?

The earlier you begin the process of sex education, the better. Sex education for children does not center on the physical acts of sex, but rather includes the broader concepts of sexuality—the physical, emotional, and social aspects. Ideally, you have had continuing conversations about sexual issues since your child's earliest years. Simply defining anatomy and using anatomically correct terms for private parts such as "penis" and "vagina" are a good start. If you wait until he or she reaches puberty or adolescence to start communicating on these important matters, the parent-child dialogue will be much more difficult. You need to become comfortable with these discussions as early as possible, so that you can lay a firm educational foundation and establish a pattern of openness and easy dialogue between you and your child *before* puberty.

Many adults had very little sex education when they were growing up. They may have learned about sex from movies or from friends, and may not have accurate information themselves about human anatomy and the biology of sex. They may be uncertain about what is appropriate during various stages of their child's development. These parents should reach out directly to their family's pediatrician with any questions so that they feel more confident when talking to their own children. Some schools include parents in their health-education courses for children, and some pediatricians offer family sex-education talks in the evenings.

When your child asks questions about sexual issues, answer with clear, straightforward explanations.

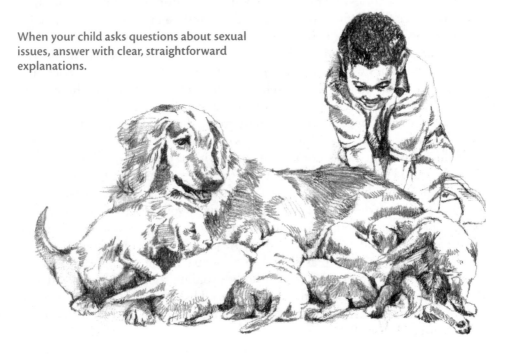

In addition to increasing their own knowledge, parents also may find a book or two they can share with their child. There are numerous books available, meant for young girls or young boys, that are written specifically for children at different ages and developmental stages. These may serve as a guide and an excellent resource especially if the parent is nervous about explaining body changes and sexuality. The discussion does not end with reading the book; rather, the book should serve as a starting point to raise further questions from your child and more conversations over time.

Some parents are afraid they will not know the answers to all their children's questions. If that situation arises, you can simply respond, "That is a good question. I am not sure," and offer to find out the information and discuss it later. Over time, as you answer their questions, both you and your children will become more comfortable with talking about sexuality.

The information that parents give can be guided primarily by the questions a child asks. Some children, however, may not ask directly for specific information, particularly if they believe their parents are uncomfortable with the topic. As a general rule, when your child asks questions, answer with clear, short, straightforward explanations. Do not overwhelm your child with more information than she asked for; instead, follow up your responses with an inquiry of your own, such as "Does that answer your question?" Parents might find themselves surprised by a sudden question regarding sexuality that seems to arise unexpectedly—a good tactic in this situation is to ask your child, "What do you think?" This will allow you a brief moment to collect your own thoughts as well as learn more about what your child's frame of reference is. Often we adults infer our adult knowledge into our younger kids' questions. Your goal during these mini-talks is to convey just the right amount of information for your child's age—not too much and not too little.

A few days later you might ask your child: "Is there anything else you're wondering about related to the discussion we had last week?" Life is busy, and sometimes the best moments to have these chats are when you're driving in the car, with screens off and put away. You have a captive audience during a car ride, for example, and the potential intensity and uncomfortable nature of the conversation are calmed a bit by the fact that you are both looking toward your destination. Similarly, chatting while playing catch or working together to put away clean laundry can be good opportunities for these conversations.

Even when questions are not posed, take the initiative and use everyday opportunities—teachable moments—to discuss appropriate sexually related topics. For example, you can bring up sexual issues when:

- A pregnancy or a birth occurs in the family.

- Your older child helps change the diaper of a brother and notices that the baby has an erection. Describe this bodily process matter-of-factly as a natural part of life.

- Relationships of all kinds are encountered in books or on television. This can prompt conversations about dating, love, same- and opposite-sex relationships, and the difference between healthy and unhealthy relationships.

- Issues arise during television viewing, such as media reports about rape or sexual harassment.

- Children mention words with sexual overtones that they have heard in the schoolyard or the playground.

- You and your child observe the sexual behavior of pets or animals in zoos, on farms, or on nature programs on TV, allowing you to discuss mating, reproduction, romance, and attraction.

To build your own confidence, you might try talking over these issues first with another adult, such as a partner or a friend. This will give you an opportunity to think about what questions may arise and help you to clarify your responses. Also, find out what your child is learning in school about sexuality so you can build upon it. Another idea is to start simply with basic anatomy and the role of different sexual organs. The conversation can branch out from there.

If you are finding it difficult to communicate with your child about sex, perhaps because of your own inhibitions and anxieties, ask for help from another adult in this educational process. Perhaps a relative or your pedia-

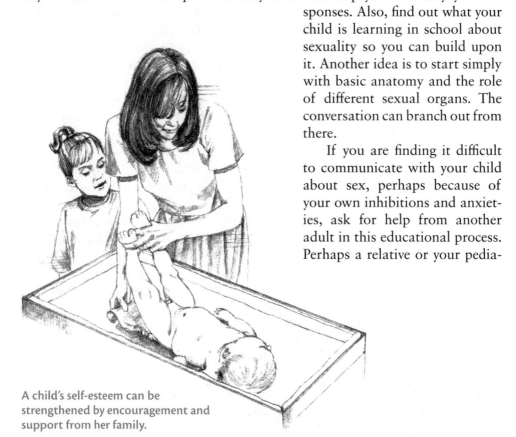

A child's self-esteem can be strengthened by encouragement and support from her family.

trician can convey the information about sexuality that your child needs during this important time in her life. In cases like this, however, you should make a special effort to convey your value system to your child; *no one* can do this better than you.

Discussing Sexuality with Your Child

The idea of a single conversation about sexuality—"the talk"—is outdated. Rather, it is important to have a series of mini-conversations with your child, keeping the discussion age-appropriate. At different stages of development your child will ask the same questions, but will be seeking different answers. For instance, questions like "Where do babies come from?" may arise several times during middle childhood, but as your child matures he or she will be able to understand more sophisticated responses.

Children ages 5–7 years: Younger school-age children have a more concrete, simple understanding of physical attributes, changes, and relationships. Keep answers to questions brief and age-appropriate. Use family news such as an aunt's new pregnancy as a conversation starter. All the details are not required at this age.

Children ages 8–10 years: As they get older, children are ready for more details. The school will likely be introducing some version of a puberty and sexuality discussion in these grades; better that your kids hear trusted information from you first. Use situations in television and movies as a launchpad for a conversation. Follow up after the school discussion to see if they have any questions.

Children ages 11–12 years: At this age, children have a more sophisticated understanding of sexuality; however, parents need to remember they still have a lot to learn and continue to require parental guidance. Use moments in movies, TV, and other media as conversation starters: for example, "What did you think of that relationship?" If you see something with your kids that you do or do not agree with, share your values with them and explain why.

What Are Your Child's Sexuality-Related Questions?

"How are the bodies of boys and girls different?"

"How old do girls have to be before they can have a baby?"

"Do you have to get married to have a baby?"

"Why do boys get erections?"

"What is a period?"

"How do people have sexual intercourse?"

"Why do some men like other men?"

These are the kinds of questions that school-age children ask. Each of them deserves a straightforward answer, perhaps beginning with a question of your own ("What do you know already?" or "What do you think?") to get the dialogue flowing and give you the opportunity to correct any misinformation. If you have a sense of your child's existing level of knowledge, you will have a point of reference from which to introduce new facts. Some children, however, will not admit to any knowledge, either because they feel uncomfortable or in an effort to get their parents to repeat and confirm what the children have heard in the past.

In the first years of life children are curious primarily about anatomical differences between males and females. Later, they may also pose questions about sexually related phenomena: "Where do babies come from?" or "How are babies made?" By age 8 or 9 they may have acquired many of these facts but have not yet tied them together in a way that makes sense to them.

Middle childhood encompasses years in which your child will experience considerable growth and development; in your discussions with your child, take into account your child's age, experience, knowledge, physical development, and emotional maturity. Here are the basic questions that your child will ask, and central themes that you should discuss together, as she moves toward puberty:

- What are the body parts related to sexuality, including their actual anatomic names and their functions? If you use euphemisms or nicknames for parts of the sexual anatomy, you will give the impression that there is something offensive or shameful about them. In these discussions it is especially important to treat the subject material as matter-of-factly as possible, as this is a natural, normal part of our bodies. Your child may already be curious about her own body, examining it and becoming familiar with her own physical sensations. You can use this natural curiosity to provide information about male and female sexual anatomy.

- How are babies conceived and born?

- What is puberty? How will your child's body change as she goes through this stage of life? (For more on puberty, see page 70.)

- What is menstruation? Both boys and girls can benefit from this information.

- What are the different ways that people have sex?

- What is masturbation? Emphasize that masturbation and self-exploration are aspects of sexuality. Help your child approach this subject (and all other parts of sexuality) without a sense of guilt. It is important to dispel myths about masturbation. (See page 117.)

- What is the function of birth control? Explain that if a man and a woman want to have sexual intercourse but do not want to have a baby, they need to use some type of contraceptive. For older kids, you can explain the basic types of birth control methods and how they prevent ovulation or fertilization.

- What are sexually transmitted infections and how are they contracted? Any discussion of sexual topics should include an age-appropriate discussion of the risks incurred in future sexual choices and behaviors.

- What does sexual orientation mean? Children become increasingly aware of relationships between people of the same sex. They may sense a social unacceptability that they misconstrue as disapproval of having feelings toward a good friend. In responding to this question, use the opportunity to reassure your child that liking and loving people does not depend on their gender and is different from liking someone sexually. (For more on gender identity and sexual orientation, see page 148.)

- What ethical guidelines should be part of your child's sexual behavior later in life? A value system is critical, helping your child place sexual issues in a context that is thoughtful, considerate, and healthy and that will encourage meaningful adult relationships. Teach your child that sex is a decision between two adults to engage in a physical activity that has both physical and emotional consequences.

■ Who has authority over one's body and safe space? Parents should introduce the idea of *consent* to their kids. A child has the ultimate authority over his own body and safe space. Younger kids, both girls *and* boys, can be taught that any area covered up by a bathing suit is only for them. The idea of consent can be introduced by not requiring a younger child to hug or kiss anyone he does not feel comfortable with; for example, a child should not be forced to kiss a rarely seen aunt at a family reunion if he does not want to. As the child grows, this idea of his having authority over his own body can be built upon.

■ In addition, parents should discuss how substance use can impair one's judgment and ability to make appropriate choices to stay safe. The subject of safety and making good choices is an important conversation to have with both girls *and* boys. (For more on substance use, see page 95.)

Common Sexual Concerns

Parent and child alike experience certain sexual anxieties as the child enters and moves through puberty. Some parents worry that when it comes to sex, all their child is thinking about is physical sexual acts. That belief is erroneous, and it interferes with communication between the generations. As your child begins puberty, he will be much more interested in looking attractive to the opposite sex, and finding and keeping a boyfriend or girlfriend, than in the act of making love.

Another misconception is also quite common among adults: many parents are convinced that if they teach their child about sex, they will be encouraging the child to become sexually active at an early age. They feel that by talking about sex, they are sanctioning it. But in fact the opposite is true. As children enter and pass through adolescence, those who are the best informed about sex are the most likely to postpone physical acts of sex, having more information at hand about what is involved in making future sexual decisions and choices. By contrast, when children do not get information from their parents, they turn to friends or other sources from whom they are more apt to receive *mis*information; that ignorance— and the inability to discuss sexuality with their parents—may lead them to earlier sexual physical acts, and a greater vulnerability to sexually transmitted infections and unwanted pregnancies. It is *mis*information or a lack of communication that gets children into trouble.

As mentioned earlier, when you talk about sexuality, do not overlook discussing your family's values. If you openly explain your beliefs—and the reasons for them—to your child, you may give your child the strength to resist peer pressure to engage in physical sexual acts before he is ready.

Gender identity and sexual orientation are important areas of development in all children's lives; for more information on these issues, see page 148. The use of social media and the dangers of "sexting" are all too real; for more on this, see page 315.

Masturbation

Masturbation is a normal aspect of childhood development of sexuality that parents find hard to respond to comfortably and appropriately. The misunderstandings and secrecy about masturbation add to both parent and child discomfort. By definition, masturbation is self-stimulation of the genitals. It is done by both boys and girls, and is normal behavior.

How common is masturbation during the various stages of childhood? Up to the age of 5 or 6 years, masturbation is quite common. Young children are very curious about their bodies and find masturbation pleasurable and comforting. Children also are noticing the differences between girls and boys, so in the preschool and kindergarten years they may be curious about each other's body, including their genitals.

From age 6 on, the incidence of masturbation in public tends to subside, largely because children's social awareness increases and social mores assume greater importance. Masturbation in private will continue to some extent and remains normal. When pubertal development begins—accompanied by an increase of sexual hormones, thoughts, and curiosity—body awareness and sexual tensions rise. Masturbation is a regular part of normal adolescence. Most young teenagers discover that masturbation is sexually pleasing and recognize that self-stimulation is an expression of their own developing sexuality.

Although the myths surrounding masturbation have been dispelled, they still persist. A child who masturbates is *not* oversexed or promiscuous. Nevertheless, many cultures still actively discourage masturbation, partly because of the general moral constraints often placed on sexual behavior.

When parents of school-age children discover their child's masturbatory play or activity, some react with embarrassment, anger, or even moral outrage; others take it in stride and recognize it as developmentally normal behavior. Ideally, this discovery provides an opportunity for teaching children about their own sexuality and about the differences between public and private activities. If you encounter your child in this situation, keep your demeanor matter-of-fact and remind your child that this activity, while normal, should only be done in private, not in the presence of others.

Excessive or public masturbation may indicate a more serious psychological or personal problem. It could be a sign that the child is stressed, is overly preoccupied with sexual thoughts, fantasies, or urges, or is not receiving adequate attention at home. Sometimes masturbation is a means of providing himself with personal comfort when he is feeling emotionally overwhelmed. Masturbation could be a tipoff to sexual abuse; children who are being sexually abused may become overly preoccupied with their sexuality, suggesting the need for further investigation.

What Should You Do?

"I caught my child masturbating. What should I do?" It is not unusual for physicians to hear this question from worried parents. However, masturbation is a part of normal human sexual experience, and children find it pleasurable. Assuming it is not excessive, meaning it is not interfering with normal routines, responsibilities, or play, it is a normal part of a child's development.

Nevertheless, make sure your child understands that masturbation, like many other things, is a private activity, not a public one. If you observe him touching his genitals in a public place, you might say to him: "It is not appropriate for you to be touching your penis [or vagina] here. It should be only done in the privacy of your room when no one is with you."

As you discuss masturbation with your child, do not label it as bad, dirty, or sinful. This will create a sense of guilt and secrecy that may be unhealthy for his sexual development. Use this as an opportunity to continue your open dialogue with your child about sexuality.

There are certain situations in which children should receive an evaluation by a behavioral pediatrician, child psychiatrist, or psychologist. These include:

- Frequent excessive daily masturbation, both at home and in public

- Public masturbation that continues even after you have talked about it with your child

- Masturbation that takes place in conjunction with other symptoms of behavioral or emotional difficulty, including social isolation, aggression, destructiveness, sadness, withdrawal, bed-wetting, or soiling (encopresis)

- Inappropriate sexual talk or other sexual activity

~ 9 ~

If Your Child Needs the Hospital

IT CAN BE terrifying for parents to see their children sick or injured. When does your child need an evaluation by the emergency room, or possibly a hospital stay? The good news is that most children don't need hospitalization. In the United States, only about 1 percent of children are hospitalized between infancy and adulthood. Of those, the majority are hospitalized for respiratory symptoms, which, while scary, usually improve. Parents should be aware of critical signs that your child requires an emergency room visit. If your child is struggling to breathe or is showing signs of dehydration (little to no urine in the past six hours, especially if associated with vomiting and diarrhea), you may need to take action. If you are unsure if you can manage your child's symptoms at home, or are concerned the symptoms indicate a condition that cannot wait until regular office hours (such as possible appendicitis; for more on this, see page 529), call your pediatrician for further advice on next steps. For more on specific conditions and their symptoms, including when medical attention may be required, please refer to Part VIII, "Medical, Mental Health, and Behavior Issues."

Going to the Emergency Room

A discussion with your pediatrician's office regarding your child's symptoms may determine that the best course of action is to visit the emergency room (ER); alternatively, your child may experience a clear medical emergency, and you have already reached that conclusion as a parent. While it can be frightening to bring your child into the emergency room for evaluation, understanding what this experience entails and being prepared can help the process go more smoothly for your family.

Wait Time

Most ERs are extremely busy places. Emergencies can happen at any time, and so personnel in the emergency room need to triage patients, meaning that they see patients not necessarily in the order they come in but rather in the order of severity of illness. For example, a patient who has had major trauma needs to be seen before someone with a minor scrape is seen.

The first thing you will do in the ER is go through triage. The nurse will take a brief history and obtain vital signs (temperature, heart rate, blood pressure, respiratory rate, and oxygen saturation) and will likely weigh your child as well. This will allow the ER to triage your child to determine how urgent the problem is. At night, even fairly sick people may be forced to wait for potentially very long periods of time. Most ERs who see children may have an average wait time of about an hour, but on busy nights it can be much longer. This is, without a doubt, one of the most frustrating things about bringing your child to the hospital. It is difficult for a parent who fears that their child is dangerously ill, rushes into the emergency room, and then is made to wait for hours before being seen by the doctor. Bring books or activities for your child to use while waiting.

If during the waiting process you feel like your child is worsening, or if there is a new symptom that develops while waiting, don't feel shy about bringing your concerns back to the triage nurse, as this development may require more urgent evaluation. You are your child's best advocate.

Types of Hospitals

There are many different types of hospitals. About 60 percent of children hospitalized in the United States are hospitalized in community hospitals, which have specific areas dedicated to children. Often, the emergency room will be staffed by a provider who sees both adults and children. Community hospitals usually do not have a pediatric intensive care, and so admit only moderately ill children; critically ill children are transported to more specialized centers. If you feel your emergency room provider doesn't have much experience with children, you might ask if a pediatric provider is available to assess your child.

Other hospitals, typically in larger urban centers, may be dedicated children's hospitals, or larger hospitals with dedicated pediatric floors. These hospitals usually have subspecialists in pediatrics, and often have a dedicated pediatric emergency room with pediatric-trained emergency care providers. If you have a child with a complex chronic health condition, a dedicated pediatric emergency room may provide you with better care, but for most typical problems, community hospitals are adequate for treating your child's illness. Your primary care provider can help you decide where to take your child for care when she is sick, and provide more information as to which facilities in your geographic area may provide more specialized pediatric care.

How to Tell Your Child's Story

Once you are seen by the doctor, you will again be asked what brought you into the hospital. In an emergency room in a children's hospital, you may be asked your child's story multiple times, as often there are medical students or higher-level trainees like residents or fellows who are taking care of your child. Retelling the story of what brought them in can seem repetitive; however, the most valuable part of making a medical diagnosis is the *history*, meaning not only what has been happening that brought you into the ER but also past medical, family, social, and surgical information.

When the doctor is asking you the history of your child's illness, it is often helpful to go through the story chronologically. You should state when things started, and then walk through the illness, telling the doctor when things started changing or getting worse. After the history of the illness, tell the doctor any previous medical problems your child had, and inform the physician about any chronic medical problems, allergies, or medicines your child is on. If any childhood illnesses run in the family, let the provider know. The physician should guide you through this conversation. Feel free to make sure your concerns are addressed. Sometimes providers focus on something that may be important but might not be your most important concern. Help to answer their questions, but also make sure your own concerns and the concerns of your child are answered.

Medical Testing

The ER physician and staff should explain to you all the tests they are ordering and why. In general, children do not require as many blood tests or imaging studies as are commonly ordered in the adult population. The need to properly evaluate the child is balanced with any risks of performing the study or procedure. For example, not every child who bumps his head needs a head CT (computed tomography, or CAT) scan; if the child is feeling well and has a normal exam, the risks of the radiation exposure of a CT scan (which is many times the amount of radiation in a regular X-ray) may outweigh any benefit to performing the test.

Ask questions before consenting to any testing on your child. In addition, when you get the test results back, make sure all your questions about those test results are answered. Sometimes, the tests are very hard for a parent to understand when printed out in a report. If you can, take notes with pen and paper or on your phone so that later on you can remind yourself of what happened.

If your child is discharged from the emergency room, make sure you keep all the paperwork and bring it with you to your child's follow-up visit with your primary care provider. Also, request that your child's pediatrician be notified about the visit, so that they have access to all the necessary information from the visit when you follow up in the office.

If Your Child Is Admitted

If the provider in the ER feels that there is more to be done, or that your child is too ill to go home, your child will be admitted to the hospital. If your child is sick or requires very close monitoring, the provider may choose to admit your child to the intensive care unit. The vast majority of children admitted to the intensive care unit do well; an intensive care admission doesn't necessarily mean that your child's illness is life-threatening. Most admitted patients are sent to the hospital's general pediatric inpatient ward. Sometimes your child isn't sick enough to be admitted to the hospital, but the doctor in the ER wants to watch your child a bit longer. In this situation, some ERs will have an "observation unit" that can house children who need to be watched for less than twenty-four hours.

Typically if your child is admitted to the hospital, the admitting nurse will ask you a long series of questions, weigh your child and obtain vital signs again, and alert the doctor that you have arrived on the floor. The physician who makes decisions for your child's care while in the hospital may be your usual primary care pediatrician, or in many hospitals there is a pediatric hospitalist, a physician specialist in hospital care, who may provide care for your child.

After the nurse obtains your intake evaluation, the doctor (or a fellow, resident, or medical student in a teaching hospital) will obtain another complete history and do a physical exam on your child. The doctor should explain to you what the plan is for the hospitalization. Feel free to ask all the questions you need to ask. Write down your questions so you can remember them and have your medical team notified of questions or concerns if necessary.

Nursing Care

For closer monitoring in the emergency department or on the pediatric unit, electrode stickers may be placed on your child. IV pumps, monitors, or several other pieces of equipment may alarm frequently. An alarm does not necessarily mean your child is in danger, and often is just a reminder to change the setting on the device. One monitor that often troubles parents is a pulse oximeter. A pulse oximeter measures the percentage of red blood cells in the body that have oxygen bound to them. "Normal" is generally over 95 percent. However, some parents are concerned if the number drifts lower than 95 percent. The doctor uses 90 percent as a cutoff and typically will provide oxygen to try to keep the number over 90 percent. Keep in mind the pulse oximeter may be inaccurate, or may not provide the whole picture of how a child is doing. Children can be 100 percent on the oximeter and be critically ill; conversely, children can be 87 percent on the oximeter and be extremely well. Try not to focus too much on any number or monitor, as no monitor is better than looking at the big picture on how the child is progressing. Ask questions of providers about how to interpret the monitors and whether to worry. The nurse or physician should provide guidance about signs and symptoms or when to be concerned about your child's health and what to look out for.

If at any point you feel your child is not doing well, ring the call button and call your nurse in immediately. Nurses are frequently checking in, but they do have other patients and can't be there all the time, except perhaps in the intensive care unit setting. It is common for new symptoms to arise that may impact your child's diagnosis or progress. As a parent, you are a critical member of the care team and your child's best advocate.

Rounds

In most hospitals, care teams will come by in the morning on rounds. This is an opportunity for the entire care team to meet and discuss the care of the patient. In a specialized children's hospital, physicians in training (interns and residents) or medical students will likely be part of the team. In smaller community hospitals, you may be seeing your primary care pediatrician or a pediatric hospitalist, a pediatrician who specializes in hospital care. Most children's hospitals engage in "family-centered rounds," which means that the care and the conversation centers around your child and your family. Rather than the medical team talking in a back room and then coming in to update you, you have the opportunity to be a part of the conversation about your child's illness. There are a lot of medical terms that the medical team uses that may be confusing to families. If you are unsure, ask the nurse or doctor to clarify what they are saying.

Common Medical Terms and What They Mean

Medical Term	What It Means
PRN	"as needed" or "if needed"
PO ad lib, NPO	Eat whenever you want, nothing by mouth (no drinking or eating)
QD, BID, TID, QID	Once a day, twice a day, three times a day, four times a day
Q4, Q6, Q8, Q12	Every four hours, every six hours, every eight hours, every twelve hours
IV, IM, SQ	Through the IV, injected into the muscle, injected just under the skin
Chem 7 (or BMP), CBC, LFTs, UA	Electrolytes, complete blood count, liver function tests, urinalysis

Daily Needs

It's important for you to be at your best for your child, and that means taking care of yourself too. The nurses can watch your child if you need to go home, pack clean clothes, shower, or take care of yourself. Parents may need to work during the day, and the hospital should provide adequate supervision of your child. Often there are people who work in the hospital who will care for your child's spiritual and educational needs, as well as their health needs. Child life providers, educators, physical therapists, respiratory therapists, occupational therapists, and others all make up important parts of the care team. Ask about games and other activities your child can play with while he is hospitalized. Sometimes hospital food isn't very palatable. If your child has a favorite food, ask your doctor if you can bring in some food from home to keep your child happy, if your child's condition allows you to do so. Sometimes a walk around the hospital or down to the cafeteria with your child can be a great break from the monotony of the hospital room. Ask your nurse if there's a garden or play room available for your child.

Discharge

Obtaining clearance to leave the hospital can be a happy relief. However, parents should ensure they understand all the necessary hospital discharge steps.

Medications

Make sure you know which medicines your child needs to continue after leaving the hospital, what their doses are, how to measure those doses, and when to give them. If your child is going home on a liquid medication, ask about flavoring the medication to help your child take the necessary doses. Have your nurses demonstrate how to perform any dressing changes by showing you during your final hours of the hospital stay.

Verify that every medication you are taking home is necessary. Sometimes children with complex chronic health needs are prescribed a confusing number of medications, some of which may be duplicates or not needed. It is important to know what side effects you should look out for when your child is taking a medicine. Medications may be scheduled or as needed for symptoms. Make sure you understand what condition or symptoms each medicine is treating.

Following Up After Discharge

Make sure you have follow-up appointments arranged and phone numbers to call for issues discovered after your child's discharge from the hospital. Sometimes specialists are consulted during the hospital stay who will want your child to follow up in their clinic, in addition to visits with the primary care doctor. If your child had surgery, the surgeon will want to have you follow up in their clinic as well. For some medical conditions, your child may follow up with a specialist for his entire childhood. Children with diabetes, for example, will follow up with a pediatric endocrinologist. Children with heart disease will follow up with a pediatric cardiologist.

Make sure you ask when you should follow up with your child's primary care provider. Make sure that the hospital team has contacted your primary care doctor and has passed along necessary information about your child's care. The nurse will review your discharge instructions at discharge. You should ask for a copy of the discharge paperwork and bring the papers to your follow-up appointment in case there is any problem in communication between the hospital team and your doctor.

If you want a complete copy of your medical records, these are usually not yet available on the day of your child's discharge, but it is your right to obtain them. You should ask for the phone number for the medical records department, and you can call after discharge and arrange to get your child's medical records if you want a copy. In most cases this isn't necessary. There may be a small fee for obtaining medical records. If your child is being transported to another facility, your hospitalist or intensivist should call that facility and verbally sign out to the facility's healthcare team, and your child's records will be transferred.

Preparation for a Planned (Elective) Surgery

Some medical situations require emergency surgery, such as appendicitis or an open fracture (broken bone through the skin). In these cases, your child's medical care progresses quickly to ensure she receives the care she needs as soon as possible. In other situations, the family has time to plan ahead for an elective or planned procedure. Examples of these planned procedures include tympanostomy tubes for recurrent middle-ear fluid or infections, tonsillectomy or adenoidectomy (removal of the tonsils or adenoids), or an inguinal hernia repair. In the case of an elective or planned procedure, your family will be able to schedule the surgery with advance notice and help your child prepare in an age-appropriate manner.

Many children's and community hospitals provide kid-friendly tours for children to see the facilities ahead of the big day. Simply seeing where things will take place will answer a lot of questions for your child and settle many concerns, as the fear of the unknown can comprise a large part of a child's anxiety about a procedure. Ask your pediatrician or surgical specialist if these tours are offered at the hospital where your child's procedure will take place, and about any other suggestions regarding preparation. In an age-appropriate way, simply "dressing up" with a hospital gown and surgical cap can serve as a good rehearsal for the big day and ease jitters. Your child will inevitably have questions after such an experience; be a good listener, answer questions as honestly and simply as you can, and if there are questions you do not know the answer to, assure your child that together you will find out.

As a parent, you may have your own anxieties about your child's condition and upcoming procedure. Children are smart and are usually aware of much more than grown-ups realize. While it is important to be honest and straightforward with your child, remember to keep discussions age-appropriate and avoid burdening your child with your own fears or even financial concerns related to the procedure. Ensure that you are able to vent appropriately and privately to a partner or other trusted adult to air your own concerns, and contact your pediatrician as needed for additional questions or consultation.

Preparing Your Child for a Planned Procedure

Children ages 5–7 years: This age group may benefit from bringing along a special beloved object from home such as a teddy bear. A parent can help distract and ease a child's fears by helping the child "examine" his teddy bear or apply bandages, for example. Give your child something to do to focus on pleasant play rather than his anxiety about the upcoming procedure. Tour the surgical facilities ahead of time if you are able.

Children ages 8–10 years: While more mature, with a deeper understanding of the world than when they were in kindergarten, children between 8 and 10 may regress under times of stress. Have open discussions with your child about the upcoming surgery to help your child air any concerns he has so he feels heard and understood. Be understanding of a regression of behavior; while it is not appropriate to chide the child "Grow up, you're a big kid now," you can instead say, "I know you are nervous about the surgery next week. Let's talk about it."

Children ages 11–12 years: Older children have a deeper understanding of what the upcoming procedure may mean. Be aware that the media has influenced a child's view of the medical establishment; keep the doors of communication open and ensure that your child has a realistic, factual understanding of what will take place, rather than an idea influenced by dramatic fictional representations in television and film, for example.

PART III

· · · · · · · · · · · ·

Personal and Social Development

~ 10 ~

Your Child's Developing Self

EACH YEAR DURING middle childhood, the little person you're raising grows and develops, finds her place in the world, and evolves into a person in her own right. As a parent, part of your function during these years is to let your child grow and become the person she is meant to be. Guiding your child toward becoming more competent, self-sufficient, and self-confident means you need to accept her for herself, a growing and learning child. As you will learn in this chapter, there are some things you can change, and some things you cannot.

Temperament

Some children are "easy." They are predictable, calm, and approach most new experiences in a positive way. Other children have more challenging traits, and are not able to manage their emotional experiences and expression with ease. When a child's personality doesn't quite fit or match that of other family members, conflict may arise. Of course no child is one way all the time, but each has his own *usual* type.

The ease with which a child adjusts to his environment is strongly influenced by his temperament—adaptability and emotional style. For the most part, temperament is an innate quality of the child, one she is born with. It is somewhat modified (particularly in the early years of life) by her experiences and interactions with other people, by her environment, and by her health.

By the time a child has reached the school years, his temperament is well defined and quite apparent to those who know him. It is not something that is likely to change much in the future. These innate characteristics have nothing to do with your own parenting skills. Nevertheless, the behavioral adjustment of a school-age child depends a lot upon the interaction between his temperament and yours, and how others respond to him—how comfortably he fits in with his environment and with the people around him.

Characteristics of Temperament

By being aware of some of the characteristics of temperament, you can better understand your child, appreciate his uniqueness, and deal with problems of poor "fit" that may lead to misunderstandings and conflicts.

There are at least nine major characteristics that make up temperament.

Activity level: The level of physical activity, motion, restlessness, or fidgety behavior that a child demonstrates in daily activities (and which also may affect sleep).

Rhythmicity or regularity: The presence or absence of a regular pattern for basic physical functions such as appetite, sleep, and bowel habits.

Approach and withdrawal: The way a child initially responds to a new stimulus (rapid and bold, or slow and hesitant), whether it be people, situations, places, foods, changes in routines, or other transitions.

Adaptability: The degree of ease or difficulty with which a child adjusts to change or a new situation, and how well the child can modify his reaction.

Intensity: The energy level with which a child responds to a situation, whether positive or negative.

Mood: The mood, positive or negative, or degree of pleasantness or unfriendliness in a child's words and behaviors.

Attention span: The ability to concentrate or stay with a task, with or without distraction.

Distractibility: The ease with which a child can be distracted from a task by environmental (usually visual or auditory) stimuli.

Sensory threshold: The amount of stimulation required for a child to respond. Some children respond to the slightest stimulation, and others require intense amounts.

Regardless of your child's individual temperament or "thermostat," use teachable moments and model appropriate behavior yourself in difficult or unexpected situations. If you have a flat tire or the pot on the stove boils over, be aware that your child's eyes are watching to see how you handle this situation. It cannot be overstated: children learn from what we *do* just as much as from what we *say*.

How Temperament Affects Children and Their Parents

Every child has a different pattern of the nine above-mentioned temperament characteristics. Many, but not all, children tend to fall into one of three broad and somewhat loosely defined categories: easy, slow to warm up or shy, or challenging. These labels are a useful shorthand, but none offers a complete picture of a child. Many parents find it more useful to think about their child in terms of the nine temperament traits, and the table on page 136 explains how the different traits may be expressed.

The *easy child* responds to the world around him in an easy manner. His mood is positive, and he is mildly to moderately intense. He adapts easily to new schools and people. When encountering a frustrating situation, he usually does so with relatively little anxiety. His parents probably describe him as a "joy to be around." About 40 percent of children fall into this category.

Another temperamental profile may reveal a somewhat *slow-to-warm-up or shy child*, who tends to have moods of mild intensity, usually but not always negative. He adapts slowly to unfamiliar surroundings and people, is hesitant and shy when making new friends, and tends to withdraw when encountering new people and circumstances. Upon confronting a new situation, he is more likely to have problems with anxiety, physical symptoms, or separation. Over time, however, he

Living with Different Temperament Traits

Here are some general strategies and solutions to help you live with a child with challenging temperament traits:

1. First, recognize that much of your child's behavior reflects his temperament.

2. Establish a neutral or objective emotional climate in which to deal with your child. Try not to respond in an emotional and instinctive manner, which is unproductive.

3. Don't take your child's behavior personally. Temperament is innate, and your child likely is not trying to create conflict. Don't blame him or yourself.

4. Try to prioritize the issues and problems surrounding your child. Some are more important and deserve greater attention. Others are not as relevant and can be either ignored or placed further down on the priority list.

5. Focus on the issues of the moment. Do not project into the future.

6. Review your expectations of your child, your preferences, and your values. Are they realistic and age-appropriate? When your child does something right, praise him and reinforce the specific behaviors that you like.

7. Consider your own temperament and behavior, and how they might also be a challenge for your child. Think how you might need to adjust yourself a bit to encourage a better fit with your child.

8. Anticipate impending high-risk situations, and try to avoid or minimize them. Accept the possibility that this may be a difficult day or circumstance, and be prepared to make the best of it.

9. Find a way to get some relief for yourself and your child by scheduling some time apart.

10. Seek professional help, when needed, from your pediatrician or another expert in child behavior.

will become more accepting of new people and situations once he becomes more familiar with them.

The *challenging* child tends to react to the world negatively and intensely. As an infant he may have been categorized as a fussy baby. As a young child he may have been prone to temper tantrums or was hard to please. He may still occasionally be explosive, stubborn, and intense, and he may adapt poorly to new situations. Some children with challenging temperaments may have trouble adjusting at school, and their teachers may complain of problems in the classroom or on the playground. When children have conflict-prone temperaments, they usually have more behavioral problems and cause more strain on the family.

Of the three types of temperament, parents are most concerned—and often exasperated—when they have a child with the attributes of a challenging temperament. Without a doubt, a child who is intense, adapts poorly, and is strong-willed can be challenging for his parents. Most mothers and fathers will feel overwhelmed, guilty, angry, or inadequate. However, once parents recognize that these characteristics are innate to the child—and, while not caused by the parents, can still be intensified or moderated by them—then parents are more likely to change their expectations and begin efforts to help the child do and feel better.

It is important to distinguish a difficult temperament from other problems. For instance, recurrent or chronic illnesses, or emotional and physical stresses, can cause behavioral difficulties that are really not a problem with temperament at all. Parents also sometimes interpret a child's style of interacting as inherently bad. However, a child's temperament is only a problem when it conflicts with the expectations of his parents, other family members, friends, or teachers. For example, if a parent is intense and ambitious, and his or her child is mild-mannered and easygoing, the parent may feel disappointed, frustrated, and angry. The child, pressured to behave in ways foreign to his basic inclinations and innate personality, may resist and cause conflict within the family.

What Parents Can Do

The problem is on its way to being resolved when you recognize and accept the reality that there is a mismatch of temperaments. Once you acknowledge that your personalities are different, any tendencies to blame either the child or yourself should ease. You need to know that nothing is wrong with your child, nor are you an inadequate parent in the way you are raising him or responding to his temperament. Your challenge is to understand your own responses to him and to adjust your expectations to meet his capabilities. You need to modify your strategies to some extent to ensure a better "fit" between you and your child. At the same time, you need to help him learn to compromise, adapt, and expand his repertoire of acceptable social responses and behavior.

How Temperamental Traits Can Be Expressed			
Tempera-mental Trait	**Positive Characteristics**	**Difficult or Challenging Behaviors**	**What to Do**
High activity level	Energetic, vigorous. Investigates his environment. Remains active even in boring circumstances.	Restless, very active. May be impulsive, reckless. Easily distracted from tasks.	Anticipate high activity. Use safety precautions if necessary. Practice distraction techniques. Provide opportunities to burn off energy and cool down.
Low activity level	Is unlikely to disrupt activities in small, cramped spaces.	Slow pace in performing tasks; often labeled "lazy." Gives appearance of drowsiness.	Provide additional time to finish tasks. Make tasks realistic within the designated time frame. Avoid criticism of child's slow pace.
Irregularity (low regularity)	May not be upset by disruptions in daily routine activities.	Unpredictable patterns of eating, sleeping, using the toilet.	Identify child's patterns and adhere to them as much as possible. Don't force the child to eat or sleep when not ready; require child to follow routines of coming to the table or going to bed, but without forcing eating or sleeping.
Initial withdrawal	Demonstrates caution in risky circumstances.	Rejection of people, food, situations. Very shy or clingy. Slow to accept change.	Introduce new things gradually, talk about them beforehand, let child proceed at own pace.

Temperamental Trait	Positive Characteristics	Difficult or Challenging Behaviors	What to Do
Slow adaptability	Lower likelihood of being affected by negative influences.	Difficulty with changes and transitions. Takes a long time to adapt and adjust.	Establish consistent and predictable daily routines. Avoid unnecessary changes and prepare the child in advance. Try multiple brief exposures.
High intensity	Child's needs get the attention of caregivers.	Expresses emotions in extremes instead of cries. Yells rather than talks. Intensity is sometimes mistaken for desire.	Learn to be tolerant. Model more appropriate responses, give general feedback, and provide alternative responses.
Negative mood	Concern may get parents involved in issues surrounding the child.	Fussy, complains a lot, appears very serious and displays little pleasure in words and actions. Parents may overestimate importance of a child's complaint.	Understand that mood is a major part of temperament. It is not your fault. Adjust expectations or demands that intensify mood. Encourage positive responses.

Once you realize that your child's behavior is, to some extent, an innate pattern and beyond his control, you can make an effort to become more patient and diminish the stress and strain your child feels. When you think of your child's temperament in objective terms rather than react to it emotionally and instinctively, you and your child will get along better. If your child has a difficult temper-

How Temperamental Traits Can Be Expressed			
Tempera-mental Trait	Positive Characteristics	Difficult or Challenging Behaviors	What to Do
Inattention and distractibility	Can soothe the child easily.	Doesn't listen. Has difficulty concentrating and studying. Gets pulled off task easily and needs reminders.	Keep tasks, instructions, and explanations short and simple. Remove distractions and competing stimuli. Practice good communication skills: Get his attention, address by name, use eye contact, repeat, clarify, and review. Provide frequent breaks and require the child to return to the task at hand when reminded. When necessary, redirect your child without anger or shame. Provide praise for completing the task.
Low sensitivity threshold	High awareness of changes in surroundings and of nuances in the feelings and thoughts of others.	Overreacts even to normal stimuli (light, noise, smells, textures, pain, social-emotional events).	Reduce level of stimulation. Anticipate problems and prepare child. Respect child's preferences when possible.

ament as a preschooler, and if you understand and respond appropriately, he will probably modify his behavior, and may not remain as difficult during his school-age years. His intensity can become part of his enthusiasm, determination, charm, and zeal as he feels better about himself and his relationship with others. For that to happen, your own attitudes and behaviors can play a major role in how he adapts and expresses his feelings.

Also, in the weeks and months ahead, avoid labeling your child as bad or difficult, or, worse, name-calling. Labels stick, and not only may family members unfairly prejudge your child, but he may come to see himself as different, undesirable, or just not fitting in. Identify your child's temperament type, but do not broadly announce this label, as the label may become a self-fulfilling prophecy. This negative self-image can further interfere with efforts—both yours and his—to improve his way of responding to challenging situations and can lead to more serious emotional conflicts.

Self-Esteem

Self-esteem plays a central role in a child's motivation and achievements in school, social relationships, and degree of resilience (the ability to bounce back from setbacks). It influences her chances of becoming involved in substance abuse and sexual activity, and her vulnerability to unhealthy or negative peer pressure.

Children develop a self-concept and self-esteem very early in life. Almost from the start, some have learned generally positive feelings about themselves, and have acquired a sense of importance and self-worth. They can acknowledge and appreciate their individual talents, achievements, and physical appearance. They can also accept their shortcomings and mistakes and realize that occasional failure is a natural part of life and learning.

Other children, however, feel quite different about themselves. They have been taught a sense of inadequacy and inferiority and have come to believe they are incapable of achieving or creating changes in their lives. They may be withdrawn and cautious, not willing to expose themselves to public scrutiny or to the risk of failure.

What Is Self-Esteem?

By definition, self-esteem is the way in which an individual perceives herself—in other words, her own thoughts and feelings about herself and her ability to achieve in ways that are important to her. This self-esteem is shaped not only by a child's own perceptions and expectations, but also by the perceptions and expectations of significant people in her life—how she is thought of and treated by parents, teachers, and friends. The closer her perceived self (how she sees herself) comes to her ideal self (how she would like to be), the higher her self-esteem.

A child's self-esteem grows from an interaction between her biological, inborn traits (such as temperament, intelligence, physical characteristics) and environmental influences (such as her parents' parenting style and economic status, and her relationships with other adults and peers). As early as the first few months of life, a child begins to develop a sense of "I," a concept of the self, and feelings of mastery over certain aspects of her environment. For instance, an infant soon learns that a cry or a smile brings an immediate and, hopefully, positive response from a parent, which reinforces her sense of trust, security, control, and self-importance. As she moves through the toddler and preschool stages, her self-concept will continue to evolve, influenced in large part by her parents' verbal and nonverbal responses to her: their praise and criticism, smiles, other facial expressions, and hugs. Other major influences include her level of independence and her sense of achievement.

By the middle years of childhood, a child needs a positive sense of self to do well in the world outside the family—that is, achieving in school and interacting successfully with her peers. Her self-concept at this age will be a major influence on her accomplishments, social interactions, and emotional status throughout childhood and adult life.

A child's self-esteem can fluctuate from day to day, or from situation to situation, although over the course of many years, it tends to remain relatively constant. In general, a child will usually seek out those activities and interactions that make her feel successful, and that can act as a buffer against stress and help her maintain a positive sense of well-being when she's not doing well. A child with high self-esteem will perceive herself as a capable individual who can set realistic goals and achieve them. A child with poor self-esteem will tend to settle for more modest accomplishments in the classroom and later in life. She may feel shame, depression, or inadequacy over what she perceives as a lack of appropriate or satisfying achievement, and the inability to earn recognition and respect from others. At the same time, her low self-esteem will make her more likely to conform to her peer group and to seek their favor, adopting their behavior and values in order to gain acceptance, a sense of belonging and self-worth. The behavior and values she conforms to may or may not be positive or healthy.

Some children have special stresses and challenges that make it more difficult for them to develop strong self-esteem. Perhaps they have a physical handicap, a chronic illness, a learning disability, or an attention problem. Or they might face discrimination because of their ethnic origin or religion. Environmental and social stresses such as poverty, a neglectful parent, alcoholism, or intense sibling rivalry can further erode a child's self-esteem. Even so, these children can develop positive self-esteem, but the need to succeed and earn the acceptance and appreciation of parents and others will be even more important than for a child without additional challenges.

Furthermore, some children appear to be very resilient and have a more positive outlook than their peers. These are children who have met and overcome hardships, setbacks, and challenges, and who tend to elicit positive responses (affection, admiration, respect) from adults. As a consequence, they are eager to explore new situations and seem able to adapt to change with greater ease. If the "fit" between parent and child temperaments is good and if parents set expectations that children can meet, the child's self-esteem is likely to be even further enhanced. Even in the face of great hardships, these children emerge with their self-esteem still intact and healthy.

You know your own child better than anyone and should be able to pick up the signs—through behavior and words—if your son or daughter has low self-esteem. Sometimes, however, you might be too close to her, or you might have difficulty seeing the world through her eyes. In cases like this, an objective third party such as a teacher, coach, relative, or friend might be able to help. Also, use the information in the box on page 144 as a guide.

Components of High Self-Esteem

Spend some time thinking about how your child deals with success and failure. Many children with low self-esteem may attribute their successes in life to luck, fate, or other influences beyond their control, thus eroding their confidence and reducing their chances of being successful in the future. When these same children make a mistake or experience failure, they again may look beyond themselves for a cause ("I had a bad day" or "The teacher doesn't like me"). This makes it harder for them to create new and more successful strategies or to seek help or advice.

What about a child with high self-esteem? She probably sees her successes largely as a result of her own efforts and abilities. She feels a sense of self-control and becomes motivated to do better when she experiences failure. She'll accept her mistakes, while realizing that she needs to make changes and work harder, and she will avoid blaming others.

For healthy self-esteem, children need to develop or acquire some or all of the following characteristics:

- **A sense of security.** Your child must feel secure about herself and her future. ("What will become of me?")

- **A sense of belonging.** Your child needs to feel accepted and loved by others, beginning with her family and then extending to groups such as friends, classmates, sports teams, house of worship, and even a neighborhood or community. Without this acceptance or group identity, she may feel rejected, lonely, and adrift.

- **A sense of purpose.** Your child should have goals that give her purpose and direction and an avenue for channeling her energy toward achievement and self-expression. If she lacks a sense of purpose, she may feel bored, aimless, even resentful at being pushed in certain directions by you or others.

- **A sense of personal competence and pride.** Your child should feel confident in her ability to meet the challenges in her life. This sense of personal power evolves from having successful life experiences in solving problems independently, being creative, and getting results for her efforts. Setting appropriate expectations, not too low and not too high, is critical to developing competence and confidence. If you are overprotecting her, if she is too dependent on you, or if expectations are so high she never succeeds, she may feel powerless and incapable of controlling the circumstances in her life.

- **A sense of trust.** Your child needs to feel trust in you and in herself. Toward this goal, you should keep promises, be supportive, and give your child opportunities to be trustworthy. This means believing your child and treating her as an honest person.

- **A sense of responsibility.** Give your child a chance to show what she is capable of doing. Allow her to take on tasks without being checked on all the time. This shows trust on your part, a sort of "letting go" with a sense of faith.

- **A sense of contribution.** Your child will develop a sense of importance and commitment if you give her opportunities to participate and contribute in a meaningful way to an activity. Let her know that she really counts.

- **A sense of making real choices and decisions.** Your child will feel empowered and in control of events when she is able to make or influence decisions that she considers important. These choices and decisions need to be appropriate for her age and abilities, and for the family's values.

- **A sense of self-discipline and self-control.** As your child is striving to achieve and gain more independence, she needs and wants to feel that she can make it on her own. Once you give her expectations, guidelines, and opportunities in which to test herself, she can reflect, reason, problem-solve, and consider the consequences of the actions she may choose. This kind of self-awareness is critical for her future growth.

- **A sense of encouragement, support, and reward.** Not only does your child need to achieve, but she also needs positive feedback and recognition—a real message that she is doing well, pleasing others, and "making it." Encourage and praise her, not only for achieving a set goal but also for her efforts, and for even small increments of change and improvement ("I like the way you waited for your turn"; "Good try; you're working harder";

"Good girl!"). Give her feedback as soon as possible to reinforce her self-esteem and to help her connect your comments to the activity involved.

- **A sense of accepting mistakes and failure.** Your child needs to feel comfortable, not defeated, when she makes mistakes or fails. Explain that these hurdles or setbacks are a normal part of living and learning, and that she can learn or benefit from them. Let your supportive, constructive feedback and your recognition of her effort overpower any sense of failure, guilt, or shame she might be feeling, giving her renewed motivation and hope. Use examples from everyday life to model these skills; if you yourself make a mistake, share the situation with your child so she can see that we are all human, adults included, and life goes on.

- **A sense of family self-esteem.** Your child's self-esteem initially develops within the family and is influenced greatly by the feelings and perceptions that a family has of itself. Some of the preceding comments apply to the family in building its self-esteem. Also, bear in mind that family pride is essential to self-esteem and can be nourished and maintained in many ways, including participation or involvement in community activities, tracing a family's heritage and ancestors, or caring for extended family members. Families fare better when members focus on each other's strengths, avoid excessive criticism, and stick up for one another outside the family setting. Family members believe in and trust each other, respect their individual differences, and show their affection for each other. They make time for being together, whether to share holidays, special events, or just to have fun.

Experiences can establish a way of responding to subsequent events and can either boost or damage her self-esteem. For instance, if a child performs poorly in school, that can cause frustration and damage her self-confidence. In an attempt to prevent further pain and failure, she may work less hard and avoid doing her schoolwork, causing even poorer performance and even more difficulties with her self-esteem. If unaddressed, this may become a repeating cycle and make her feel, think, and act like a non-achiever, living up to this new self-image.

This cycle also can work in positive ways. If a child performs well and her success is acknowledged, her belief in her own abilities will grow, and she may feel motivated to work harder and achieve even more as she responds to the intrinsic pleasure and external rewards of success. As that occurs, her accomplishments will increase, instilling in her even stronger feelings of control over her life. Pushed along by her own desire to improve, she will keep trying and succeeding, and her self-confidence will grow even more. She soon feels, thinks, and acts in a way that fits her self-image.

Keep in mind that throughout childhood, your child and her attitudes toward herself will be molded by your own expectations and responses. If she gives school her full effort, she brings home a report card with B's, and you praise her effort and work ethic, she will feel good about herself and what she has achieved. However, if you react with disappointment and overly focus on the end result, not the effort—"Why didn't you get an A in math?"—her self-esteem will suffer. Be sensitive to the power of your own reactions and words.

Signs of Low Self-Esteem

To help you determine if your child has low self-esteem, watch for the following signals. They could be everyday responses to how your child relates to the world around him, or they might occur only occasionally in specific situations. When they become a repeated pattern of behavior, you need to become sensitive to the existence of a problem.

- Your child avoids a task or challenge without even trying. This often signals a fear of failure or a sense of helplessness.

- He quits soon after beginning a game or a task, giving up at the first sign of frustration.

- He cheats or lies when he believes he's going to lose a game or do poorly.

- He shows signs of regression, acting babylike or very silly. These types of behavior invite teasing and name-calling from other children, thus adding insult to injury.

- He becomes controlling, bossy, or inflexible as ways of hiding feelings of inadequacy, frustration, or powerlessness.

- He makes excuses ("The teacher is dumb") or downplays the importance of events ("I don't really like that game anyway"), rationalizing to place blame on others or external forces.

- His grades in school have declined, or he has lost interest in usual activities.

- He withdraws socially, losing or having less contact with friends.

- He experiences changing moods, exhibiting sadness, crying, angry outbursts, frustration, or quietness.

- He makes self-critical comments, such as "I never do anything right," "Nobody likes me," "I'm ugly," "It's my fault," or "Everyone is smarter than I am."

- He has difficulty accepting either praise or criticism.

- He becomes overly concerned or sensitive about other people's opinions of him.

- He seems to be strongly affected by negative peer influence, adopting attitudes and behaviors like a disdain for school, cutting classes, acting disrespectfully, shoplifting, or experimenting with alcohol or other substances.

If Your Child Needs Help

The most important component of self-esteem comes from the success of doing and achieving. Kids' competency and self-confidence grow through their success in mastering challenges and activities. The lifelong rewards of early success and competency are self-confidence and self-esteem. If you or your pediatrician or other professional have concluded that your child could use help with her self-esteem, start with some positive steps of your own. You can become the most influential person in getting your child's self-concept back on track.

First, review the various components of self-esteem described above, which will help you identify and better understand your child's particular needs and develop helpful strategies and solutions. Do not protect her from difficult situations, but rather help her brainstorm how she can confront issues in a manner that will yield more success than in the past. Assist her in dealing with the problem at hand—for example, an issue with a particular school subject. Help her identify changes she wants to make or skills she wants to improve upon, and then assist her in setting up challenging but realistic goals and a timetable for achieving them.

To meet these goals, develop a plan of action with her. For instance, if the goal is to improve reading, she should commit herself to spend extra time with her books, starting with an extra fifteen minutes per day and increasing that gradually. Teachers and family members should be available to provide the child with support. At the same time, however, avoid the temptation to run the show, superimposing your own directives over the entire process; instead, give your child as

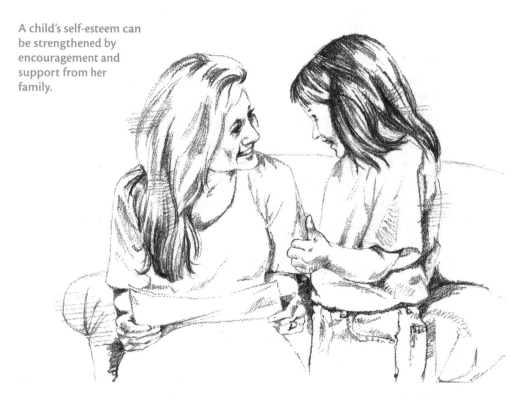

A child's self-esteem can be strengthened by encouragement and support from her family.

much control and responsibility as possible. This will build competence, confidence, and trust, and demonstrate your respect for her and her abilities.

At the same time, find other areas of strength in your child and build upon them. For example, make sure she has opportunities to do things she is good at doing. Single out something from which she derives pride and pleasure, nurture it, help her develop it, and let her appreciate her achievement. These experiences will show her, more than words, that she is capable of accomplishment.

In the weeks ahead, assess your child's feelings about herself from time to time. If there still seems to be a problem with her self-confidence or self-esteem, repeat some of the interventions mentioned above if they still appear appropriate but simply need to be tried again or in a slightly different manner. Alternatively, consider different strategies if she is not making progress, all the while reaffirming your faith in her ability to succeed. Consider modifying goals and expectations if they have been too difficult to meet. When she ultimately reaches a goal, give her praise, and if it seems appropriate, offer her a reward (non-monetary rewards such as experiences are ideal in that they strengthen self-esteem and family bonds). Reassure her of your faith and confidence in her ability to attain what she sets out to accomplish. As her efforts continue to pay off, she will feel encouraged and motivated by her successes, and her sense of personal competence will grow.

Here are some additional suggestions:

- Spend time with your child. Find activities you can do together that will make her feel successful—and that are fun, too, without winners and losers. Attend her soccer games and music recitals. Show her that you are interested in her and what she accomplishes. By giving time and energy to your child, you will convey a powerful message of love and acceptance.

- Treat your child as an important person. Encourage her to express herself, listen without judging, accept her feelings, and treat her with respect. Family mealtimes, even if it is breakfast at the start of the day, offer an opportunity to listen to your child.

- Whenever possible, allow your child to make decisions and assume more responsibility in her life. Demonstrate your trust in her.

- Build close family relationships, and make your child feel that she is contributing to the family unit.

- Do not expose your child to, or confide in her about, adult topics or family/marital tensions that will cause her stress. Try to minimize her anxieties related to family crises and changes, providing her with as much continuity and stability as possible.

- Encourage your child to provide service to others—perhaps through Scouts or a similar type of program—in order to increase her sense of community, her feeling of belonging and being appreciated, and her sense of importance and personal worth.

- Teach your child to praise herself. She should feel pride in her accomplishments.

- Tell your child how much you love her—without any conditions or strings attached. Although parents' actions and efforts convey love indirectly, children also need to hear the words "I love you."

Boosting your child's self-concept will not happen overnight. It may take months or years, and it will be an ongoing process. If your child is not responding to your attempts at helping her, however, and worrisome or serious problems persist, talk to your pediatrician about the need for professional assistance.

No matter what your child's self-esteem may be, your goal should continue to be to help her feel as good as possible about herself. Remain sensitive to what she is feeling, recognize and acknowledge her efforts and gains, and remain flexible and supportive in the way you approach her difficulties. Accept your child as the person she is, and help her feel good about herself and the person she is becoming. Keep in mind that the single most important factor in maintaining a child's self-esteem is the presence of an adult who demonstrates respect and acceptance and who provides support that conveys the message "I believe in you."

Gender Identity

"Gender" and "sex" are two different terms with two different meanings. When we are born, we are assigned as a boy or a girl based on our physical characteristics, which is our *sex*. When children are able to express themselves, they will identify themselves as a boy, or a girl, or at times something in between; this is referred to as their *gender identity*. Most children's gender identity matches their biological sex, but other kids feel a disconnect from what they have been termed and how they feel inside. How can parents help promote healthy gender development in kids?

By the second birthday, toddlers have a sense of the differences between boy and girl, and by the fourth birthday, kids have a sense of their own inherent gender identity. While society may unfortunately still foster older ideas about boys playing with blocks or trucks and girls selecting dolls or playing house, all children need the opportunity to explore different gender roles and different styles of play.

As a parent, ensure that your child's environment reflects an array of gender roles and encourages opportunity for all. Gender-neutral toys such as building blocks are a great idea, and *both* boys and girls enjoy action figures and dolls. Select from the library or purchase children's books that show women and men in diverse and non-stereotypical gender roles such as male nurses, female police officers, and stay-at-home dads. Allow your kids to make their own choices as to who their playmates will be, boy or girl, and what sports and activities they choose to participate in.

Younger kids typically express their gender identity through their clothing, hairstyle, preferred name, social behavior and manner, and social relationships. A child's gender identity—the sense of being a girl or a boy—*cannot* be changed.

Gender Stereotypes

Over time, society increasingly recognizes that stereotypes of masculine and feminine behaviors and characteristics are inaccurate. In the past, girls were expected to play with dolls or cooking toys, and be more passive. Boys were expected to play with building blocks and action figures, and to show more aggressive behaviors. Thankfully our expectations of "what girls do" and "what boys do" has changed. Girls excel at sports and school subjects traditionally thought of as masculine. Boys can participate in artistic subjects once traditionally thought of as feminine. All children show some behaviors that were once thought of as typical for the opposite gender—no one shows exclusively male or female traits—and this is normal and appropriate.

When a child's interests and abilities are not aligned with outdated societal expectations, he may be subjected to discrimination or bullying. It is natural for parents to want their child to be accepted socially. However, children need to feel comfortable with, and feel good about, themselves. If your son doesn't have an interest in sports participation, for example, there are many other opportunities and areas in which he can excel. Each child has his own strengths, and at times they may not conform to society's or your own expectations, but they will still be a source of his current and future success.

Do not attempt to force your child into the mold of traditional gender behavior; rather, help him fulfill his own unique potential. Don't focus your attention on whether your child's interests and strengths coincide with the socially defined gender roles of the moment. Instead, love your child for who he is, let him know you love him for who he is, and allow him to evolve in his own way.

Gender-Nonconforming and Transgender Children

Some children have a gender identity that is different from their sex assigned at birth, and many children have interests and hobbies that may align with the other gender. Some kids, however, do not identify with either gender. They may feel like they are somewhere in between, or that they have no gender.

For some young children, expressing a wish to be or identifying as another gender may be temporary; for others, it is not. Some children who are gender-nonconforming in early childhood grow up to become transgender adults, consistently identifying with a gender that is different from their birth sex; others do not. Many gender-nonconforming children grow up to identify with a gay, lesbian, or bisexual orientation.

It is impossible to predict how a child will end up identifying herself later in life. This uncertainty is one of the hardest things about parenting a gender-nonconforming child. In all situations, it is important for parents to make their home a place where their child feels accepted, safe, and loved unconditionally. Research suggests that gender is something we are born with; it cannot be changed with interventions. Research also suggests that children who are persistent, consistent, and insistent about their gender identity when it is different from their birth sex are the ones who are most likely to become transgender adults. It is important to support and follow the lead of the child. This may mean you will not have an answer for quite a long time, which can be difficult for parents.

Sometimes a young child who strongly identifies with another gender does change how she identifies herself. The most common time for this to occur is about 9 or 10 years old. Often it is unclear if this change means the child has learned to hide her true self due to social pressures, or if the child went through a "phase." However, a 12-year-old male who has consistently identified as female since preschool will most likely remain transgender throughout life.

There may be a particular period when a child's gender identity can come into question. At times, a child who never exhibited anything outside expected gender expression or identity may start feeling differently as his or her body changes. Finding out your child is transgender can be very confusing for parents, who may wonder if this is a phase or if their child is truly transgender. In these cases it may be helpful for your child to connect with a counselor experienced with transgender youth.

While it is not understood why some children identify with a gender different from their assigned birth sex, the cause is likely both biological and social. There is no evidence that parenting is responsible for a child having a gender identity that is not in line with his biological sex. Experiencing childhood trauma will not cause a child to become gender-nonconforming, transgender, or homosexual. There is nothing "wrong" with your child. However, children perceived as "different" may suffer from teasing or bullying. If this is happening, speak with the child's teacher and the school. Continue to support, love, and accept your child as she is.

At some point, a child who is persistently gender-nonconforming may choose to transition, or begin to live as her self-identified gender instead of the sex assigned at birth. The transitioning process is different for everyone, and is often initiated by the child. Many specialized children's hospitals have a gender development program; talk with your pediatrician to find out what your family's options are. These programs utilize a thorough multidisciplinary approach to address the myriad needs of the child, and include adolescent specialists, endocrinology or hormone specialists, psychologists, urology specialists, ethics consultants, social workers, and school consultants.

Sexual Orientation vs. Gender Identity

Sexual orientation refers to the person someone falls in love with or is attracted to. Sexual orientation becomes evident in later childhood, while gender identity refers to the way one identifies him- or herself in early childhood. While sexual orientation and gender identity are different paths of development, children who are gender-nonconforming often grow up to identify as gay or bisexual, and many gay or bisexual adults recall gender-nonconforming behavior in childhood. Like gender identity, an individual's physical and emotional attraction to a member of the same or the opposite sex cannot be changed.

Sexual Orientation

An individual's physical and emotional attraction to a member of the same or the opposite sex is a biological phenomenon. Whom an individual grows to love in later years is deeply ingrained as part of them. As a parent, your most important role is to offer understanding, respect, and support to your child. A nonjudgmental approach will gain your child's trust and put you in a better position to help him as he develops. Acceptance and support for your child is paramount in all situations, but especially if your child discloses her orientation to you.

Your own child's sexual orientation may be established by the middle years. At these younger ages, however, as there is little opportunity to test and act out this orientation, it may not be evident to the family until adolescence or even later. Meanwhile, keep in mind that many children try out different ways of relating to their peers, and these can be confused with sexual orientation.

The greatest difficulty for children is the social pressure they feel to behave heterosexually, and the discrimination they may experience because of their sexual orientation. They may feel isolated from their peers and even their family, impacting their self-esteem and confidence.

Related Mental Health Issues

All gender-nonconforming kids, regardless of how they identify themselves later on as straight, gay, lesbian, bisexual, or transgender, are at risk for bullying from peers and for mental health issues. Unfortunately, many teen suicide attempts are linked to gender and sexuality issues. Parents play an important role in understanding, accepting, respecting, and supporting their child. Supportive families reduce a teen's risk of suicide. Be aware of any warning signs of anxiety or depression. Assist your child to find LGBTQ organizations and resources so they feel more connected. As a family, celebrate diversity, and point out role models who stand up for the LGBTQ community. Reach out for education and support yourself as a parent if you feel you need more information.

Growing up provides challenges for all kids, but gender-nonconforming children face particular issues navigating school, family, and the community. Look for age-appropriate kids' books, parenting books, and national and international organizations that support families undergoing similar issues. Visiting a mental health professional and participating in a support group setting may be helpful for further support and minimizing risks of anxiety and depression.

~ 11 ~

Developing Social Skills

GOOD SOCIAL SKILLS are necessary for forming and fostering interpersonal connections with family, friends, and peers. When kids can relate to others, it boosts feelings of self-esteem and security, and allows children to adjust to inevitable transitions and life changes. Social skills are developed in the home, in the classroom, on the playground, and in the community. When a child is able to interact well with others, she will develop and maintain resilience when encountering stress, and will be better able to compensate for life's inevitable ups and downs. Conversely, inadequate or inappropriate social skills—and the peer rejection that they may cause—can contribute to social, behavioral, emotional, and academic problems.

What are social skills? They are the verbal and nonverbal behaviors that occur during everyday social interactions. Some are innate; most are learned. Usually, children learn their social skills at home, with friends in the community, at school, or in places of worship.

As children grow, they spend an increased amount of time outside the family, not only at school but also in a variety of peer-group organizations, such as youth sports programs and after-school activities. Time spent with other children gives the opportunity to learn good social skills and highlights the need for such skills.

Does Your Child Have Problems with Social Skills?

If you suspect that your child has difficulties with social interactions, the following questions might help pinpoint the problem.

Does your child have difficulty:

- Entering and joining a group?

- Keeping a friend?

- Dealing with teasing and provocation?

- Effectively managing major conflicts?

- Successfully participating in group activities?

- Responding to failure or disappointment?

- Responding to success?

- Meeting the expectations of peers, parents, and teachers?

- Considering other people's feelings?

If Your Child Has a Problem

As a first step, you can ask some general, open-ended questions of your child that might allow him to raise social issues that concern him. With his help, identify the specific difficulties he is experiencing. Be sure to focus on specific behavior in a calm, supportive way. Even if his poor social skills irritate you or other family members, it is important not to make him feel ashamed or insecure.

Quite often, in order to maintain their self-esteem or avoid pain and embarrassment, children will deny that a problem exists in their lives, no matter how obvious. Even when a problem is acknowledged, they may have difficulty accepting responsibility for it and for its resolution. But the first, necessary step toward making the situation better is for both of you to acknowledge that a difficulty really exists, although it may take several attempts on your part.

Once the problem is identified and acknowledged, then there are actions you can take to help your child overcome his difficulties. Social skills can be learned. Be sure he really understands what the problems are, explaining them (without blame) in words that make sense to him. Avoid predictions of doom and gloom, and instead maintain an optimistic and hopeful outlook.

Other suggestions to nurture your kids' social skills:

- The Golden Rule applies to most situations. Treat others the way you wish to be treated. Remind your child of this both in your home family environment and outside the home. Model this rule by your actions yourself; if you slip (we are all human, after all), own up to your misstep and use the situation as a learning opportunity with your child, explaining that we all have a chance to make things right.

- Join a Scouting club, athletic team, park district program, or other extracurricular activities that your child is interested in.

- Teach him to think in terms of actions and consequences. If he alters his behavior in a particular way—for example, if he is willing to share his toys and games with the neighborhood children—help him see the positive consequences of that action, including a greater likelihood that he will be accepted and liked by his peers.

- Help him identify alternative behavior to replace the actions that are causing the difficulty. For example, if he tries to resolve conflicts by hitting other children, discuss more productive, socially acceptable ways of approaching the same situation, such as taking turns, walking away, or knowing when to back off before things heat up. Physical contact is not acceptable.

- Relate your child's particular problem—and its solution—to circumstances he is likely to face in the future. Help him anticipate situations that may arise, and discuss or even practice how he will respond to them. Remind him that everything will not necessarily always proceed according to plan, however, and that he will need to be flexible and adapt to unexpected turns of events.

- Remember that social skills are not developed overnight, but are learned through practice, observation, discussion, and more practice until they become automatic and natural. You and your child may find that practice works best when done in a role-playing situation, where a parent, sibling, or trusted friend plays the role of the child in order to demonstrate an alternative or appropriate behavior. Then the "players" switch roles so the child can practice and rehearse.

- Encourage your child to bring a playmate or classmate to your home, where you can observe their interactions and teach them some appropriate social behavior. Teaching children that "to have a friend you must be a friend" can be very powerful when opportunities are made to practice at home.

- Help your child develop a skill or interest that will assist him to fit in with peers. This should be done in a way that suits your child and does not force him to change in ways that make him feel uncomfortable.

- Highlight your child's strengths and talents, say that they make you proud of him, and explain how they might be used to help overcome his social difficulties.

- Encourage participation in multigenerational interactions. Family gatherings and volunteering as a family will expose your child to both older and younger people, increasing her breadth of experience and furthering social skills with non-peer-age groups. As time goes on your school-age child should feel more comfortable interacting with people outside of her age group.

Understanding Your Child's Age-Appropriate Social Skills

Children ages 5–7 years: At this age, children make friends quite easily. A same-age neighbor makes for an excellent playmate. The prior preschool years of parallel play have evolved into a more mature, imaginative, socially dynamic play. Games such as tag and hide-and-seek are favorite interactive ways to play for kids in this age group.

Children ages 8–10 years: As they get older, kids become more selective about who they prefer to spend time socializing with. School classmates and sports teammates are natural choices. Kids these ages should feel comfortable speaking with teachers, coaches, and other grown-ups, as well as their peers.

Children ages 11–12 years: Eleven- and 12-year-olds have increasingly significant relationships with friends. In the school setting, kids these ages should take increased self-responsibility communicating with teachers regarding school assignments and issues that may arise. Texting and social networking may become more prevalent for some kids; this should be done with involved parental supervision and guidance (for more on this, see page 315).

Should You Seek Professional Help?

Sometimes other problems are causing or contributing to your child's poor development of social skills. These might include family discord and stress, medical problems, emotional difficulties such as depression or anxiety, or your child's speech and language difficulties or attention deficits. If you suspect that problems like these are making things worse, seek out advice from your pediatrician or school social worker.

To deal with your child's specific difficulties with social skills, consider involving her in formal social skills training programs, which are available through school social workers, behavioral psychologists, or behavioral pediatricians. They are frequently offered in small group settings, so that children with similar problems can support one another as well as learn successful strategies for dealing with their own areas of concern. In general, those who fare best in these groups tend to be insightful and open to new ideas, have a good intellectual understanding of their situation, and are willing to discuss or role-play their problem with other children who are learning to cope with similar difficulties. Often local school districts' social workers run a "lunch bunch" program or similar idea to get kids together in a small group to communicate and exchange ideas. Whether your child works with a therapist in a group or an individual setting, the professional should regularly assess your child's progress as she continues to meet new and more challenging situations.

Peer acceptance is one of the most gratifying experiences for children. By contrast, peer rejection or ridicule can take an enormous toll on a child's self-esteem and sense of security. As you help your child, remember to remain sensitive and supportive at every step. Set expectations at a realistic level; offer lots of praise, encouragement, and rewards for efforts and even small improvements. Your child's greatest reward for these efforts will be the gift of friendship.

Friends

Through friendships, children can broaden their horizons beyond the family unit, begin to experience the outside world, form a self-image, and develop a social support system.

During the preschool years, play provides positive social encounters and increasing amounts of cooperative activity, which are the foundations of friendship. Aggressive behavior increases between ages 2 and 4 but then declines. Rules and social roles become increasingly important, and gender differences in social activities may become more obvious. The stability of friendships also increases as children approach school age, and girls seem to develop more intense relationships with a few other children than do boys, who scatter their affection across a larger number of kids.

Between the ages of 5 and 12, making friends is one of the most important missions of middle childhood—a social skill that will endure throughout their lives. Developmentally, school-age children are ready to form more complex relationships. They become increasingly able to communicate both their feelings and their ideas, and they can better understand concepts of time—past, present, and future. At this age they are no longer so bound to the family or so concerned mostly about themselves but begin relying on peers for companionship, spending more time with friends than they did during the preschool years. Day by day they share with one another the pleasures and frustrations of childhood.

Friends play many roles in a child's life, serving as companions, confidants, and allies, sharing advice and feelings, and providing stability and support in difficult times. Friends also supply feedback that allows children to measure, judge, and make adjustments within themselves, while answering the nagging and important question "How am I doing?" In some natural sequences, children move through stages in which their friendships first emphasize common activities and similarities in outlook, then are characterized by shared values and rules; finally, as puberty approaches, they focus on understanding others, self-disclosure, shared interests, and stronger emotional bonds.

Even so, children differ in the rate at which they develop social skills. Also, some kids desire and need friends more than others. While certain children may be quite content spending most of their time by themselves, with family members, or with just a single best friend, others may be much more gregarious, forming and maintaining many friendships. A child's preferences and needs may change from year to year and even from month to month. In most cases there is no reason for concern when a child decides to limit the number of his friends, unless he also seems depressed or is being rejected by his classmates. Children also form friendships with siblings, especially in large or close families, or when families are isolated from other children and families. These sibling friendships may replace outside friends and the need for them.

Late in the middle years, peer influence is very evident. Friendships often evolve into highly exclusive cliques in which children strongly influence one another. At most schools there are a variety of cliques, each with its own hierarchy of members. Kids' attraction to particular friends may be based on anything from personality to extracurricular interests, from athletic ability to appearance. In these preadolescent years, kids in tightly knit inner circles may feel quite secure with one another, creating their own group identity by looking and talking alike. These kids often feel a strong pressure to dress and talk in a particular way, listen to certain music, and wear their hair in a specific style. This peer pressure begins to compete (and sometimes clash) with the influence of parents and their values.

Preadolescents also tend to be quite judgmental, labeling others and at the same time becoming increasingly concerned about what their friends think of them. If a peer is even just a little different, they may conclude, "He's terrible; I don't like him."

In the early elementary school years, friends are frequently of the same gender. During the latter years of middle childhood, however, girls and boys begin to spend a little more time together. Girls may gossip with their girlfriends—and boys with their boyfriends—about whom they like and who is cute; even so, at this age there is no real dating, even though kids may talk of "going together." Sometime during adolescence, they will finally begin to pair off in a more serious way. Social networking and the internet have made it possible to interact with peers twenty-four hours a day, seven days a week; kids this age need the guidance and involvement of adults to help them make good choices. For more on this, see page 315.

Choosing Friends

A number of factors play a role in determining whom a child befriends. Some research shows that the friends a child chooses tend to share mutual traits with him or possess characteristics that he would like to have. Thus, as a child's preferences and goals change—which they inevitably do as he grows—he will make new friends to satisfy his evolving needs and desires and fit his own self-image.

Children also select friends with similar temperaments and patterns of play. Shy children tend to be attracted to others like themselves; loud and boisterous children usually choose boisterous friends. Children interested in the same activities and hobbies are drawn together as well.

Particularly in your child's early years, you, as a parent, often will arrange opportunities for him to spend time with playmates of your choosing. With the passage of time, however, he will begin making more choices of friends on his own, and you need to know with whom he is spending time, actively monitoring (if not supervising) that play.

A number of factors can come into play as your child selects his friends. If he feels good about himself, and if he has been loved and respected within the family, he is more likely to make good choices of friends. If you and your spouse relate to each other well, and if your child has caring and supportive relationships with his brothers and sisters, he will have seen and experienced positive examples of how people can relate, and he will carry these impressions over into his own friendships, including the friends he chooses. On the other hand, if those family experiences have not been supportive and confidence-boosting, he is likely to seek out peers who have similar types of troubles.

Take some time to help your child understand why he chooses the friends he does. This is an opportunity to discuss his own values, feelings, and behaviors.

A healthy friendship is one in which both children are on an equal footing. Neither child should dominate the other or make all the decisions on what activities to pursue. They should share and make an effort to please each other. They should also be capable of problem-solving on their own: if one boy wants to play with a particular toy that belongs to his buddy, they will probably work out a schedule so that each can have a turn. Or they might devise alternative activities that they can do together.

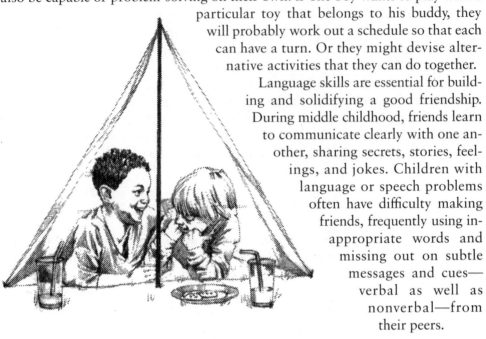

Language skills are essential for building and solidifying a good friendship. During middle childhood, friends learn to communicate clearly with one another, sharing secrets, stories, feelings, and jokes. Children with language or speech problems often have difficulty making friends, frequently using inappropriate words and missing out on subtle messages and cues—verbal as well as nonverbal—from their peers.

A "Best" Friend

In middle childhood some kids concentrate their social activity on a single best friend. In these relationships children usually match themselves with someone with whom they feel completely compatible, someone who is capable of meeting their needs for companionship, approval, and security.

These can be wonderful friendships, the kind that seem as though they will last a lifetime—sometimes they actually do. Even though parents often worry that exclusive friendships can be confining and stifling, and that their child has too much invested in this single relationship, most experts disagree. Sharing experiences, thoughts, and feelings with one special pal can often be more satisfying than spending time with a large group, as long as these two friends are having a positive influence on each other and are not excluding themselves from a broad range of experiences.

Dealing with Negative Peer Influence

What should you do if your child wants to play with the neighborhood trouble-maker? What if he starts hanging out with a child who lies, destroys property, or bullies other children? What if he begins expressing values or attitudes you do not like? What if he adopts behaviors that are worrisome?

Dealing with negative peer influence is a challenge, but there are solutions. Some parents may demand that their own child stop spending time with this "bad influence," but this may not be the best strategy. Typically, children adamantly defend such a friend, and they may trivialize or rationalize his faults or shortcomings. They may ignore their parents, finding a way of seeing this playmate anyway. And if they do abide by their parents' wishes, other problems may ensue, since the children's own judgment and ability to make wise decisions independently are affected.

In most cases a better strategy is to reinforce positive friendships with children whose behavior and values meet with your approval. Encourage your child to invite these children over to your house to play. Arrange activities that are somewhat structured, mutually enjoyable, and time-limited, such as bowling, bicycling, or watching a sporting event. Also, arrange summer events (camp, special weekend trips) that bring the children together.

Speak calmly and rationally when you explain why you would prefer that your child not spend time with a particular friend, focusing on specific behavior rather than generalizing or criticizing their character. Make it a point to have this friend over to your home so that you can observe the friend dynamic; often these kids come from troubled homes, and it is possible your home could be a safe haven for her. This approach will teach your child to think more logically and assume responsibility for his actions, and show that you trust his growing capacity to make the right decisions. For more information on decision-making on social media, see page 315.

Children Without Friends

At one time or another, most children enjoy spending time alone. Perhaps after a long day at school or a busy weekend, they prefer just to relax by themselves, reading a book or playing a videogame. As normal as this type of behavior is, there may be cause for concern when a child has no friends, and especially when she feels lonely or socially inadequate. She may not get invited to parties, often sits alone during school lunch, is not picked to be part of a team, and receives few, if any, invitations to play with other children.

Most children want to be liked, yet some are slow in learning how to make friends. Others may long for companionship but might be excluded from one group or another, perhaps picked on because of the way they dress, poor personal hygiene, obesity, or even a speech impediment. Kids are often rejected by peers if they exhibit disruptive or aggressive behavior. Still other children may hover on the fringes of one clique or another but never really get noticed and spend most of their time alone. In some cases, children do not have opportunities to make friends, which requires time and energy. They are too programmed in highly structured activities, live far away from school, live in areas without children's facilities or activities, or are bound tightly to their families.

A child without friends is, for parents, a difficult and painful dilemma. The problem is not uncommon; as many as 10 percent of school-age children say they have no best friend. These children may feel lonely and socially isolated and, as a result, have emotional and adjustment difficulties or fail to master the social skills so necessary for success with peers or adults.

To help your child resolve these social dilemmas, you will need skill and sensitivity. If your child senses that you are agonizing over—or are too intrusive toward—the problems in her social life, she may become overly anxious or defensive, perhaps even feeling that she has let you down by her inability to make friends. In response to your attempts at intervention, she may withdraw or deny that any problem exists. If she says, "Everything is just fine, Mom," she still may be aching for some friendships.

As a parent, try to discover why your child is not happy with or is rejected by

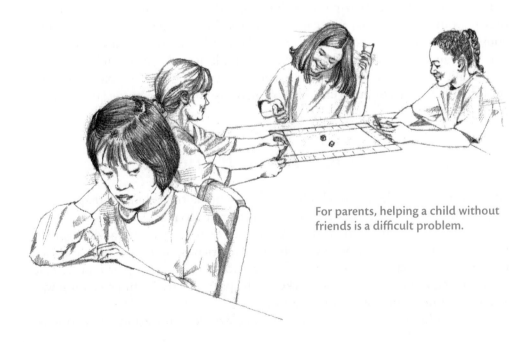

For parents, helping a child without friends is a difficult problem.

peers. From your adult perspective, your child's world may seem quite simple, but it is actually quite complex and demanding. For instance, on a playground your child may have to accomplish many tasks: entering a group, maintaining conversations, coordinating play, dealing with teasing and other forms of provocation, and resolving conflicts with others. Those are a lot of issues to handle, and if she is not adept at them, she may have difficulty making or keeping friends.

There are a variety of child-centered reasons she may not have friends, including being rejected, being neglected, or simply being a shy child. Rejected kids are overtly disliked by their peers and are constantly made to feel unwelcome. They often tend to be aggressive or disruptive and very sensitive to teasing. They may be bullies and rule-violators, or they may be so unsure of themselves that they invite the rejection of others. They might also be rejected because of their impulsive and disruptive behavior. Some of them may have attention deficits or hyperactivity.

Neglected children, on the other hand, are not overtly rejected and teased but are often just ignored, forgotten, not invited to parties, and the last ones picked for a team. These kids may be perceived as loners but might be passive and detest their isolation. Others may actually prefer to be alone. This latter group might be respected and admired by others but simply feel more comfortable in solitary pursuits or in spending time with parents, siblings, other adults, or even pets. They may also lack the social skills and self-confidence necessary for them to enter social arenas, often because of limited social experiences. Or they may be more shy, quiet, and reserved than most of their peers.

Shyness

Although childhood shyness is commonplace, it concerns many parents, especially those who place great value on sociability. Some children become shy because of life experiences, but most are born that way. For some middle-years children, social situations and interactions can be terrifying. When they come in contact with new children, they rarely feel at ease. Typically, they are unwilling or unable to make the first move, preferring to abandon a potential friendship rather than reach out to the unfamiliar. A few of these timid children may be emotionally distressed, but they are in the minority. In fact, some children are just naturally withdrawn and slow to warm up in new situations (for more on temperament, see page 131).

In some cases, shyness can be disabling. Extremely shy children often do not adapt as well as most of their peers in the classroom and on the playground. The longer this pattern exists, the more difficult it is for children to change. Shyness can increasingly lead to purposeful avoidance of social settings and withdrawal, and ultimately create an inability to function effectively as a social adult. If your child's shyness becomes debilitating, it may be caused by an anxiety disorder or a

Why Some Children Don't Have Friends

Children may have social problems for a wide variety of reasons, some of which are outside their control—and yours. Following are some of the factors that might be contributing to your child's difficulty in making or keeping friends.

CHILD-RELATED INFLUENCES

Temperament (difficult, shy)

Attention problems/hyperactivity

Learning disabilities

Social skill problems

Communication skill difficulties

Delayed physical, emotional, or intellectual development

Physical handicap

Chronic illness, frequent hospitalizations, school absenteeism

Poor gross motor skills, limiting participation in group activities

Emotional difficulties (depression, anxiety, low self-esteem)

Poor personal hygiene

Unattractive physical appearance

Child chooses or prefers to be alone

Child derives social satisfaction and friendship mainly from family members

Cultural values do not fit those of peers

PARENT-RELATED INFLUENCES

Parenting style (too authoritarian, too permissive) adversely affects child's social development

Parent keeps child too busy with programmed activities, chores, or jobs that limit time, energy, or opportunities for developing friendships

Parent is overly critical or negative of child's choice of friends

Parent has poor social skills; child does not have a good role model

Parent has depression or mental illness

Parent has substance abuse problem

Parenting style includes domestic chaos or violence

Parents experience marital stress, tension, abuse

Parent overprotects child or imposes excessive limits on activities

Parent has difficulty adjusting to child's individuality or special needs

SOCIAL-ENVIRONMENTAL INFLUENCES

Family lives in rural, isolated area

Family residence is far from school

Neighborhood has few other children

Family goes away all summer

Family experiences financial stress and frequent moves

Family has cultural or language differences

Community has few opportunities or programs for children to gather and socialize

Danger of violence in usual play areas prevents children from interacting

Child's peer group perceives differences in dress, values, and behavior

temperament pattern and an evaluation by a child mental health professional would be helpful. Be wary of your child spending too much time on the internet; it is dangerous for children to replace "in real life" relationships with an inappropriate presence on the internet.

Most shy children, however, do well in relationships and in social settings once they are past an initial period of adjustment. Children who have difficulty establishing and maintaining relationships even after the ice-breaking period merit more concern and attention. Eventually, most children who are shy learn to conquer their tendency. They function in ways that are not obviously timid or reticent, although they self-identify as an introvert.

The Influence of Parenting Styles

Parents have their own temperaments, social skills, and parenting style that can influence a child's social abilities and her acceptance by peers. If you are highly critical, disapproving, rejecting, or aggressive, your child will tend to mimic your style and behave in a hostile and aggressive manner with her peers. By contrast, if you are generous, accepting, and patient, your child probably will adopt these same characteristics and fare much better in making friends.

Some experts have categorized parenting into three styles:

Authoritarian parents tend to overcontrol their children, instituting a set of absolute rules and standards. As they emphasize a high degree of control, they may de-emphasize warmth and trust. They also tend to assert their power by restricting privileges and even withdrawing love or approval. This parenting style may cause the child to feel rejected and isolated. She may develop only adequate social skills and will tend to remain dependent on her mother and father.

Permissive parents are at the other end of the spectrum. They demonstrate considerable warmth and affection, are generally very accepting, exercise a low level of control over their children, and make few demands upon them. Their children tend to become moderately independent and achieve modest degrees of social success.

Authoritative parents fall between these two extremes. While exercising considerable control, they also exhibit warmth and affection and seem to have appropriate expectations for their children. As their kids move through the middle years of childhood, the parents recognize the growing maturity of their children, encourage appropriate levels of responsibility, and use reason and negotiation in resolving differences. Their children tend to be independent and socially successful.

The way you relate to your child also can be influenced by the child herself. If your child is temperamentally difficult, for instance, you may react by becoming more anxious, aggressive, negative, and controlling, and less nurturing and less likely to respond positively. As a result, your child may grow up insecure and lacking appropriate social skills, and she may experience difficult interactions with peers.

Social Influences

Although children sometimes feel they are the sole cause of their lack of friends, that is not the case. Friendship is a two-way, dynamic process that depends on how children perceive one another. In middle childhood, kids tend to see one another in absolute terms, often lacking appreciation for more subtle individual differences or unique characteristics—a situation that sets the groundwork for rejection or neglect.

Often, an unpopular child develops a self-image or a reputation among her peers that is difficult to alter. Even if the child makes improvements in her social style, labels and peer perceptions are hard to change. Children may decide to cling to their biases, and thus even when the unpopular child has finally moved into a group, she may not be fully accepted or welcomed. So although technically she may no longer be an outsider, she still may experience feelings of loneliness, isolation, and diminished self-esteem.

While some unpopular children can change their behavior, others cannot and continue to behave in a way that interferes with their ability to make friends. Some kids simply have difficulty acquiring the new social skills they need. Others actually are not even aware that they are having trouble with relationships. Still others have come to expect rejection as part of their lives, and these expectations become self-fulfilling prophecies keeping them from behaving in ways that would promote friendships. Sometimes several of these influences are at work at the same time, reinforcing one another.

When families live in rural, isolated areas far from school, there may be few opportunities for children to socialize after school or on weekends. Some communities do not have activity programs in which children can participate together. A family's financial stress, or frequent changes of jobs and homes, can add to the difficulty of making friends.

What Parents Can Do

When your child seems to be lacking friends and is hurting because of it, you need to get involved as soon as possible. As a first step in helping your child overcome her loneliness and isolation, you and your child need to acknowledge that a problem exists. In a sensitive, supportive manner, talk about this situation together. Although denial, sadness, embarrassment, or rationalization are normal responses, you and your child need to get beyond them.

Maintain open communication at home. Encourage your child to talk openly about her concerns and difficulties regarding friendships. She is much more aware of her social scene than you are, so be a good listener. By being a good listener you are modeling good communication skills for your child; relationships are a back-and-forth, an exchange of communication. At the same time, this is an extremely sensitive subject, and problems may be difficult for your child to acknowledge. Her own insights and understanding of the group dynamics may be limited.

Avoid downplaying the social problems that your child is having with her peers. When your child is in pain, if you offer only simple reassurance, you may communicate that you neither understand nor care. For example, if peers are calling her a wimp or a nerd, do not advise her just to ignore them. That is like asking an adult not to be concerned when she loses her job. Be accepting, nonjudgmental, and sympathetic.

Find balance between empathy and responsibility. In many cases your child may be able to solve her social problems without your direct intervention. If she is being excluded from the basketball games at the playground on Saturday afternoons, for instance, nothing could be worse for her stature among her peers than for you to show up and insist that she be allowed to play. ("Look who needs her mommy to stick up for her!") Also, if you constantly rescue her, she will become overly dependent on you, or resent your well-intentioned efforts, rather than find solutions on her own. Ask your child plenty of open-ended questions along the lines of "What do you think about that?" or "What could you do about that?" Kids need practice developing independent skills in these areas.

Get information from school. Ask your child's teacher at school how she interacts with other students. The teacher may have impressions of whether your child comes on too strong or whether she is withdrawn. You may find that she has some eccentric habits that place her at the receiving end of jokes or bullying among her peers. The teacher may have some suggestions on what your child can do to make friends or identify other children with like interests. Also, a group of students with similar needs might benefit from a few sessions with a qualified professional.

Initiate a plan. With this information in hand, you might be able to focus on specific problems and guide your child in appropriate directions, perhaps developing a strategy for entering into a group activity and practicing how to start and maintain conversations and deal effectively with minor and major conflicts. Spend a few minutes talking with her about the perspective of other children—what they might think of her and what they consider important. By encouraging her to talk with you about her struggles with friendships, you will have the opportunity to troubleshoot with her to develop strategies to get along. And if you maintain and nurture other areas of gratification and success, you can help your child become resilient and persistent in her attempts to gain success in the social domain.

Direct your child. A child in this position needs help and guidance to find social events or initiate activities. Guide her into situations where she is likely to meet other kids and develop friendships. Encourage her to invite someone in her

Peer Relationship Skills

Successful peer interactions require a variety of skills and special ways of interacting. Good communication with your child will help him develop interpersonal skills outside the family.

Coping with failure and frustration	Comforting someone
Coping with success	Sharing
Coping with change and transitions	Making requests
Coping with rejection and teasing	Self-disclosure
Managing anger	Giving a compliment
Using humor	Expressing appreciation
Forgiving	Coping with loss
Apologizing	Sticking up for a friend
Refusing to accept a dare	Doing favors
Thinking up fun things to do	Asking for help
Expressing affection	Helping others
Avoiding dangerous situations	Keeping secrets
Defending himself	

class to spend a few hours at your home, or to accompany your family on a fun outing.

To increase your child's likelihood of success, suggest that she spend time with peers whose temperaments and interests are similar to her own. Pick the friends your child seems closest to, and those who seem to have a similar temperament, and provide them with opportunities to spend time together, first in relatively brief, structured activities, and then in progressively less structured ones. Short visits and structured activities are usually the easiest first steps. More active girls, for instance, tend to have greater camaraderie with equally active playmates. Encourage her to build one or two special friendships. Really, as long as children have *one* good friend, that is a good place to be in.

As a starting point, invite your child's friend to go bowling or to a sporting event, a movie, or a play—something where the two of them won't have to engage in much conversation face-to-face but can do something together side by side. Let them warm up gradually with an activity that has a definite end, rather than an open-ended day at the beach or "spending the afternoon." Usually if the activity itself is pleasurable and time limits are brief, the odds of success increase dramatically. Unstructured activities can follow if the initial encounters are successful and might be at a selected place—a park or a playground—or simply be at home without designated things to do.

As these friendships develop, get to know your child's playmates better. Encourage your child to invite them over to your house to play. Make contact with the parents of her friends. Keep the lines of communication open between families.

Identify your child's strengths or interests. Encourage your child to use her strengths to make friends. If she has a good sense of humor, for example, she might be able to take advantage of it in a class play or other situation where she is likely to be appreciated by peers. If she likes animals, she might meet others with the same interest and go to the zoo with them or watch nature and wildlife videos together.

Social activities. Encourage your child to avoid situations that are likely to lead to embarrassment. Help her take advantage of her strengths, selecting activities where she can excel. Or involve her in individual noncompetitive sports activities. Ask your child if she would like to sign up for a Scouting program or other group activity, an excellent way to meet and share experiences with a group of children the same age. Look into the group composition and activities of the Scout troop beforehand, making sure that your child fits in with the group. Be cautious of activities that are competitive and in which conventional friendships are not emphasized.

For shy children, a summer camp can also bring them out of their shell. Finding the right camp is critical. For a child who is very shy, or who has never been away from home before and may experience homesickness, a day camp may be best for the first camping experience. Consider your child's interests; there are camps that specialize in computers, writing, and nature study, among many other areas of interest.

Seek professional help. When your child has serious difficulties making friends, and when your own initial efforts at helping her are unsuccessful, seek the help of your pediatrician, the school social worker, a child psychologist, or another professional with expertise in behavioral problems. These professionals might suggest programs to help your child develop her social skills. Child counseling, peer groups, or family therapy can often help point a child in the right direction toward developing positive friendships. Parent training might be part of these therapeutic efforts, helping you to recognize, reinforce, and reward your child's positive behavioral changes. Other problems (like attention deficits, learning disabilities, or emotional problems) might be contributing to social difficulties. Children with these problems can benefit from professional help.

~ 12 ~

Dealing with Prejudice

UNFORTUNATELY, PREJUDICE IS still commonplace in the world. Bigotry based on race, sex, ethnicity, religion, gender identity, sexual orientation, or physical or mental disabilities impacts the lives of children and their families. Our children are growing up in a time when the racial and ethnic composition of our country continues to evolve. In many areas of the nation, groups of people previously characterized as racial or ethnic minorities make up the majority of the population.

In addition to experiences in day-to-day life, children are exposed to different cultures through the media. They are learning and forming opinions about people and events all over the country and the world, which is a great opportunity to help children learn to understand and value diversity.

Children's encounters with prejudice are not confined to ethnic and racial stereotypes and bias. Every day, children are exposed to the way some individuals are valued more or less because of their gender or age. Young children are aware that their feelings, opinions, and beliefs receive less consideration because of their youth. As children approach adolescence, they also become increasingly aware of the more subtle prejudices and intolerances tied to differences in social class, religion, sexual orientation, gender identity, or physical and mental disabilities.

Children can suffer from a climate of prejudice. Prejudice creates social and emotional tension and can lead to fear and anxiety, and possibly hostility and violence. Prejudice and discrimination can undermine the self-esteem and self-confidence of those being ridiculed and make them feel unaccepted, unworthy, and undeserving of affection. When that happens, their school performance often suffers and they may become depressed and socially withdrawn, which can lead to self-harm or causing harm to others.

It is critical that you help your child understand diversity in a positive way. Prejudice is learned at a very young age from parents and caregivers, family, other children, and people and institutions outside of the family. By about 4 years of age, children are aware of differences among people, primarily in characteristics like appearance, language, and names, but later they are aware of religious and cultural distinctions as well. To some extent, children begin to define and identify themselves through their understanding of these personal differences. This is normal.

As children try to make sense of these individual distinctions, they may hear and accept simplified stereotypes about others. When that happens, they not only develop distorted views of the children and adults they encounter in daily life, but they may start to deny and overlook the common, universal human elements and traits that would bring people together. As a result, intolerance may develop where there should be friendship.

Taking Action

As a parent, don't ignore the prejudice to which your child may be exposed in the media or in her own experiences. Keep in mind that you serve as the most powerful influence and role model for your child, and more than anyone else, you can mold her attitudes and her behavior toward others. Here are some guidelines to follow:

- Your actions toward the people in your life will lay the foundation for how your child relates to his peers and others. Examine your attitudes and the way you feel about people with traits and characteristics different from your own. Consider the different roles, relationships, and responsibilities within your own household, and what forms of age or gender discrimination may occur there. If you want your child to be free of prejudice, you need to demonstrate that attitude in your words and deeds. Encourage positive values toward diversity and harmonious and cooperative ways of living. Love and respect your child, so he can come to value and respect others.

- Nothing is more powerful in dispelling myths and stereotypes than person-to-person contact. Bring diversity into your own life. Make your friends

How Parents Can Help Children Embrace Diversity

Children ages 5–7 years: At this age children have a simpler view of their peers and the world. The younger kids are when they are exposed to others of different racial, ethnic, cultural, and physical backgrounds, the more likely the children will appreciate and embrace diversity in many forms.

Children ages 8–10 years: As children grow older, they should continue to learn about how other parts of the world live. A daily newspaper subscription with a news source that includes world events is a great eye-opener for kids this age. The internet is an excellent tool to learn about the diversity of the world in which we live. A subscription to the print version of *National Geographic* or *National Geographic Kids* is a great way to expose kids to other cultures and ideas.

Children ages 11–12 years: These days 11- and 12-year-olds are increasingly using technology, but do not underestimate the value of print newspapers and magazines to teach kids about the greater world. Internet and social media users tend to view the content they seek; a print daily newspaper with world coverage educates readers about events and issues they may not have realized were taking place. If the internet or social media is preferred, consider email subscriptions to kid-friendly world news sources.

and coworkers of different races and cultural backgrounds regular participants in your family's activities. Let your child see that you accept people of different physical and mental abilities. Let your child experience that there are more similarities than differences among people. It is valuable to expose him to cultures and holidays different from his own: for example, with the cooperation of friends and neighbors, gentile children can attend a bat mitzvah or Passover Seder, while Jewish children can go to a church service or baptism. But your child should understand that these are only limited aspects of the differences and diversity that surround him.

- Children initially focus on differences in physical appearance. In language appropriate for your child's age, explain why people have different skin and eye color, hair type, and other features. Discuss how differences in appearance are inherited from mothers and fathers. Talk about the diversity of your own child's ethnic heritage. At the same time, point out the similarities among all people, such as the need to be loved, the need for self-respect, and feelings of happiness and sadness, anger and pain, which everyone has at some time.

■ Discuss your family's history of immigration to this country, or more recent moves to new neighborhoods and the adjustments that this required

How Schools Can Defuse Prejudice

In addition to academics, schools help kids learn about the diverse world in which they live. Schools can promote understanding and cooperation among people from a variety of backgrounds and cultures.

■ Do learning and problem-solving tasks emphasize cooperation and team play? Children should not be placed in situations where differences in gender, race, ethnicity, physical or mental abilities, economic status, and academic ability are stressed, or are even allowed to be expressed in a negative, divisive way. Team spirit can conquer feelings of difference and separateness that children experience among themselves.

■ Does the school have a curriculum that covers the different races, religions, and cultures of present-day America? Is your child continuously exposed to the achievements and contributions of all Americans and cultures?

■ Does the school take advantage of ethnic holidays—Chinese New Year, Cinco de Mayo, Kwanzaa, etc.—for children to actively learn customs and traditions with which they may not be familiar?

■ Do teachers have open discussions in class about discrimination and negative feelings toward others? If an incident involving prejudice has occurred at school or in the community, is it used as a springboard to discuss these issues in a sensitive, age-appropriate, non-stigmatizing way that emphasizes the common human qualities of people?

for the family. Talk to your children about their unique qualities, and the characteristics, feelings, and dreams you and they share with people all over the world.

■ Discuss the issue of prejudice with your child. Many schools have curricula that promote discussions of diversity and prejudice, and as a parent, you have the opportunity to reinforce this at home. Make it clear that diversity should be valued and that discrimination in any form is unacceptable. Your child should understand that teasing, insulting, rejecting, or diminishing another person based on race, religion, background, origin, sexual orientation, physical or mental abilities, economic status, gender identity, or appearance will not be tolerated. Explain that there is no need for your child to build himself up by putting others down.

■ If you sense that your child has negative attitudes toward others, or you witness or hear about any intolerant or discriminatory behavior on his part, do not ignore the situation. In a timely fashion, address these prejudices by discussing why your child feels the way he does. Let rational thinking defuse the emotional intensity of prejudice. Remind your child of the Golden Rule: treat others as you wish to be treated yourself.

■ Help your child understand the erroneous basis of stereotypes and hatred. Call attention to negative stereotypes when they appear in the media, including the internet, social media, videogames, television (both programs and commercials), newspapers, and magazines.

■ When choosing experiences for your child—including camps, schools, child care, and extracurricular events—seek out diversity in racial and ethnic backgrounds among the other children participating.

■ Actively work to reduce prejudice in your life and community. Establish a household in which all members are valued and respected. Participate in your child's school to ensure that diversity is valued and reinforced. Join political and civic organizations and attend multicultural events, both to change the world in which your child lives and to demonstrate your commitment to addressing the prejudices that exist.

■ If your child personally experiences prejudice, she will probably feel hurt and angry. However, due to social circumstances or her own stage of development, she may feel unable to express these emotions. You need to encourage her to vent her feelings, and you must acknowledge the validity of these feelings before trying to discuss the situation with logic and reason. A child whose personhood has been attacked through prejudice needs to be supported and have her self-esteem bolstered by her family and friends. From there, you can discuss the roots of prejudice with her, and how the two of you believe she should respond.

PART IV

Behavior and Discipline

~ 13 ~

Communication and Your Child's Behavior

A CHILD'S FAMILY instructs and gives guidance about personal values and social behavior. Behavior refers to one's verbal and nonverbal communications—the conduct, actions, and words that children use and exhibit. A child's behavior is a signal with which they express their thoughts, feelings, needs, and impulses. It is judged as to whether it meets social, cultural, developmental, and age-appropriate standards. Behavior can be positive or negative, impulsive or planned, predictable or unpredictable, consistent or inconsistent, and it can elicit a wide range of positive or negative responses from others.

The term "discipline" refers to a framework that helps kids understand what is, and is not, acceptable behavior. While the word "discipline" often carries negative connotations, parents should keep in mind that it helps kids learn and internalize codes of conduct that will serve them well for the rest of their lives. Discipline also helps kids develop positive interpersonal relationships, and it provides an environment that encourages learning both in the home and at school.

Children, especially in the younger years, cannot always directly communicate their thoughts and needs through *spoken* language. Parents can learn much about their child by what he *does*, in addition to what he *says*. Through his behavior, your child may be trying to communicate messages such as "That's too difficult for me . . . I'm afraid of failure . . . I'm tired . . . I'm afraid of being rejected . . . I want you to play with me . . . I need you . . . I love you . . . I want you to pay attention to me." This holds true for children approaching middle school age as well.

Attention is one of the most important things that children desire and seek from their parents. Receiving the attention kids need sends the message that they are loved, valued, accepted, and respected. Children will go to great extremes for the feeling of security and unconditional love. Kids quickly learn which kinds of behavior obtains a response from parents; if positive behavior doesn't work, they will often turn to negative behaviors. Even if their misbehavior gets them a negative reaction such as being scolded, to a child's eyes any recognition is better than none.

Behavior does not occur in isolation. It is a form of communication, a way to express needs and feelings, and is influenced by a child's desires, temperament, and ability to adapt, as well as by her parents' parenting style, family situation, and various stresses and transitions—from a minor illness to starting a new school year.

During the school-age years, children are developing rapidly and trying to understand the world around them, face new demands, deal with success and failure, and communicate with their siblings, parents, and peers. In many cases these transitions can lead to problems. Just as the middle years offer endless opportunities for children to learn and to meet new challenges, they also provide an equal number of chances for them to make mistakes, to achieve and succeed, and to question or challenge parental values, rules, and attitudes. Consistent, appropriate parental discipline is a way to teach children what behavior is appropriate in which circumstance, or how to interact in a socially acceptable manner.

In this sense, "discipline" does not imply punishment or scolding. It means "to educate," and it provides a framework for acceptable behavior. Proper discipline teaches children to live in a safe, civilized, and harmonious manner with themselves and others. There are some essential elements to disciplining well, including correctly understanding the child's needs and abilities (going beyond the concrete, actual behavior), communicating effectively, and using positive and negative reinforcement appropriately. (See Chapter 15, "Your Child's Behavior and Discipline.")

The Perfect Parent Does Not Exist

The idea of perfect parents who raise happy, well-adjusted, problem-free children is a myth and simply does not exist. In truth, there is no such person as a perfect parent—or a perfect child. Rather, parents should strive to do the best they can given their own specific set of circumstances, based in reality.

Problem behavior is common among school-age children and takes up a significant portion of a parent's time. At any one time, on average, school-age children have a handful of traits or behaviors that their parents find challenging. These behaviors may include not complying with simple requests, avoiding chores, spending too much time watching TV or playing videogames, engaging in sibling rivalry, or having difficulty completing homework. Other common problems for parents are dealing with a temperamentally challenging child, or guiding a child who either wants too much independence or hasn't achieved enough autonomy. Parents also sometimes encounter the dilemma of a child who prefers friends or activities not approved of by the parent.

As a parent, you need to recognize that it is normal to feel worried, confused, angry, guilty, overwhelmed, and inadequate because of your child's behavior. That is part of being a parent. It is futile and self-defeating to try to be perfect or to raise perfect children. Think back to how you behaved, or misbehaved, as a child, about how your parents dealt with your behavior, and how you felt about their disciplinary techniques. They were not perfect, but neither was anyone else. Do not try to overcompensate for their shortcomings by trying to be perfect yourself, and by getting caught up in statements like "I'm not going to make the same mistakes my parents made."

All parents and all children make mistakes in their attempts to communicate and deal with one another and in trying to solve problems. Parents need to trust themselves and their instincts. Parents tend to have good intuition and knowledge of their own children. They often know more than they think they do, and they should not be afraid of making mistakes. Children are resilient and forgiving and usually learn and grow through their mistakes. Parents tend to be just as resilient and forgiving.

However, parents who "live for their children" are putting themselves in a very vulnerable position, setting themselves up for possible disappointment, frustration, and resentment. They are also being unfair to their family. Parents should not expect to receive all their personal fulfillment from their children or from the parenting role. Parents need other activities to fulfill their self-images, and other sources of love and nurturing. They need time to be adults and time for themselves—and a break from children and parenting responsibilities.

As a parent, you need to develop your own philosophy—one with which you feel comfortable—within a flexible and adaptable framework. Take into account your own expectations, parenting style, and temperament, and how each fits with each of your children and your partner, and their own unique preferences and temperaments. Your approach and philosophy will vary from child to child, mainly because of their own particular attributes. (See "Nature vs. Nurture," page 289.)

Along the way, remember that professional help is available if problems ever become too intense, exceed your own coping capabilities, interfere with activities of daily living, or cause secondary difficulties such as a decline in school performance, increased family stress, or serious emotional problems. A good start is by discussing the issue with your primary care pediatrician. Take comfort in the fact that in the majority of cases, children turn out well. Along the way, keep your sense of humor, trust your instincts, and seek help and advice early rather than late. While parenting is a great challenge, it can also be one of the most rewarding and enjoyable experiences of your life.

Development and Behavior

To help you better understand and deal with some of the challenging—yet often normal—behavior of childhood, you should understand the general developmental trends in school-age children. All children desire recognition, success, acceptance, approval, and unconditional love. Younger children seek them from their parents in particular. While older children (ages 10 and up) continue to have these same needs from a parent, they also increasingly desire recognition and acceptance from their peers and other adults.

At the same time, school-age children have a growing need for privacy, autonomy, and separation from their parents. To some degree they will gradually move away from the family—physically, socially, and emotionally. This is a normal part of growing up; a principal goal of raising children is to help them eventually navigate the world outside the family as an individual. For many parents, this evolving relationship can be painful, confusing, and the source of tension and behavioral conflicts.

As they grow up, children also experience a variety of challenges and transitions. Some are predictable and part of the life of every child; some will be unique to that child's experience. There are no certainties in life, but one certainty is that changes and transitions *will* occur, and kids need to develop resilience and adaptation skills. Children face transitions such as entering school, learning new subjects, changing classrooms and teachers, making new friends, trying new activities, and moving to new homes or cities. They might also include certain losses, like losing a pet or a friend. The illness or death of a family member or loss of a parent through divorce can be especially traumatic (for more on death, see Chapter 34; for more on divorce, see Chapter 30). These times of transition can be painful for school-age children, and parents need to provide the appropriate support.

Developmental Variations and How They Affect Behavior

You should be aware of two less typical patterns of behavior that your child might exhibit, which reflect variations in development to some extent, or an inability to cope with challenges. First, extremely well-behaved children may be overly anxious to please, and very needy of attention, love, and approval, or fearful of rejection. Sometimes these children are attempting to care for, defend, or protect a parent by being very well-behaved. They may be overly cautious, shy, overprotected, or feel insecure and incompetent. They also may have few friends and interests that are appropriate for their age.

Another worrisome pattern is characterized by self-defeating behavior, such as the child who deliberately does poorly in school, breaks rules, or continually places herself in no-win situations. These kinds of behavior may stem from the child's need to assert her own power, to gain control of her life, or to reject parental authority, pressure, or expectations. They also may arise from a fear of failure

Understanding the Stages of Development

A child's developmental stage is a key component of behavior. A parent's behavioral expectation must always be in alignment with what the child is capable of:

Children ages 5–7 years: The younger school-age child does well with concrete instructions. Similar to the preschool years, instead of saying "no" or "don't do that" repeatedly, tell your child what she *should* do. As an example, if your 6-year-old is fidgety in the grocery store checkout lane, instead of saying "Stop touching all the candy," say "Stand here next to me and keep your hands in your pockets." Better yet, have your child help you put the groceries on the checkout conveyer belt! An engaged child enjoys helping and is less likely to get into mischief.

Children ages 8–10 years: Now that they are a little older, children are able to sit patiently for longer periods and understand more complex social situations, yet still require guidance and good modeling of social skills by the adults in their world. Be mindful of screen time, as an excessive amount can hamper kids' ability to appropriately interact with others, maintain eye contact, etc. For more on media use, see page 315.

Children ages 11–12 years: On the cusp of the teen years, children continue to mature in their social skills and behavior. Your expectations for your sixth-grader should be on a different plane than the expectations you had for her in first grade. Be mindful of screen usage, as this can interfere with IRL ("in real life") relationships and communication.

Three Types of Behavior

Some parents find it helpful to consider three general kinds of behavior:

1. Some kinds of behavior are wanted and approved. They might include doing homework, being polite, and doing chores. These actions receive compliments freely and easily.

2. Other behavior is not sanctioned but is tolerated under certain conditions, such as during times of illness (of a parent or a child) or stress (a move, for instance, or the birth of a new sibling). These kinds of behavior might include not doing chores, regressive behavior (such as baby talk), or being excessively self-centered.

3. A third kind of behavior cannot and should not be tolerated or reinforced. This includes actions that are harmful to the physical, emotional, or social well-being of the child, the family members, or others. These unacceptable behaviors may be forbidden by law, ethics, religion, or social mores. They might include very aggressive or destructive behavior, overt racism or prejudice, stealing, truancy, smoking or substance abuse, school failure, or an intense sibling rivalry.

or rejection, or from a need to rationalize failure or to avoid the uncertainty of taking on a new task. Quite commonly, these children have low self-esteem and lack self-confidence. (See "Self-Esteem," page 139.) This latter group of children finds it emotionally safer and more comfortable to accept the certainty of failure rather than risk the uncertainty and anxiety of attempting success. They also often blame themselves when things go wrong or when they feel rejected or unloved. They tend to think in absolute and fatalistic ways, feeling that "now is forever"—that is, if their life circumstances are unpleasant now, they will be so forever.

These children also may have difficulty seeing the world from the perspective or viewpoint of others. For instance, a parent may be having her own difficulties and is thus unable to give much love or positive feedback at a particular time. Children take this change very personally and may respond by feeling rejected, or they may inappropriately blame themselves for their parent's disregard. If a child has persistent behavior issues and does not seem to be able to bounce back after a transition such as moving homes or the birth of a sibling, discuss the situation with your pediatrician.

Evaluating Behavioral Problems

Parents often have difficulty telling the difference between variations in typical behavior and true behavioral problems. The difference between typical (a term preferred to "normal") and atypical behavior is not always clear; usually it is a matter of degree or expectation. A fine line often divides typical from abnormal behavior, in part because what is typical depends upon the child's level of development, which can vary greatly among children of the same age. Development can be uneven, too, with a child's social development lagging behind his intellectual growth, or vice versa. In addition, typical behavior is in part determined by the context in which it occurs—that is, by the particular situation and time, as well as by the child's own particular family values and expectations, and cultural and social background. A family should worry if a child's behavioral issues are persistent and occur in multiple settings, such as both in the home and in the school environment.

Understanding your child's unique developmental progress is necessary in order to interpret, accept, or adapt his behavior, as well as your own. Remember, children have great individual variations of temperament, development, and behavior. In addition, your own parental responses are guided by whether you see the behavior as a problem. Frequently, parents overinterpret or overreact to a minor, normal, short-term change in behavior. At the other extreme, they may ignore or downplay a serious problem. They also may seek quick, simple answers to what are, in fact, complex problems. All of these responses may create difficulties or prolong the time for a resolution.

Behavior that parents tolerate, disregard, or consider reasonable differs from one family to the next. Some of these differences come from the parents' own upbringing; they may have had very strict or very permissive parents themselves, and their expectations of their children follow accordingly. Other behavior is considered a problem when parents feel that people are judging them for their child's behavior; this leads to an inconsistent response from the parents, who may tolerate behavior at home that they are embarrassed by in public.

The parents' own temperament, usual mood, and daily pressures will also influence how they interpret the child's behavior. Easygoing parents may accept a wider range of behavior as typical and be slower to label something a problem, while parents who are by nature more stern move more quickly to discipline their children. Depressed parents, or parents having marital or financial difficulties, are less likely to tolerate much latitude in their child's behavior. Parents usually differ from one another in their own backgrounds and personal preferences, resulting in differing parenting styles that will influence a child's behavior and development. Kids who are cared for by extended family members when the parent is working will realize that there is a separate set of rules in this environment that may or may not be consistent with the routine established by the parent.

When children's behavior is complex and challenging, some parents find reasons not to respond—for example, by rationalizing or fearing that responding will impact their relationship with their child. Our job as parents is to nurture the future adult that the child will evolve into; keeping this in mind will help us to make the right choices in how to proceed with issues. If you are worried about your child's behavior or development, or if you are uncertain as to how one affects the other, consult your pediatrician as early as possible, even if just to be reassured that your child's behavior and development are within a typical or normal range.

Your Child's Development and Behavior: Points to Keep in Mind

1. Even among children of the same age, there is a range of what is typical in the way they develop socially, emotionally, intellectually, and physically.

2. A child's maturity level may be different for the various qualities he is developing, including social skills, athletic abilities, and learning capabilities.

3. The variations described above may be permanent, forming a child's own unique profile; or they could be evolving and thus be subject to change.

4. The way a child develops can influence his behavior, and vice versa.

5. The particular parenting style of a mother and father, as well as the child's environment, will affect the child's behavior and development.

~ 14 ~

Communicating with Your Child

COMMUNICATION IS MORE than the exchange of information. When parents and children communicate, they are understanding one another and learning about the others' thoughts and feelings. While many people tend to think of communication primarily as talking, the most important part of it, and perhaps the most difficult to learn, is listening.

The initial communication between parent and child occurs in infancy. A baby's smile, seen by the parent, is an invitation to talk and smile back. At this stage, engaged parents are good observers. Soon, parent-child sharing of messages moves beyond nonverbal communication to sounds and spoken words. Not only do children and parents exchange information, but their communication quickly becomes a way of sharing emotions and giving support. Families that communicate well share a full range of experiences—the happy and good parts of life, and also sad times, problems, and their solutions.

To be effective communicators, you and your child must practice and develop skills together. Successful communication not only allows any topic or feeling to be shared but uses nonverbal as well as verbal ways of expressing oneself.

Life can get hectic, and especially during the school year, family schedules can be chaotic. During the course of a busy weekday, especially if one or both parents work outside the home, it can be a challenge to establish good communication on a regular basis with all family members. Add in after-school extracurriculars and sports, and the best conversations may actually happen in the car. Some busy families elect to make breakfast the main family meal each day, providing a designated time for all family members to come together to the same table. Alternatively, ensuring one-on-one time at bedtime with each of your children provides a regular safe space in which you and your child can communicate. Bedtime is often a time in which kids feel safe to share events of their day, feelings of concern, or whatever needs to be expressed. Whether there is a specific issue of importance to discuss or nothing in particular, regular face-to-face time keeps the conversations flowing. Regular time to talk about seemingly little aspects or minutiae of life opens the door for future, more meaningful conversations with your

Get the Conversation Started

All too often, the query "How was your day?" is answered with a single word: "Fine." Try some creative questions to really start a conversation and learn more about your child's world. Many families play "Apples and Onions" (alternatively, "Highs and Lows") at dinnertime to reconnect after a busy day. Everyone takes a turn and states their "apple," the best part of their day, and their "onion," their least favorite part of the day. These games typically lead into sharing more stories and effortless conversation.

Children ages 5–7 years:

What is your favorite thing to do at recess?

What was the funniest thing that happened today?

Children ages 8–10 years:

Tell me something about your day I don't know yet.

What was the nicest thing you did for someone else today?

Children ages 11–12 years:

What new thing did you learn today?

What would you rate your day today, on a scale of 1 to 10, and why?

child. There is an expression: when your kids are younger, be sure to listen to your kids about all the "little stuff," because as they grow older, then they will tell you the "big stuff"; to your kids, all along it has always been "big stuff."

As with other aspects of parenting, it is possible that you communicate with your own child in much the same way that your parents did with you. When it comes to communication, your parents were your models—and in many families, parents were not necessarily good models. Try to remember what was positive and negative about their ways of communicating, and see if you can find echoes of that in your own style. You may need to train yourself to break old habits of poor listening and damaging criticism. As you do, not only will you communicate better with your child, but you will also be providing a model of more positive behavior, so that she will become a better communicator.

Communication Beyond the Family

The communication skills your child learns will affect the way he interacts not only with you but also with the world at large. These skills will help your children to negotiate, solve problems, and learn from others. Communication can also be used to praise, punish, express feelings, and provide insights and understanding.

The *way* you communicate is part and parcel of *what* you communicate. Done well, communication is how you convey love, acceptance, respect, and approval to your child. Providing praise, for example, is not just saying words. It requires that you understand how your child thinks about himself and his behavior, and knowing when and in what way you can share with him your pride, so that he is best able to hear you and accept what you are trying to say. Successful communication is a two-way process. If you consistently communicate well with your child, he will know that you respect him and value him as an individual person. Not only will this nurture your relationship with him, but it can help him grow, develop, and live up to his capabilities. (See "Self-Esteem," page 139.)

Make an effort to communicate this acceptance through both words and actions. You can demonstrate your feelings in nonverbal ways through your body language, including your facial expressions, hugs, and gestures. Be positive and accepting in the way you talk with your child. Offer praise frequently, and be as specific as you can ("You worked hard on that difficult problem in your math homework tonight"). Let him know how much you appreciate him as he is: "I was so proud just watching you run in the track meet today" or "I love to watch you swim."

You can also demonstrate acceptance by *not* involving yourself in some of your child's activities. For example, if you just let him paint without giving him advice on what colors to mix together, this will convey the message that he is doing just fine on his own. In much the same way, you can listen quietly to your child at times, without interjecting your own thoughts and comments that might contradict or correct him.

The Components of Communication
Listening Skills

An essential part of the communication exchange with your child is receiving messages from her. They can be verbal messages (questions, requests) or nonverbal ones (actions or nonactions). Listening is a learned skill, and with effort you can become better at it. In the process you will be setting a good example for your children, and they will become better listeners too.

Active listening is the central component of communication. When you become an active listener, you are telling your child that the channels of communication are open. You are recognizing that your child has a need or a desire to share her feelings and thoughts, and that you are receptive.

There are several skills and techniques involved in active listening that will decrease the likelihood that you will be judgmental or critical. These skills allow you to help your child get in touch with what she is really feeling and thinking, analyze it, and put it in perspective so that problems do not seem bigger than they really are. It will also build a bond between you and your child, and make her more receptive to what is on your mind.

To become an active listener:

- Set aside time to listen. Block out distractions as much as possible. Put away phones and turn off screens. In order to hear and understand what your child has to say, you have to want to do so, and want to help your child with any concerns she has at the moment. Some parents and children find they can communicate best just before bedtime, or when driving together in the car. Make it a habit to put away phones and other electronics regularly to encourage face-to-face conversations, especially at mealtimes and in the hour before bedtime.

- Put aside your own thoughts and viewpoints, and place yourself in a frame of mind to receive information from your child. Give her your complete attention, and try to put yourself in her place so you can better understand what she is experiencing. You value her thoughts, and you are sensitive to her point of view.

- Listen to, summarize, and repeat back to your child the message you are hearing. This is called reflective listening. When appropriate, gently state what you think she may be trying to say. Do not just parrot what you hear, but go beneath the surface to what your child may be thinking and feeling. Remember, the spoken words may not be the true or complete message.

The underlying messages may include the feelings, fears, and concerns of your child. Assign these feelings a name or label ("It sounds to me as if you are scared [or angry, or happy]").

- Accept and show respect for what your child is expressing, even if it does not coincide with your own ideas and expectations. You can do this by paying attention to what your child is communicating, while not criticizing, judging, or interrupting.

- Create opportunities for your child to solve the problems she may be facing. Ask her, "What do you think?" to encourage problem-solving skills. As she grows, she should be taking increasing responsibility for identifying and troubleshooting life's inevitable bumps.

The process of active listening will help your child understand her feelings and be less afraid of the negative ones. It will build bridges and create warmth between you and your child. It will also help her solve her own problems and gain more control over her behavior and emotions. And if your child sees you as an active listener, this will make her more willing to listen to you and to others.

Talking Techniques

As you talk to your child, you should try to make it a positive dialogue, rather than impose judgment or place blame. That usually means choosing "I" messages rather than "you" messages, especially when attempting to change or encourage certain behavior.

"I" messages are statements like "I have trouble finding things on my desk when it hasn't been straightened up by the last person who used it" and "I need more quiet when I am trying to read." These "I" statements communicate the effect of a child's behavior or actions upon the parent. But they are less threatening to a child than "you" messages, even though they still convey an honest feeling or message. They also communicate how a child's behavior affects her parents and encourage her to take responsibility for straightening up Dad's desk or helping clean up the kitchen. They communicate trust—showing the parents' willingness to express their own feelings and their belief that their child will respond in a positive, responsible way.

By contrast, "you" messages are statements like "You should never do that" and "Why don't you pay attention?" These messages are more child-focused and are more likely to create a struggle between you and your child, and they might put your child on the defensive, encourage personal counterarguments, and discourage effective communication.

Even worse are "put-down" messages that judge or criticize an individual. They might involve name-calling, ridiculing, or embarrassing the child. These messages can have a serious negative impact on them and their self-esteem. If a child has made a poor choice, criticize the *action*, not the *individual*.

With "I" statements, however, children do get the message in a more positive light. They often say things like "I didn't realize that the noise I was making was bothering you" or "I'm glad you told me you were so tired. I'll help you with an extra chore or two." Children often readily assume more responsible roles if they are made aware of the situation and the feelings and needs of others, and are not put down in the process.

As you communicate with your child, be sensitive to your tone of voice. It should be consistent with your message. Do not let your emotions confuse the message you are trying to convey. Be as consistent as possible with all your children. You should have the same communication approach and style with every child, although the unique aspects of each relationship and each child's temperament may require some modifications.

Communication Dos and Don'ts

Here are some points to keep in mind as you communicate with your child:

- Listen actively.

- Make and keep eye contact.

- Look for the underlying messages in what your child is saying. What is the emotional tone or climate?

- Show respect for his ideas and feelings. Stay away from sarcasm, hurtful teasing, blaming, belittling, and fault-finding.

- Use "I" messages and avoid "you" messages and put-downs.

- Be honest.

- Be sensitive to the times and places that are good for talking. If your child comes home from school tired, give him some time to rest or have a snack before you communicate what may be on your mind. If you come home tired, take a rest yourself. Choose a quiet, private area in which to talk.

■ Praise or reward your child from time to time when he shows good listening habits. He may be motivated to listen more carefully and follow through on what you are saying if his efforts are recognized.

If you and your child have ongoing problems with communication, ask your pediatrician for guidance. She can evaluate your child for problems that may be interfering, such as language and attention deficits, or family issues. Your pediatrician might also be able to refer you and your child to a family counselor who can work out the difficulties and improve your communication skills.

Causes of Poor Communication

If you are having difficulty communicating with your child, see if the problem might lie in one of these areas.

■ Do one or both of you do a poor job of interpreting the messages of the other?

■ Is there a poor fit between the communication styles or temperaments of parent and child?

■ Do you have communication shortcomings that turn your child off? For instance, middle-years children sometimes complain that their parents nag, become judgmental, or do not make an effort to understand their child's point of view. If these sound like familiar complaints, you may have to work on your own listening and talking skills.

■ Does your child have attention-span problems that may make it difficult for her to concentrate long enough to receive a message? Is she too impulsive, and does she talk before she thinks? If you have these problems, there is a chance your child may have them too.

■ Does your child have a memory deficit, perhaps related to her attention problems, in which messages are received so superficially that they do not get placed into her memory? Or do memory problems prevent her from knowing what to say or finding the right phrase, or make her just a bit late with a response? Keep in mind that worry and sadness can interfere with attention and memory.

- Does your child have language or speech disabilities that make it hard for her to understand what you are saying, or to express her own ideas and thoughts in words? Does she have a speech problem that makes it difficult for her to communicate verbally?

- Do you or your child have other worries, stresses, or preoccupations that may be interfering with your communication?

- Are you choosing the right time and place to communicate?

- Does the pace or intensity of the conversation overwhelm your child's ability to listen and respond?

~ 15 ~

Your Child's Behavior and Discipline

EFFECTIVE DISCIPLINARY APPROACHES teach the child to regulate his or her own behavior, keep him or her from harm, and reinforce the behavior taught by the child's parents and caregivers. Good communication and reasonable expectations are the cornerstones to nurture a child's healthy development of appropriate behavior. Communication is a two-way street, and children who feel heard and respected respond well to praise and other forms of positive reinforcement. If there are aspects of a child's behavior that need modification, it is important to understand why the behavior occurs; this takes time, effort, consistency, and good communication. As with many parenting and child-rearing issues, there is no quick-fix solution.

It is often helpful to remember what circumstances were in place just before your child's unacceptable behavior occurred. Where were you and your child? What were each of you doing? Who else was present? What was said, by whom, and in what tone of voice? What would have been an acceptable response or action by your child? Carefully observing the situations in which the problem behavior occurs and talking about these questions with your child can be a way to begin understanding better why the behavior occurs. With that new knowledge, it may be easier to help your child behave in ways that you appreciate. Often a child has one specific behavior pattern that parents find especially troubling and challenging to handle. Sometimes a parent's initial interventions may not have been successful, and occasionally they may even have made things worse.

What can parents do? Consider, for example, a child who regularly bullies a younger sibling. This child needs to be told in a calm, matter-of-fact manner that while disagreements and arguing are normal and inevitable, bullying is not permitted. Explain and even demonstrate appropriate, alternative behavior (arguing, sharing, taking turns). She then needs to understand that if she is again aggressive toward her brother or sister, she will be given a warning and then will lose a privilege (no media use for a day; not having a friend over to visit). Praise the child when she is playing nicely with her sibling or if she exhibits one of the appropriate alternative behaviors you demonstrated. If the bullying behavior recurs, carry out the consequence or punishment that has been promised.

When it comes to discipline, learn from both your child's mistakes *and* yours. If you do not handle a situation well the first time, try not to worry about it. Think about what you could have done differently, and try to do it the next time. If you feel you have made a real mistake in the heat of the moment, wait to cool down, apologize to your child, and explain how you will handle the situation in the future. Be sure to keep your promise. This gives your child a good model of how to recover from mistakes. No one is perfect.

Positive Reinforcement

When you catch your child exhibiting good behavior, recognize it and reward it in a timely fashion. Positive reinforcement can include demonstrations of affection, words of praise, eye contact, points, or special experiences or activities. Give them specific feedback about specific behavior: for example, "I like the way you shared your toys with your friend."

Rewarding your child's good behavior on a consistent basis is more challenging than you might first imagine. It requires dedication and good observational skills on the part of the parent. However, without positive reinforcement, other efforts to change behavior, such as punishments, are unlikely to work. (See "Positive Reinforcement" on page 200.)

Demonstrating Good Behavior Yourself

Parents' actions are more powerful than their words. Parents should demonstrate the desired behavior. Help out someone else with a task. Do what you say, say what you mean, and mean what you say. Keep actions and words as consistent and positive as possible. When you slip up and don't match your behavior to your own expectations, show your child how you are able to learn from your mistakes and try to do better the next time. We *all* have room for improvement!

Special Time

Special time is regular, guaranteed, unconditional, and uninterrupted time that a parent spends with a child—a time when they interact without the parent being judgmental or directive. Children of all ages want parents to pay attention to them and to feel loved and capable. Special Time is one way to fill these needs. It is a "time in," an opportunity for parents and children to spend time together.

Special time should:

- Be given to each child every day regardless of behavior or mood.

- Be called "special time" or another favorite name so the child knows she is getting it.

- Be an activity of the child's choice (within reason). Older children may want to carry out an activity over several sessions.

- Engage the child in an interactive activity, although occasionally a passive activity such as watching nature or cooking videos together is okay.

- Be a time that is convenient for both parent and child; the time of day can vary.

- Be a consistent, fixed, short, and predetermined amount of time (to avoid boredom and fatigue) depending on age and interest (ten to thirty minutes). Measuring the time with a timer can avoid conflict when special time is over.

- Not be saved up and used to extend the time on the next day. Parents should avoid promising special time but not fulfilling that promise.

- Be without interruption of any kind, except true emergencies. This time should be special and recognizable for the child.

- Be adjusted. If the child is aggressive or disruptive during special time, she should receive a timeout or another consequence with the timer still running. If both parent and child want and agree to cancel or shorten special time, they should do so.

Punishment and consequences need to be *appropriate* and *proportional* to the behavior, as well as to the child's age and abilities. Positive reinforcement should occur in a timely fashion, linked with behaviors to be encouraged. Negative consequences similarly need to occur soon after the behavior in order to connect the behavior to the consequence and reduce the problem in the future. A child's punishment should be to lose a privilege that day or the next, not the next month. Effective disciplining and rewarding require that the parents be in agreement, or at least not interfere with or undermine each other's priorities or efforts.

Special One-on-One Time with Your Child: Suggestions by Age

Special time does not need to be a trip to an amusement park or shopping for material possessions. Children remember most the *experiences* they share with a parent.

Children ages 5–7 years: Younger kids love to help parents on simple errands around town. Your second-grader can help count apples to bag at the grocery store, and your first-grader would love to mail a package at the post office.

Children ages 8–10 years: How about a simple lunch just with you? This meal does not have to be fancy; having you all to himself is exciting enough. Put away electronic devices and other distractions, and just talk.

Children ages 11–12 years: As children begin to move toward adolescence, they may become less inclined to have spontaneous chats. Put away all electronic devices during meals to encourage conversation. A simple car ride across town without distractions may provide a great opportunity to talk.

For some behavior, parents can implement a behavior modification program. This approach involves modifying both the child's and the parent's behavior. It works by setting appropriate expectations for meeting goals and time guidelines, encouraging and rewarding positive behavior, and discouraging negative behavior.

Even if you plan to carry out a behavior modification program on your own, you might find it helpful to consult a pediatrician or another behavioral expert for advice and support.

Setting Expectations

Does your child fully understand what you expect of her? Some guidelines to keep in mind when setting and communicating expectations:

- Expectations need to be stated clearly and explicitly and must be achievable and reasonable.

- There needs to be an agreement between what parents expect and what the child expects.

- Parents and child should set short-term goals that can be achieved steadily in a step-by-step manner. These goals should ensure success that will satisfy both parents and child.

- Set goals for one to three behaviors at a time. Parents often have difficulty being consistent with positive reinforcement and punishment when they set too many goals at one time.

- Acknowledge the child's genuine efforts, even when she doesn't fully meet expectations. Small increments of change are important and more realistic.

- Be willing to reconsider and adjust when the child is consistently unable to meet parental expectations.

- Parents should set up realistic, short-term time schedules for implementing specific behavioral goals. For example: "By the end of two weeks, Sophia will be picking up her clothes four days a week" (as opposed to never picking up clothes).

- The family meeting provides an excellent forum for a discussion of appropriate expectations, methods of achieving goals, and rewards and punishments. To minimize misunderstandings, someone should write down the major points of agreement. (For more on family meetings, see page 268.)

Positive Reinforcement

Some children need more than recognition and praise. Positive reinforcement can be effective in middle childhood, especially once you have clearly defined the specific, positive behavior goals you expect. Here are some effective strategies:

■ Make or devise a chart that specifies the desired behavior, as well as the time of day or the situation in which it should be demonstrated. The calendar should cover an entire week or, for some behavior, a longer period. It should allow the activity or goal to be rated each day. Decide how many points an incidence of positive behavior will earn. In a summary column, total up the points. (Tokens, such as paper stars pasted on the calendar, tend to work better for early school-age children; points and contract systems work better for older children.) Small rewards may be given for a predetermined number of points at the end of each day or week, with larger rewards reserved for a longer period of time or a greater number of points. Keep this behavior chart in a conspicuous place so it can serve as a source of positive reinforcement and pride.

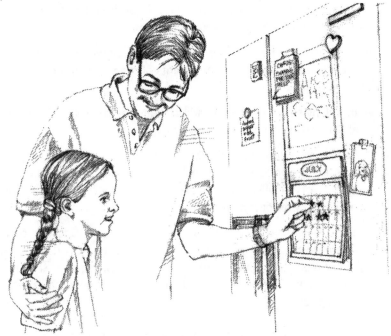

- Make a list of the rewards your child will receive for a particular number of points. Rewards should be meaningful to your child, and she should participate actively in their selection. Be very clear about how many points or days or weeks of changed behavior it takes to earn a reward.

- It is important to keep close daily track of your child's progress. Keep her enthusiasm level high by reinforcing behavior as frequently as possible.

- Keep in mind that the chart should be used as a measure of success. Avoid penalties and demerits that are humiliating, or that discourage your child from even trying. Use other forms of mild punishment, such as timeouts. (See page 204.)

Gradually, this program can be phased out as children internalize their behavior. At that time, children usually lose interest or forget to ask for their points.

Extinction, or "Active Ignoring"

This approach entails briefly removing all attention from the child. It is particularly effective with children who are whining, sulking, or pestering. As part of this technique, parents provide appropriate alternative behavior for the child to use; when he adopts this new behavior, he receives parental attention again. If you usually talk to your child when he is whining or pestering you and you decide to try "active ignoring," some children will initially whine more loudly or try to pester you more vigorously. If this happens, continue to actively ignore the child. Once your child learns that whining or pestering will not get you to respond, the frequency of whining and pestering will decrease.

A Behavior Contract

A contract between a parent and child can be an effective means for changing behavior, particularly for a child who is age 10 or older, an age when children want to negotiate, feel more empowered and independent, and show more initiative and responsibility.

First, identify a problem that is of mutual concern, even if it is only a potential or anticipated problem. Sometimes contracts are most effective before a particular conflict or problem arises. Do not impose the contract on your child. He should be a participant in developing it. Children have definite and firm thoughts, opinions, and feelings and are capable of quite sophisticated negotiations if given the opportunity.

First the child and then the parents should state their needs, desires, and responsibilities. Then both child and parents should state what they feel are appropriate rewards, punishments, or consequences of the child's behavior. Next, parents and child should negotiate an agreement, probably a compromise or middle ground on which they can all agree. Then the contract should be written. It should clearly describe what the child and parents intend to do—for example, what activities are permissible, and what actions will be taken if the contract is breached or is successfully completed. Make sure all the actions in the contract are things that you, as the parent, are willing and able to do.

Post the contract in a prominent place so that it can serve as a reminder, as a stimulus for positive reinforcement, and as a marker for achievement and progress. If your child feels embarrassed by having it displayed, put it in a private place. It should be reviewed (and modified as necessary) on a regular basis for a specified length of time, usually until goals are reached.

Consequences

Your child needs you to be her parent, not her friend. Hopefully, you do not feel the need for your child to like you every minute; parents who have this need are destined to be ineffective, frustrated, and disappointed. By setting appropriate behavioral boundaries, you will clarify who is in charge, create the values, and show the parental guidance children want and need. Children need to be loved and to love, and therefore it is necessary to focus on and punish only the specific *action*, not blame or criticize the child herself, which may make her feel ashamed, inept, and undeserving of love.

Consequences may be an important element in changing a child's behavior, but they are most effective when the child is also receiving frequent praise and positive reinforcement. There are various types of consequences, and the one chosen must fit the need or the deed. While children have a need for parental control, that control should vary for different ages or stages of development. The form of discipline that you use with a 6-year-old may not work or be appropriate when that child is 10.

Children may feel guilty about inappropriate behavior or failing to do the right thing, and a mild, appropriate punishment often relieves them of that guilt. Like everyone else, children have the right to make mistakes and learn from their experiences.

Natural Consequences

As a result of the child's own actions, certain consequences or reactions naturally happen, unless someone intervenes. For example, not taking care of a toy may result in that toy's becoming unusable. Going outside without mittens may result in cold hands. Running on an uneven surface may result in a fall. Remind your child about these consequences and use these opportunities to teach them.

Logical Consequences

In certain situations, a natural consequence may be too dangerous. For instance, bike riding in the street may result in an accident or injury. So instead, the parent provides a punishment or consequence that is logical and demonstrates a reasonable relationship between the behavior and the consequence. For example, tell your child that if she does not pick up her toys, you will put them away for the rest of the day. When you use this method, it is important that you mean what you say and that you follow through in a timely fashion. You should not yell or scream; be firm and respond in a calm way.

Withholding Privileges

Withholding privileges is when you tell your child that if she does not cooperate, she will have to give something up she likes. The penalty should be something meaningful to the child. For instance, when a child does not care for her pet, she may lose screen time privileges. These behavior penalties should be calmly discussed before they are instituted. Rules and expectations should be clear, preferably laid out in advance, and not presented as a surprise or as a threat. If you use this technique, never take away something your child truly needs, such as a meal. Choose something that your child values that is related to the misbehavior. For children younger than 6 or 7 years, withholding privileges works best if done right away. For example, if your child misbehaves in the morning, do not tell her she can't watch TV that evening. There is too much time in between, and she probably will not connect the behavior with the consequence. Be sure you can follow through on your promise. Kids are smart, and empty threats will not make an impact on your child's behavior.

Timeout

This is an effective way of dealing with a child's impulsive, aggressive, or hostile behavior, which often includes hitting, having tantrums, throwing toys, name-calling, interrupting, humiliating, or directly disobeying a request to stop a particular action. It is not useful for a child whose only recognizable problem behavior is excessive sulking, crying, or whining. For these children, it is important to discover the root or purpose of these behaviors, and "active ignoring" (described on page 201) may be helpful. Occasional crying or whining may be emotional expressions of frustration or disappointment that are normal and should be allowed.

A timeout removes the attention children are getting for their behavior and thus does not reinforce the behavior. It also allows parent and child alike to calm down, lessening the chances of angry encounters and power struggles. It permits parents to focus on the rational, specific behavior and allows interactions to return quickly to normal.

Here are some other points about timeouts to keep in mind:

- Discuss the use of timeouts—and the specific problem behavior that prompts them—with the child ahead of time so that expectations are clear. Changes in behavior may need to be measured so both of you will know if timeouts are succeeding.

- Employ timeouts immediately after the specific behavior occurs. Use the rule of "ten plus the child's age"—that is, send the child to a timeout within ten seconds of the bad behavior, with no more than ten words being said (calmly). Timeouts should last about one minute per year of life, up to age 11 or 12.

- Send the child to a preselected place that is safe, boring, and away from the busy areas of the house. Do not use a location the child finds entertaining or frightening. For each minute of protesting going to timeout, you can add a consequence.

- Use a portable timer (such as an egg timer; in this case it may be wise to use a timer other than the timer on a smartphone) that she can see or hear ring at the conclusion of the timeout. If the child leaves the timeout location before the time is up, place the child back in timeout without any discussion.

- Talk to your child after the timeout, when you are both calm, and explain the particular behavior that prompted the timeout. If the child is still angry or pouting, give her more time to calm down. Do not act angry or apologize, and do not ask her to apologize.

- Timeouts may require some practice before they become an effective means of modifying behavior.

- If a child repeatedly leaves timeout early, damages the room, or continues the same behavior repeatedly despite the timeouts, the family should seek professional help.

When Timeout Fails

When timeouts fail, consider the following:

- Are you using timeout correctly and consistently?

- Review the steps you took to begin the timeout. The two most common errors parents make in timeouts are talking too much and getting emotionally upset and angry.

- Are your expectations realistic for your child and for the specific situation?

- Are there changes you can make in the environment that would reduce conflict? For example, must your child do homework right before dinner, when she is hungry? Is your child tired or already irritable, and in need of some quiet time before she is ready to take on a task?

- Would your spouse or another adult be more effective in doing timeout with your child or working through a disagreement with her in a particular situation?

- Are there transitions, new stresses, or other changes in your lives that are affecting you or your child?

Physical Punishment

Parents may ask, "Should I spank my child?" Spanking may relieve a parent's frustration for the moment and extinguish the undesirable behavior for a brief time; however, it is the least effective way to discipline. It is harmful emotionally to both parent and child. Not only can it result in physical harm, but it teaches children that violence is an acceptable way to discipline or express anger. While stopping the behavior temporarily, it does not teach alternative acceptable behavior. It also interferes with the development of trust, a sense of security, and effective communication; spanking often becomes the method of communication. It also may cause emotional pain and resentment.

Many parents occasionally lose their patience and, in anger or fear, may spank their child. For instance, if a child runs out into the street, a parent may sweep the child up and, in a moment of anxiety for the child's well-being, spank her to emphasize the parent's sense of urgency or worry. In fact, it is the parent's expression of disapproval that is the effective deterrent in this situation, not the spanking act itself. For more on the AAP's stance on spanking, see the box opposite.

The Noncompliant Child

Younger children (ages 5 to 8) often flatly refuse to comply with a reasonable request. They may say "No!" or they may simply ignore their parents' requests.

Before imposing any punishment upon the noncompliant child, make sure you have given him a specific, clearly stated, reasonable request, such as "Jason, please pick up your toys and put them on the shelf before dinner." Broad statements like "Clean up your room" or "Straighten things up" are too vague and general. If the child is preoccupied, distracted, or seems confused by the order, call him by name, make eye contact at his height level, and state the command in as simple a form as possible, using a calm, rational voice. (See Chapter 14, "Communicating with Your Child.")

Wait ten seconds and maintain steady but not intimidating eye contact with the child. If he begins to obey your command, praise him right away for this specific behavior. If he does not obey, tell him you will give him another ten seconds and then he will need a timeout. In this case it is appropriate to use timeout as a threat or warning. If the child exceeds the ten-second limit, impose the timeout right away.

Once the timeout is over, return him to the task and repeat the command in a clear, calm, task-specific manner. If he refuses again, repeat the timeout, adding an extra minute or two. This may need to be repeated several more times. If timeouts seem not to be working, you will need to reconsider how they are being used (see "When Timeout Fails," page 205).

Behavior Problems Outside the Home

If your family is taking a trip, visiting relatives, or embarking on other adventures, sleep and eating routines will not be on a normal, routine schedule; these changes can impact a child's behavior. Positive reinforcement for good behavior continues

WHERE WE STAND

The American Academy of Pediatrics does not recommend spanking. Although many Americans were spanked as children, we now know that it has several side effects.

- Even though spanking may seem to "work" at first, it loses its impact after a while.

- Because most parents do not want to spank, they are less likely to be consistent.

- Spanking increases aggression and anger instead of teaching responsibility.

- Parents may intend to stay calm but often do not, and then regret their actions later.

- Spanking can lead to physical struggles and even grow to the point of harming the child.

It is true that many adults who were spanked as children may be well-adjusted and caring people today. However, research has shown that, when compared with children who are not spanked, children who are spanked are more likely to become adults who are depressed, use alcohol, have more anger, hit their own children, hit their spouses, and engage in crime and violence. These adult outcomes make sense because spanking teaches a child that causing others pain is okay if you're frustrated or want to maintain control—even with those you love. A child is not likely to see the difference between getting spanked by his parents and hitting a sibling or another child when he doesn't get what he wants.

to be the cornerstone of discipline. Ensure that meal patterns are appropriate and that sleep schedules are respected as best as possible. Anticipating problems and taking preventive steps and action are good ideas.

Decide upon the type of age-appropriate and achievable behavior you want your child to exhibit in these situations, and then discuss it with your child in terms of what you both expect ahead of time. If your child is having greater difficulty in some specific situations away from home, you might modify your expectations accordingly. Do not put your child in situations that you know she cannot handle. You may find that the most helpful approach is to use immediate praise when good behavior is exhibited. Be willing to utilize timeouts or behavior penalties in public situations. The use of logical consequences is also often helpful.

Some parents have difficulty implementing timeouts away from home, and in cases like this you and your child may have to take a timeout together. In a restaurant a timeout may require that you and your child sit in the car for a while. In a mall she might sit on a bench while you stand beside her; in a park or at the zoo, use a bench or a rock as a place for a timeout. If you are driving, stop the car at the side of the road and sit quietly until she settles down. For older children you might use a delayed timeout when you arrive at a hotel, a restaurant, or a rest stop.

Suggestions for Changing Behavior

1. Be selective about disciplining, and keep things in perspective. Prioritize your top behaviors that need attention and primarily focus on those. Any behavior that causes physical or emotional harm to a child or others is not acceptable and should be a top priority.

2. Avoid these common mistakes:

   - Parents may inadvertently punish good behavior or at least fail to reinforce good effort. For example, if their child improves her grades, raising them all to C's, they may ask, "Why didn't you get B's?"

   - They may reward or reinforce bad behavior. This often occurs when a child continually whines and pleads and then finally gets her way.

   - They may fail to reward good behavior. For instance, a child might wash the dishes and the parents fail to praise her for accomplishing this task.

   - They may fail to stop a child's bad behavior, or they may rationalize it. Perhaps one sibling is hurting another; the parent may respond, "Well, she deserved it," or "She needs to learn to fight back."

3. Reward and punish specific behavior. Focus on the behavior, and do not criticize the child as a person. Instead of "You are such a bad child," it is preferable to say "That was a rude thing to say."

4. Use punishments sparingly, and only when you are in control of your emotions. Physical punishment is harmful and not productive (see page 205).

5. Especially during times of transition (for example, parental job loss, or the death of a grandparent) children can experience physical and emotional stress, which can result in behavioral problems. Be sensitive to this issue, and do your best to support your child during these times.

6. Some children exhibit behavioral problems because they have not been taught or have not experienced appropriate alternative behavior. Teach them other, more acceptable ways to behave and respond ("If I shouldn't do this, then what should I do instead?").

7. Look beyond the concrete behavior the child is exhibiting, and understand what she might be trying to tell you. Recognize that sometimes a child's worrisome behavior is a signal that she or the family is in pain. She may be the designated family "messenger," and her behavior may be a cry for help for the entire family.

8. Recognize the state of your own emotions and your coping ability when confronting your child's behavior. That state may range from feeling competent and secure to feeling depressed and helpless. This recognition and self-awareness will help you decide if you need help or not.

9. Seek professional help when you think it is necessary. The earlier the intervention, the better the outcome. This professional input can also often provide reassurance that you are doing the right thing.

Dealing with Your Own Feelings

Your child's difficult behavior can no doubt make you feel angry, resentful, unappreciated, inadequate, or guilty. These negative emotions can interfere with effective parenting and good parent-child communication. You should not deny your feelings, and you need to learn to share them effectively and appropriately with another adult—a partner, friend, relative, or professional.

Here are some suggestions for dealing with your own emotions or anger:

- Accept the fact that children can make parents feel angry, resentful, and guilty at times.

- Recognize that parents are entitled to these feelings without feeling even more guilty, angry, inadequate, or full of shame.

- Express your feelings without attacking or condemning your child: for instance, "It hurts my feelings when I prepare dinner and nobody comes to the table."

Successful child-rearing is easier if parents also understand how and why they react to their child's behavior as they do. Often parents respond to their children in much the same way they were treated by their own parents. Even when parents intend to raise their children differently, ingrained patterns persist, and these patterns become especially evident during times of stress in the family. Alternatively, some parents deliberately respond at the other end of the parenting spectrum from what their own parents would have done a generation ago. Sometimes particular memories are so powerful that they influence how you interpret something your child has done. Perhaps your child's behavior reminds you of a childhood playmate or a relative about whom you have strong feelings. It is natural, but incorrect, to generalize from a single behavior and react as though your child will behave in other ways or suffer the consequences that you observed in your past. Understanding your own temperament and experiences can be a helpful tool in raising your child.

~ 16 ~

Managing Common Behavior Problems

Disobedience

As kids grow up, they will test adult guidelines and expectations. It is one way for children to learn about and discover their own selves, express their individuality, and achieve a sense of autonomy. As they stretch their independent wings and engage in minor conflicts with their parents, they discover the boundaries of their parents' rules and of their own self-control.

Sometimes, however, these conflicts are more than occasional disturbances and become a pattern for how parents and children interact. Misbehaving can have a variety of causes. At times, it is due to unreasonable parental expectations. It might be related to a child's difficult or intense temperament, or to school problems, family stress, or conflicts between his parents.

In some instances, these children have demonstrated a persistent pattern of disobedience throughout their development, beginning in their early years. They may resist authority by talking back to their parents and misbehaving. They may stubbornly tell their parents no when asked to do something. In many cases this behavior occurs only at home; at other times it is a pattern with all authority figures (teachers, sitters, grandparents) in all settings.

Other kids who are generally cooperative and agreeable may suddenly become disrespectful and disobedient during middle childhood. This is usually a sign that they are experiencing transitions or that new stressors are occurring. Transitions such as the start of a new school year can be a challenge; families may see an increase in the frequency of their child "acting out" at home during these periods. Their hostility is directed toward the nearest target (the people closest to them), and is a way of coping with and expressing the stress they feel.

Some children may have a lengthy history of being out of control and uncooperative. When children have been disobedient for longer periods—routinely talking back to and having outbursts aimed at their parents and others—there is often conflict and disorganization within the family as a whole. This might include harsh punishment and family relationship problems, including physical aggressiveness between family members. The children may reject their parents' authority, feeling that their mother and father disapprove not only of their behavior but of them as people. These children learn to be unhappy with themselves, and their self-esteem can suffer greatly. Gradually, if the family relationships continue to deteriorate, the children become even more angry, sad, hostile, and aggressive.

Many misbehaving children do not adequately communicate the reasons for their sadness or discomfort, or their parents are unable to understand what they are trying to express. This breakdown in communication sometimes occurs if the child is not receiving enough parental attention, perhaps because his parents are preoccupied with their own lives, careers, or even addicted to their own screens and other electronic devices. (See Chapter 14, "Communicating with Your Child.")

For some children, aggressive and disobedient behavior is a response to violence they see within the family. To children raised in abusive environments, aggressive behavior may seem like a reasonable way to deal with anger or frustration or may seem like the way to solve problems between people. Many families with disobedient children resort to physical abuse as one of their techniques for disciplining. But physical punishment leads to more aggressive behavior by the children, and a vicious cycle is established. Children raised in this type of setting are at much greater risk for lifelong problems with interpersonal relationships and authority. (See Chapter 51, "Child Abuse.")

As a parent, you need to keep in mind that middle childhood is a vulnerable period of life. Young school-age children are quite egocentric, thinking that all events that happen around them have something to do with themselves. For example, in families where there is marital conflict, children may misinterpret this problem, concluding that they themselves have been bad and have upset their parents. In the process their self-esteem may suffer, and they may be more prone to reacting inappropriately to the events around them.

What Parents Can Do

When you have a chronically disobedient child, examine the possible sources of his inner turmoil and rebelliousness. If this has been a persistent pattern that has continued into middle childhood, closely evaluate your own family situation: How much respect do your family members show for one another? Do they respect one another's privacy, ideas, and personal values? How does the family work out its conflicts? Are disagreements resolved through rational discussion, or do people regularly argue or resort to violence? What is your usual style of relating to your child, and what forms does discipline usually take? How much spanking and yelling is there? Do you and your child have very different personalities and ways of getting along in the world that cause friction between you? Is your child having trouble succeeding at school or developing friendships? Is the family undergoing some especially stressful times? Are you mindful of your own usage of electronic devices, and make it a point to put away electronic devices so that the family can come together to communicate?

If your child has only recently started to demonstrate disrespect and disobedience, tell him that you have noticed a difference in his behavior and that you sense he is unhappy or struggling. With his help, try to determine the specific cause of his frustration or upset. This is the first step toward helping him change his behavior. In response to your child's ongoing disobedience, you must examine your style and pattern of parenting, including your own background. How were you raised? How consistent are your disciplining efforts? Do you reward cooperation, or just react to disobedience and conflict? Are you and your partner supportive of each other? Do the two of you agree about discipline?

If you react to your child's talking back by exploding or losing your temper, he will respond with further disobedience and disrespect. By contrast, communication will improve when you remain calm, cooperative, and consistent. He will learn to be respectful if you are respectful toward him and others in the family. If he becomes disobedient and out of control, impose a timeout until he calms down and regains self-control. Have your child apologize for any disrespect he shows toward you or others.

When your child is obedient and respectful, compliment him for that behavior. Reward the behavior you are seeking, including cooperation and resolution of disagreements. These positive efforts will always be much more successful than punishment.

When to Seek Additional Help

For some disobedient children, you may need to obtain professional mental health treatment. Here are some situations where outside counseling may be necessary:

- If there is a persistent, long-standing pattern of disrespect of authority both at school and at home.

- If the patterns of disobedience continue in spite of your best efforts to encourage your child to communicate his negative feelings.

- If a child's disobedience or disrespect is accompanied by aggressiveness and destructiveness.

- If a child shows signs of generalized unhappiness—perhaps talking of feeling blue, unliked, friendless, or even suicidal. Any thoughts of self-harm are a medical emergency and must be brought to the attention of a professional immediately.

- If your family has developed a pattern of responding to disagreements with physical or emotional abuse.

- If you or your spouse or child uses alcohol or other drugs to feel better or cope with stress.

- If your reaction or your partner/spouse's reaction to the behavior is violent.

If relationships within your family show signs of difficulty and a lack of cooperation, then family therapy may be indicated. By dealing with and resolving these problems at a young age, you can minimize and even prevent more serious struggles that may emerge as your children reach adolescence. The key is early identification and treatment.

Aggressive Behavior

An aggressive child is one who hits, bites, bullies, demands, or destroys. Although aggression is a part of human nature, most people learn to manage and control their aggressive impulses and to channel them into appropriate and socially acceptable activities.

Aggression is particularly likely during times of threat, anger, rage, and frustration. As an important task of early childhood, kids must develop the ability to manage aggression and replace it with more socially acceptable responses. By the time most children reach school age, their coping skills are sophisticated enough, and their range of social skills broad enough, that they can generally remain calm and cooperative even in the face of stressful or unpleasant circumstances. Such appropriate behavior does not prevent them from competing and striving toward competence.

Some elementary school children have not yet mastered the skills needed to manage their aggression effectively. Their behavior ranges from hitting to throwing to having tantrums. By kindergarten, children whose aggressive behavior is a threat to their peers and to themselves should receive professional help. Other children, usually between ages 6 and 9, occasionally regress and exhibit aggressive behavior when they are under extreme stress. Typically, boys have more problems with aggression than girls; this is due to a combination of factors, from the innate aggressive tendencies of boys to the fact that our society continues to encourage and accept more aggressive behavior from boys. Excessive videogaming can lead to aggression as well.

Socially immature children may express their negative and hostile feelings in destructive ways. They may have bouts of aggression that damage property (such as their own toys or the property of others), throw objects, turn over furniture, break lamps, or kick walls. These behaviors are usually triggered by frustration, anger, or humiliation. Some children who have failed to receive sufficient positive attention for their more socially desirable behavior develop a habit of resorting to negative behaviors to get parental attention.

Sometimes these children exhibit even more serious antisocial behavior—so-called conduct disorders—such as setting fires, being cruel to animals, hurting other people (physically or emotionally), or lying habitually. As kids grow older, this pattern may evolve to include vandalism and truancy and is often associated with alcohol and other drug abuse. These kinds of worrisome behaviors occur only rarely in some children, but they have serious implications for later functioning, and their presence should prompt an evaluation by a specialist in child behavior and emotional problems.

What Causes Aggressive Behavior?

As with any kind of behavioral difficulties, there are many complicated reasons for aggressive or destructive behavior. Some children, because of inherited personality traits, are more predisposed to aggression. Children with intense temperaments experience more problems with aggression. (See page 131 for a more complete discussion of temperament.) Others who are very active, strong-willed, or impulsive have more trouble learning to control their aggression.

Your child's environment—family, school, and peers—can shape his responses to stressful situations and greatly determine the way he handles anger and displays aggressive behavior. Imitation is one of the most powerful influences upon a child's development, and children learn to handle themselves by watching and copying how adults and other children control their own aggressive impulses. If you and your spouse act aggressively toward your children, toward each other, or toward others with whom you come into contact, or if you permit fighting and destructiveness by your children, they will learn that this behavior is acceptable.

Sometimes a child is aggressive because he has failed to learn self-control. Children develop self-control by learning from their parents what are acceptable limits to their aggressive impulses. If parents are permissive, have set no limits, and have let their kids do whatever they wish, a child may have issues with self-control.

Sometimes parents use inappropriate means—physical punishment, for example—when responding to their children's negative behavior. These parents may erroneously believe that a spanking, or a similarly aggressive and abusive response, is a proper reaction when a child fights or misbehaves. However, physical punishment will not help a child learn to control his negative emotions or hostile behavior; rather, it teaches him to be aggressive when he is angry. Physical punishment is rarely if ever effective. Rather, it usually occurs when a parent is unable to manage his or her own anger or frustration effectively and thus inappropriately resorts to aggression. When a child's aggressive behavior is met with more aggressive behavior from a parent, things usually get worse, not better (see "Where We Stand," page 207.)

Aggressive behavior can have other causes too. Children may become more aggressive and destructive when they feel overwhelmed by stress, including family problems like marital discord, divorce, unemployment, financial distress, parental illness, or a move to a new city. When a child has been abused physically, sexually, or emotionally, or has been neglected, his aggression may be a cry for help. Some children may lash out in frustration or anger if they feel they have not lived up to their parents' expectations. Sometimes, although rarely, aggressive behavior has its roots in medical problems such as head injuries or hyperactivity.

Child psychiatrists, when trying to deal with aggressive behavior, believe it is important to distinguish between children who have never learned to control their aggressiveness and those who previously had good self-control but have since regressed. The first situation is more difficult to treat, since the child has never developed any control over his aggression and so must learn new skills. In the second circumstance, the child's symptoms may be a sign of a new and powerful stress in his life. Treatment for these children is aimed at helping the child deal with the stress that may be provoking his aggressive behavior.

Aggressiveness with Peers

When a child exhibits aggressive behavior at home—perhaps throwing toys or screaming at siblings—his parents can intervene immediately and help the child learn better self-control. If the child has learned how to manage this aggression at home, he is better prepared to deal with the inevitable conflicts that arise with peers. Many children, however, still struggle with their aggressiveness upon entering school. Parents find the situation more disturbing and more difficult to manage if their child is fighting or intimidating *other* children, either at school or on the playground.

In some families, however, parents encourage fighting as a way for a child to assert his manhood, settle conflicts, and "stand up for himself." This pattern of aggressive behavior and response becomes self-perpetuating and can lead to lifelong problems with relationships and social rules. Parents need to teach their children socially appropriate ways to manage themselves in conflicts with peers.

Aggressive behavior and bullying can occur online as well; for more on this, see page 322.

What Parents Can Do

When your child is consistently fighting with or bullying his peers, or exhibiting destructive behavior, he should be evaluated by a mental health professional. Meanwhile, here are some strategies you should consider:

1. Express disappointment in the specific behavior you disapprove of, without implying that your child himself is bad. Discuss in depth the situation that occurred, exploring the reasons why he is bullying and other options for action with your child.

2. Help your kids see how it might feel to be bullied by others. The Golden Rule is an excellent rule for all of us: treat others the way you wish to be treated.

3. Help him understand that no one likes a bully. Explain how bullies develop reputations that can result in a loss of friends and difficulty making new ones. Tell him that the sooner he alters his behavior, the better, since long-standing reputations are hard to change.

4. Online bullying is unacceptable and should result in the loss of technology privileges and closer parental supervision. For more on media use, see page 315.

5. For a child prone to fighting, insist that he learn to resolve conflicts without physical force. As a starting point, do not permit conflicts at home to be settled by physical means. Teach all of your children to use their words instead to resolve differences. Work with them so that instead of acting out, they stop, consider what they are feeling, and then turn their feelings into words. Take a breather if need be to defuse the situation. Reward them for settling conflicts without fighting.

6. Do not become intimidated by your child's anger, nor avoid conflicts that may arise with him. Instead, take charge of these situations in a consistent way, aimed at helping him control his aggression.

7. Establish effective ways of promoting self-control in your child at home. Timeouts work for most children—telling them they must stay in a designated location, preferably not their bedroom, until they get themselves back under control. This will provide them with a safe environment as they learn to manage themselves better.

8. If any destruction of property has occurred, your child should be responsible for correcting the situation. For example, if he destroys a sibling's or a neighbor's toys, he might need to increase the number of chores he does around the house, earning money to replace what he has broken. He should also apologize to the other party.

9. Reward your child (with praise or star charts, for example) as he learns to express his anger and frustration in more acceptable ways. Positive reinforcement will be the most important way to change his behavior.

10. Explore whether your child's school offers courses in conflict resolution, or if such opportunities exist with other community organizations. The school social worker is a good contact person for this question.

11. Develop an attitude of hopeful expectation that your child can learn to manage his own frustration and anger. If you are doubtful that he can control himself, look within yourself to determine why. Remember, parental attitudes help shape your child's behavior.

12. Examine your family's style of expressing anger and resolving conflict. If the family exhibits a style similar to that of your child with his peers, the key to helping your child rests with changing these family patterns.

When to Seek Additional Help

If your own efforts at assisting your child or family to control aggressive behavior are not working or seem unlikely to do so, ask your pediatrician for a referral to a mental health professional or behavioral pediatrician who can help. The earlier these professional interventions occur, the greater the likelihood of success.

Temper Tantrums

Occasional tantrums are quite normal for children from ages 1 to 4, and these outbursts subside for most children by the time they enter school. Normal psychological development tends to provide most children with better self-control and make them considerably more cooperative by school age. Even when they are upset, school-age children generally can express their frustration and anger in words, with reasonable control.

For some children, however, temper tantrums persist into the school years and occur with regularity. Their parents ask why the child has not yet developed more socially appropriate ways of communicating anger and frustration. To answer this question, pediatricians often recommend that parents first evaluate what kind of role models they have been—how they themselves respond to anger, and how they have taught their children to react. When parents are prone to exaggerated, disruptive outbursts and fits of temper, their children often are too. When parents are explosive—having tantrums of their own in their relationships with others—that is the type of behavior they are teaching to their children.

Other factors can come into play as well. Some parents may have unrealistic expectations of their children's behavior. Asking children to sit quietly for long periods of time, to do tasks beyond their physical or developmental abilities, or to accept responsibilities or parents' decisions that are clearly unfair are examples of situations that will be frustrating and can trigger an outburst. Expectations should be kept age-appropriate and developmentally appropriate for the child.

Because of their innate temperament, some children have a lower threshold for feeling frustrated and a greater tendency toward intense negative expressions of displeasure. (See "Temperament," page 131.) Children with strong wills have more difficulty managing their anger and negative emotions and a harder time learning self-control. However, with proper guidance and support, they can learn to suppress their more explosive behavior.

In some situations, a tantrum is a way for a child to get attention from her parents, who respond to their kids only when she is demanding. In the eyes of a child, any attention at all, even negative attention, is better than no attention. When a family is under continual stress and strain—perhaps because of financial troubles, alcoholism, marital conflict, poverty, physical or sexual abuse, or moving to a new town far away from friends and family—children may react with more frequent temper tantrums.

Sometimes school-age children have gone tantrum-free for several years only to develop tantrums later on. If this sounds like your child, consider whether these symptoms are being provoked by a new, overwhelming stress occurring at school, at home, or in the neighborhood. As a parent, consider the sources of this stress and try to help your child transition more effectively.

What Parents Can Do

Many parents have difficulty deciding how to respond to a child's temper tantrums. Here are some suggestions:

- Recognize that some children have a harder time expressing their frustrations, or have more difficulties to overcome.

- Avoid having unrealistic expectations of your child. Keep expectations age-appropriate and developmentally appropriate for your individual child.

- When your child is out of control, ignore the temper tantrum so as not to create a "reward" for her inappropriate behavior. She may be trying to get attention, and if so, *any* response, positive or negative, can reinforce her outbursts. Ignoring the tantrum provides the child with an opportunity to learn self-control.

Sometimes, however, you may be unable to ignore her tantrums, perhaps because she comes running after you, is destroying toys or hitting a sibling, or is a danger to herself. In cases like these, insist that she go to another room for a time-out away from others until she can bring herself under control. Physically escorting her to a designated timeout area, preferably not her bedroom, may be necessary. (See Chapter 15, "Your Child's Behavior and Discipline.")

In general, parents should remain as calm as possible and avoid becoming involved in the tantrum by controlling their own frustration and anger. They should also avoid physical confrontations, which can escalate to frightening levels and even end up with someone, usually the child, getting hurt.

After your child and you have calmed down, sit and talk with her about what provoked the outburst. Emphasize the importance of communicating her negative feelings through words, not actions, and discuss more positive ways to respond. You might find a reward system useful, offering praise when your child solves conflicts without throwing a tantrum.

When to Seek Additional Help

Your pediatrician usually can guide and support you through the resolution of problem behavior. In certain cases, some middle-years children can benefit from consultation with a child psychiatrist or psychologist because of their temper tantrums. You should consider seeking professional help in any of the following situations:

- The tantrums become a pattern whenever your child feels frustrated or angry.

- The tantrums occur frequently, such as several times a day.

- Your child has tantrums outside the home, perhaps at school.

- The tantrums result in destruction of property or physical harm to your child or others.

- The tantrums are becoming unbearable for the parents and are interfering with a normal, happy parent-child relationship.

In any of these situations, address the problem at once. Temper tantrums do not necessarily go away on their own. You need to try to understand what your child is experiencing—and perhaps change your own response to the outbursts—so that she can learn to control her negative feelings effectively, with your guidance.

If these symptoms continue into adolescence, they can become even more of a concern. With the added pressures of the teenage years, and the expanded repertoire of behavior available to teenagers along with their increased physical size, tantrums can become increasingly worrisome, dangerous, and difficult to manage.

Stealing

Much to their dismay, parents often discover that during the middle years of childhood their kids might steal, lie, or cheat. These episodes might be an isolated circumstance, or part of a larger trend. This behavior can be a surprise to parents who often respond with embarrassment or anger. However, these childhood behaviors, although unacceptable, are a normal part of the developmental process of young children. They are a part of learning about themselves and the world around them and developing their personal morals, ethics, and conscience.

From ages 6 to 12, children are increasingly psychologically and physically independent from their parents. They are more heavily involved with school and their peers and are developing a new sense of themselves at a greater distance from the watchful guidance of their parents. They are facing new challenges to maintain friendships, compete with peers, and meet the demands of teachers and fellow students. Thus, at a time when pressures can be great, and when they have not yet fully adapted to the rules of society, they may find dishonesty to be an expedient way of coping.

Before age 6, children may not have a clear sense of what belongs to them and what does not. Three- and 4-year-old children take toys that others might be playing with, simply because they want them. If that behavior is not responded to by parents or others, it may progress to taking toys that belong to other children when they are not looking. The behavior clearly then becomes stealing. After age 6, children are much more likely to be aware that they are doing something wrong when they take things they know are not theirs. Commonly, the first stealing incident occurs at about age 7.

In the preschool and kindergarten years, children are occupied with learning about social order and, especially, the significant relationships within the family; these are times of family intimacy. However, by the time children reach ages 6 to 8, they have developed some sense of independence from their family and have a heightened feeling of being in charge of themselves. As they enter school and their peer relationships become more important, they have an increased desire to belong, to show off, and to compete with others. At the same time, children develop feelings of possessiveness and an interest in their belongings and collections, their rooms, and their activities at home. All these needs intensify at about 7 years old.

Children of this age often take an object from a teacher, from a friend's home, or from the friend himself. Perhaps they feel deprived—they want something for themselves that they do not have—and they impulsively take it. Or they may steal money from home to share with their friends at school or to buy candy for themselves and their friends. Children may also secretly take something from a store.

Stealing may fill an emotional void. Stealing may also be a way of responding to feeling deprived, or a way of getting something a child wants that he feels would otherwise be unavailable. Sometimes stealing is an expression of anger or hostility. Child psychiatrists theorize that children who have stolen feel some sense of deprivation, envy, anxiety, or resentment. There is another peak incidence of stealing at about age 13. This, too, is a period of rapid change—physically, psychologically, and socially—and stealing may again become a way to impress friends. Peer (and gang) pressure can also sometimes coerce children into acts such as stealing. In particular, dares can lead to stealing.

Sometimes stealing occurs repeatedly or is associated with a multitude of other behavioral or emotional difficulties. In this context, stealing is much more troubling and indicates that the child is in need of professional help.

What Parents Can Do

When you discover that your child has stolen something, it is important that your child understand that stealing is wrong. You may remember how ashamed you yourself felt if you were ever caught stealing as a child. Your child needs to learn the same lessons, although most experts say that intensely embarrassing or ridiculing him is not beneficial. Simple explanations are best.

In most cases it is probably best not to ask your child directly whether or why he has stolen something; this will only tend to prompt a series of lies as he tries to save face. Rather, be straightforward and acknowledge that you know the theft has occurred. It is important to establish some restitution, a way to make things right. Your child needs to return the object that was taken, either to the store, his friend, or the school. You might wish to accompany him and encourage him to apologize, stating that he will never do it again.

Afterward, have a talk with your child. Rather than implying that he is a bad person, try to discover the underlying reasons for the stealing. Explain that while children understandably want things, it is wrong to take the possessions of others. In most situations, if the stealing incident is handled directly and immediately, it will not recur and your child will learn from it.

When an older child approaching or entering adolescence has stolen, again you should offer him an opportunity to explore and discuss his behavior, especially addressing stresses he is experiencing. In some situations, you may respond to stealing episodes with a serious discussion about peer pressure and its influence upon his behavior. At this age, stealing is often indicative of a personal or social difficulty and may require professional help. You should seek outside assistance through a child psychologist or mental health worker in the following situations:

- Your child repeatedly steals from home or school, from parents, or from others.

- Your child is "buying" his peer relationships by stealing.

Lying

Children younger than age 6 often have difficulty distinguishing between reality and fantasy. Hence, for them there is often an uncertain boundary between truth and fiction. After about age 6, however, children clearly can differentiate truth from fantasy. As a result, when a child lies she knows she is being deceitful.

Many pressures can cause a child to lie. Most frequently, when a child has been brought up in a loving and responsible home, she will first lie when she is confronted with having done something wrong and feels afraid of disappointing her parents or being punished by them. Already feeling guilty, she will try to protect herself from what she thinks will be harsh discipline. In many cases, parents of children who lie have high standards of behavior and expectations. These children know right from wrong, and when they are in what they view as a difficult situation, they lie in an attempt to save face.

Context is important. Sometimes children lie when they are under significant stress to meet impossible demands. Thus, children who are struggling at school and cannot keep up with their studies may feel overwhelmed and lie about having completed all their homework. Because of circumstances like these, lying should be interpreted in relation to the surrounding events.

Remember, *lying shows that a child is aware that she has done something wrong*. By attempting to protect herself from parental disappointment and disapproval, she is demonstrating that her conscience is working. Parents who overreact and become extremely negative may push their child into a position of feeling that she needs to lie again and again to protect herself.

Children in middle childhood also might become confused in a home where there is a double standard about lying—that is, where she is forbidden to lie but her parents sometimes tell "white lies," distorting the truth for their own convenience. When a child has always been told to be honest, witnessing a parent stretching the truth on the phone or telling white lies to neighbors can be confusing. Children often have a hard time differentiating among the subtleties in situations like these. "The Boy Who Cried Wolf" is a good story to look at together that examines the consequences when one's words cannot be trusted.

What Parents Can Do

If you discover that your child has lied, let her know immediately that you are aware she is not telling the truth. Harsh punishment is usually not very effective. Instead, make the following points with both your words and your behavior:

- "I want you to tell me only the truth, and I will always tell you the truth, so that we can always believe each other."

- "You will get in much less trouble if you tell the truth instead of lying."

Also, remember that your own actions and your own style of telling the truth are probably the most important ways you can teach your child the importance of honesty.

When to Seek Additional Help

A child who has a history of chronic lying should be seen by a counselor or mental health professional. Chronic liars often have had difficulty establishing a true conscience that can clearly differentiate between right and wrong. These children also may be crying out for help because of disturbances in their family life or outside the home.

Cheating

In our culture, with few exceptions, competitiveness is commonplace and in fact is rewarded. Children learn that losing is bad, and especially in the early school years, they have a strong wish to do well. A great parenting strategy to buffer against cheating is to praise a child's *effort* rather than the *outcome*. This sends a message to the child that the process and the work put into a project is more important than the results themselves.

As children play games with one another, cheating will frequently occur. In the early years there is a lot of breaking of rules and conflicts in these peer struggles. Watch how children play board games or card games, and you will recognize the competitiveness and social learning taking place and sometimes digressing into cheating. As children become older and approach adolescence, however, this behavior is much less tolerated by peers, and thus some children become labeled as cheaters. A sense of fairness has a higher value in these older peer relationships.

If you are confronted with a situation where your child has cheated, you need to consider many factors, including the degree of pressure that he is under to win or do well, and his own background regarding competition. Children tend to cheat, or set their own rules, when they are engaged in games or schoolwork that is too complex for them to handle. If you or others in his life expect him always to perform exceedingly well, then cheating can become almost a self-defense mechanism under the strain of this pressure. He may feel he has no other outlet than to cheat as a means of achieving success. For this child, the end becomes much more important than the process.

Consider the example that your family environment is providing for your child. If you or your spouse cheat from time to time—perhaps declining to return too much change given to you at the grocery store, or maybe even talking about fudging on your income taxes—those are the moral values you are teaching. Be sensitive to the examples you set; you can be an important role model for the prevention of cheating. To a large degree, your child's willingness to cheat is related to the values with which he is being raised.

What Parents Can Do

For a child in the middle years, parents need to identify and deal with any cheating episodes in order to teach him right from wrong. For example, if he is caught cheating at school—a common phenomenon—sit down with him and discuss the seriousness of this infraction. Talk about the kinds of stresses and pressures he may be feeling, including your own expectations for success. Excessive punishment for these misdeeds is rarely helpful.

Playing family games where chance is involved can teach children to compete with one another without cheating. These games can guide your child toward appropriate conduct and healthy competition.

When to Seek Additional Help

A child who has a chronic cheating problem, or who gets so labeled at school, may need further help. Often cheating is a symptom of an internal emotional struggle or peer problems that should be addressed. You can find assistance from your pediatrician or a mental health counselor.

Swearing

Swearing—the use of profanity or "dirty" words—is almost a developmentally normal behavior for children during middle childhood and early adolescence. For these children, swearing is often a sign of being worldly wise and unafraid to be a little "bad." Profanity is used to impress friends and can become a part of peer relationships. Quite frequently, younger children do not know the meanings of the words they are using, but they will say them anyway simply because they have heard others use them.

Fortunately, this phenomenon of cursing seems to lose its attraction and abate as children become more mature. Until then, however, kids often delight in shocking their parents with the swear words they have learned away from home. Bear in mind that parents who swear in the home are teaching their children to do the same and should not be surprised when their kids copy their behavior.

At times swearing is part of a larger behavior problem including other personal and social difficulties. These kids may be more prone to swear and rage at other people—a different phenomenon than using a few swear words during times of frustration. Profanity directed at another individual should never be tolerated.

What Parents Can Do

Here are some suggestions to help you manage the problem of swearing:

- If you feel it is appropriate, establish a rule that "no swearing will take place in our home." Do not under any circumstances tolerate swearing that is aimed at someone in anger. If this occurs, a child may be sent immediately to her room for a timeout.

- Minor swearing in frustration can be a natural human behavior. Although perhaps inappropriate, it is commonplace in some families. If that is your own personal style, you will find it hard to teach your child something different.

- When your child swears, do not overreact with your own outbursts. We parents are human; if you slip up and swear yourself, own up to that, admit that it was inappropriate, and tell your child you are working on fixing this behavior in yourself.

- On occasion, you may feel that your child is using profanity in an attempt to provoke a response from you. In these instances, ignoring her may be the most effective strategy.

- Reward your child for expressing her frustration appropriately without swearing. Star charts and money are helpful approaches. For example, use a jar of nickels that she can earn at the end of two weeks; for each day that she doesn't swear during this time, two additional nickels will be placed in the jar; but each time she swears, nickels will be removed. Your child will catch on quickly. If you have a swearing habit yourself, you should join in with your child with your own jar.

When to Seek Additional Help

In and of itself, swearing is not a sign of emotional disturbance. However, if there are other problems—chronic lying, chronic stealing, or difficulty with peers—then swearing may be just another symptom of a psychological or social disturbance. In this situation, talk to your pediatrician about counseling—either individual or family therapy.

Running Away from Home

"Running away" has been glorified in the media as if it were an adventurous tradition of seeking a better life. The reality is much more sobering. In most cases, children are not running *toward* a specific new situation but rather are running *away* from existing problems—and thus may be issuing a cry for help.

Not only do runaways leave anxious and worried parents behind, but they may enter a world of gangs, drugs, prostitution, malnutrition, and truancy. They are quite vulnerable and at a much higher risk of becoming involved in early sexual behavior, sexual exploitation, or alcohol and other drug use. They may end up living on the street, in a homeless shelter, or in jail.

Most children who run away and are reported to the police as missing are between ages 13 and 15. However, some younger children threaten to, or actually do, leave home. Lonely children are at risk for developing inappropriate relationships online. This is yet another reason to monitor and be aware of your child's online activities. Kids may have online conversations with others who may encourage the child to run away or even provide a plan or place to go if the child does run away. For more on media safety, see page 315.

When a child runs away, there has often been a crisis in the family. The child himself may be in some sort of trouble that he feels he cannot face for fear of severe punishment. Or there may be family stresses that can range from marital difficulties to alcohol-related problems to physical or sexual abuse—situations from which the child feels an overwhelming need to escape. Sometimes children are made to feel that they are a burden for their parents or the cause of the family's difficulties; children then run away to relieve their families, as well as to punish them.

On the other hand, some children run simply because they are looking for a good time. Impulsively and without planning, they will flee with a friend or two, seeking the thrill of life on the run. Often these children have already experienced various difficulties, perhaps conduct problems or substance abuse.

Some children who run are loners, without many friends and with little support at home. Rather than running away with a friend, these loners often flee by themselves. They are driven by a feeling that there must be a better world out there.

If Your Child Threatens to Run Away

As a part of normal development, some children will talk of running away when they face conflicts with parents. If your child threatens to leave home, talk with him. Ask about any stresses and problems he may be experiencing. At the same time, be aware that these threats can sometimes be little more than a child's attempt to manipulate you. Perhaps he is trying to avoid chores or responsibilities. Or maybe he is attempting to relieve guilt feelings over having fought with you or having done something for which he is ashamed. If a situation has occurred in which the child and parents have been at odds, the child may feel that the only resolution is to hurt his parent by threatening to run away. Be aware of your own vulnerability to your child's manipulation, and remain in control of your emotions. In cases like these, the child will rarely leave home, but his threats should be heard as a last-ditch effort, one designed to turn the tide in the parent-child conflict, changing his parents' attitudes in a direction more sympathetic to his own.

If a child says he is going to run away, his parents should use their judgment on how to react. If he has never left home before, the threat may not be a serious one. Sometimes parents become very upset by their child's threats and try to talk him out of running away. However, arguments aimed at changing the child's mind are usually counterproductive. In effect, they acknowledge that the child is in control, something few children actually want. In addition, by focusing on the threat to leave, parents are ignoring the larger problem of the underlying issues that have caused the situation.

If your child lives in a two-household family and threatens to go live with his other parent, you might feel insecure about how you are faring as a parent or guilty over something you think you might have handled wrong. It is possible that your child may be trying to manipulate your thoughts and behavior. At some time, most children of separated parents either threaten or request to live with the noncustodial parent. Try to understand your child's actions and appreciate his point of view. Talk over the situation with him, but let him know that until he's much older, the decision about where he will live remains his parents' decision. Do not make a hasty decision regarding living with the other parent, particularly during times of conflict. Consider these important decisions calmly and carefully. For your own peace of mind, remember that most of these conflicts eventually resolve themselves.

If Your Child Runs Away

What should you do if your middle-years child does actually run away? Of course, your most immediate efforts should be directed toward locating your child and returning him home. Runaway children often will wind up spending the night at a friend's or a relative's home, so check there first. Then enlist the aid of the police, school, friends, and family. Be prepared to tell the police the last time and place you saw your child, who he was with, and what he was wearing. Having a child missing is a frightening experience, so turn to a spouse, a friend, or a relative to help and support you through the ordeal.

Some runaways use a runaway hotline to contact their parents before the more stressful step of a face-to-face reunion (such as the National Runaway Safeline at 800-RUNAWAY). After your child is found or returns, you need to seek out the reasons that led him to run away. What kinds of stresses has he been feeling at home or in school? What was making him frightened or unhappy? What kinds of negative peer pressure or threats has he had difficulty handling? The answers to these questions must be confronted and resolved, or running away may recur. When these issues are discussed and acted upon, you and your child may see some beneficial effects from his decision to run away, even if the overall experience was negative.

When to Seek Additional Help

If your child has threatened to run away but never has done so, he may not require outside help. However, if these threats have become a pattern and an ongoing way in which he deals with conflicts, then he, and possibly the entire family, may benefit from an evaluation. Your pediatrician can refer you to the most appropriate type of professional help—whether from a child psychiatrist or psychologist, a behavioral pediatrician, or a social worker. This therapy should attempt to help you and your child understand and resolve the misunderstandings and conflicts in your household. The reasons for running away are often complex, and need to be fully explored by examining both internal personal distress and external threats. Crises must be resolved, and the family's lines of communication must be reopened. Running away is always a cry for help, and the underlying issues must be confronted and resolved. Treatment will often take time and commitment by the family to truly understand what their child is experiencing in his world.

~ 17 ~

Seeking Professional Help

A VARIETY OF specific kinds of child behavior may indicate an underlying behavioral, developmental, or emotional problem. You should consider seeking professional help when problems are interfering with your child's or the family's ability to function well in day-to-day life. Problems that are persistent, severe, or cause significant stress to the family (or to your child's teachers or coaches) need attention. If you note behavior that is not age-appropriate for your child—for example, a 6-year-old who will not speak to her teachers, an 8-year-old who is having nighttime urinary accidents, or a 10-year-old who has excessive separation anxiety—speak with your child's pediatrician.

When to Seek Help

Help is warranted when your child demonstrates:

- Behavior that is not age-appropriate

- An inability or great resistance to respond to your initial, appropriate interventions, so that behavioral and emotional problems are repeated without resolution

- Worrisome changes such as new sleep problems, sudden alterations in mood or behavior, intense self-stimulation, sexual promiscuity, runaway behaviors, sudden interest in adult sexual topics, use of alcohol or drugs, complaints of chronic pain such as stomachaches or headaches, poor school performance, declining relationships with peers or family members, repeated victimization, or diminished self-esteem

- Severe anxiety reactions, in which your child is panicked and cannot be calmed down, including phobias and extreme separation difficulty

- Risky behavior that threatens the safety of the child or others; these might include intentionally harming an animal, setting a fire, or beating up a classmate at school

- Suicidal actions, including talk about killing herself or especially where there has been an attempt at suicide

To find a competent professional and an appropriate treatment or therapy, start by talking to your child's pediatrician. Pediatricians are trained in the recognition of mental health problems and can assist in the management of many common behavior problems. Discuss with him or her the problems your child is having and the reasons you are considering further evaluation and treatment. Because your pediatrician likely knows your family and your child and understands some of the difficulties you and your child are facing, she may be in a good position to either evaluate your child herself or, alternatively, recommend the specific kind of counselor or specialist your child may need.

Your pediatrician should be familiar with many of the mental health professionals in your community, including their particular expertise and professional interests, and can refer you to the most appropriate professional who can best deal with your child's problem. School principals, teachers, or friends may also supply names of professionals. Reassurance from individuals who are satisfied with their experiences may help you feel more comfortable and confident that a professional is competent and trustworthy. Share any suggestions you have received with your pediatrician when you discuss treatment options.

When making your decision, also consider the time and cost of the treatment, and the distance you must travel to get there. Mental health therapy concentrates on social, emotional, and behavioral problems and is usually provided on a frequent (weekly or every other week) basis. Sessions typically last an hour and the fee is calculated on a per-hour basis. Evaluate your insurance coverage to determine whether some or all of the cost of this care will be reimbursed by your insurer. Some insurance policies require prior authorization from your child's physician before it will cover mental health treatment. If you belong to a health maintenance organization (HMO), you may have to use the HMO's own mental health specialists. Some insurance companies have their own mental health clinics; others allow patients to choose any professional they would like. Review your insurance coverage before you begin searching for a mental health provider.

When you tell your child about your decision to seek counseling for her, she may resist the idea. She might feel there is a stigma attached to this type of care ("I'm not crazy, am I?"). Or she simply may not understand what will take place during the sessions. *Before* your child begins seeing a mental health professional, talk with her about the reasons for this care. Share with her that you are aware of the struggles she is having and the pain she is experiencing because of her symptoms. Emphasize that counseling is to help her develop strategies to overcome her current challenges, and that you will ensure that the therapist is a "good fit" for your child. Tell her that the therapist will help her get along better with her classmates, conquer her phobias, or whatever the specific problem and goals may be. Emphasize that the entire family will be getting help to deal with any family issues that may be involved. Assure her that any individual counseling will be confidential within appropriate limits. Do not make her feel as though she alone is to blame, or that she alone has a problem or is the "sick" one. As the treatment process begins, your child should undergo a medical evaluation to ensure that she has no associated or contributing medical issues such as sleep problems.

Mental health professionals often have specialized training or expertise in specific areas. Families should consult with their pediatrician to ensure that an individual mental health provider has experience with the diagnosis and treatment of the particular problem that *your* child is experiencing, ideally *before* the treatment experience begins. This information can often be determined with a simple phone call to the mental health provider's office (or, alternatively, consulting the practice website) to determine if the provider has training and experience with your child's specific issue.

Approaches to Counseling and Therapy

Successful therapy requires that children feel safe and respected. Treatment should begin with at least one or two assessment sessions in which the therapist gathers background information and meets you and your child. During this time additional information may be acquired from the schools or other people who know your child. During this initial period, it is important that the child and the therapist establish a good connection and rapport; touch base with your child to see how sessions are progressing from her perspective.

After the initial sessions, recommendations and a treatment plan should be discussed. Following that will be several sessions devoted to helping you and your child develop strategies to help with specific issues. Following these strategy ses-

Types of Mental Health Professionals

Many types of professionals and agencies are available for mental health consultation and treatment.

Psychiatrists. General psychiatrists are physicians (MDs or DOs) who have gone to medical school for four years and then have had four years of training in general psychiatry. Child psychiatrists specialize in the mental health of children and have had two additional years of special training after the four years of general psychiatry. They have also been trained in neurology and child development.

If there is no child psychiatrist available, your pediatrician may know of a general psychiatrist with a special interest in working with children. Most child psychiatrists have had experience with psychotherapy such as cognitive behavioral therapy (CBT) or can make an educated referral for the child.

Psychiatrists are able to prescribe medications that may be helpful for particular kinds of disorders, including attention deficit hyperactivity disorder, depression, anxiety, and obsessive-compulsive disorder.

Psychologists. They may have either a master's degree (MS) or a doctoral degree (PhD, EdD, PsyD) in psychology or education. They have been trained in human development and behavior, and in the treatment of learning, behavioral, and emotional difficulties. Part of their training included supervised work providing therapy for children or adults. Psychologists have special skills in evaluating and treating emotional problems and learning disorders. Some have had special training in family or marital counseling.

Behavioral and developmental pediatricians. They are pediatricians (medical doctors) who have had four years of medical school, three years of pediatric residency training, and additional fellowship training after residency specifically in child development and the emotional and educational problems of children. They treat children with behavioral and emotional problems and a wide range of developmental difficulties, from attention problems to mental retardation. Pediatricians can also prescribe medications for a variety of disorders.

Mental health counselors. Several types of practitioners fall into this category. Licensed clinical social workers with master's degrees in social work (MSW) are among the most common; they have had four years of college and two years of postgraduate training in counseling children and families. School counselors are educators who work directly with children in school settings, providing guidance and counseling, and making referrals when necessary. They have had four years of college and additional training in counseling children with behavioral problems.

Community mental health resources. Many community agencies provide mental health services or can make appropriate referrals. They often are associated with county health departments, religious organizations, or nonprofit counseling agencies. Colleges and medical centers also may offer a variety of mental health services available to the public.

sions, you and your child may be seen less frequently to monitor his progress and to help deal with anticipated or unforeseen problems that may occur. In the initial evaluation of your child's behavioral problems, his teachers may be of help, since behavioral difficulties often occur in school and sometimes stem from problems with learning or attention and the frustrations they can cause.

Depending on the type of problem, one or more methods may be used:

■ The counselor works directly and only with the child. This child-centered treatment is what most parents expect, but it is often not completely effective.

■ The counselor works with the child and the parents, sometimes together, sometimes individually, to better understand the potential causes of the behavior, the nature of the problems, and parenting techniques, and to implement new strategies.

■ The counselor works with the parents to help them understand and resolve personal problems such as marital stress, financial difficulties, and emotional problems that may be causing or contributing to the difficulty. Specific parenting management techniques can be helpful.

■ The counselor works with the entire family in a family-systems or family-centered approach that seeks to deal with behavior problems and improve communication.

The duration of the therapy may range from weeks to over a year, depending on the needs of the child and family, the therapist's skill, the response to therapy, and its costs.

Therapies for children can be grouped into the three general categories that follow. Each has a distinctive aim and perspective on the child, and there are many variations within each of them. Some therapists employ and blend parts of different therapies into their own individual therapeutic style.

Cognitive behavioral therapy (CBT) helps the child develop better ways of acting and reacting. Its aim is to change the child's behavior, to allow him to see the world differently and think about and be aware of his actions and how they affect him and others. It uses behavior modification techniques to change his expectations and responses. Some common elements of CBT include graduated exposure, thought-stopping, and fading. It is usually carried out by pediatricians, psychiatrists, psychologists, or social workers and can last for varying lengths, but usually several months. CBT typically requires additional training above that required for the provider's particular license.

Parent management training helps parents develop strategies and techniques to navigate both expected and unexpected developmental transitions. These can be learned in group family sessions as well as from parenting books devoted to the topic. Techniques involve positive parenting steps to modify behavioral trends of anger, aggression, and temper tantrums, for example. Group parent training programs emphasize that the parent-child relationship is a two-way street, and these methods have been validated by investigative research to improve positive relationships and child behavior.

Family-system therapy looks at the family structure and its subunits (marital, sibling, parent-child). In this approach, a child's behavioral problem is seen as a reflection of a dysfunction, stress, or a larger problem within the family. While the child is identified as the patient, in fact the whole family is the patient. The aim is to change and improve the child's and the family's relationships, communication, and behavior. Therapy can last several sessions or many years and requires a trained family therapist.

Because school failure or underachievement is such a common concern, an additional category of treatment is **school problem therapy.** Learning disabilities or difficulties usually have several causes, and a complete assessment may require the skills of a psychologist, an educator, and a pediatrician. With school issues, it is particularly important that the child's school has input into the process. They may find that emotional and behavioral problems have contributed to learning difficulties or, conversely, that learning problems may have caused emotional and behavioral troubles. (See Chapter 40, "Learning Disabilities.")

Psychodynamic therapy helps the child look inward, to reflect on his experiences, feelings, and reactions. Its aim is for the child to gain insight into and understanding of his behavior and emotions, especially those of which he may not have been conscious, and to change them in some fundamental way. Some therapists are *nondirective*, meaning that they may encourage a child to play and talk about whatever comes to mind while they listen for clues as to what may be at the root of the child's difficulties. This type of therapy is sometimes necessary to understand a child's deeper and more personal problems. Central to this approach is providing the child with an opportunity to form a relationship with the therapist. In this context, the therapist can observe the child's problems firsthand and work with the child to overcome them. Other therapists are more *directive* and guiding, leading children into discussions of specific problematic issues. Psychodynamic treatment requires a highly skilled therapist such as a child psychiatrist, psychologist, or trained social worker. It may be more effective with older (middle school age) children who are reflective and insight-oriented.

Which style of treatment is best for your child? It depends primarily upon his particular diagnosis and issues. Certain children, perhaps because of their personalities, fare better in particular settings and may make more progress with a practitioner who directs and structures the sessions thoroughly. Successful therapy requires that children feel safe and respected. Your pediatrician can help direct you toward the most appropriate style of therapy for your child.

Parents should be cautious of treatment techniques that are not backed by published research that supports the technique and its outcomes (physicians call this "evidence-based medicine") but, rather, rely on testimonials. Most legitimate therapies do not rely on previous patients to "market" or "sell" their brand of therapy, do not "fully guarantee" successful outcomes, and do not require full payment prior to the start of treatment. Be aware that most quality mental health providers are either discouraged from or not allowed to advertise their programs; if parents investigate options online, look for published research as opposed to flashy websites to find quality providers.

Parental Anxieties

If you are like many parents, you may have to overcome some personal obstacles that cause you to be reluctant to seek mental health treatment for your child.

Many parents feel anxious and uncertain about seeking out this kind of help. These doubts are often fueled by feelings of parental guilt and responsibility for the child's challenges. Sometimes parents may be reluctant to seek therapy because their child's behavior reminds them of their own issues growing up. Other times parents may recognize that the child's symptoms are a response to discord between the parents, or to violence or alcoholism in the home, and they prefer not to confront these problems. They may also fear being lectured to or criticized as inadequate or incompetent parents. Keep in mind that in most situations, the main focus of the therapy is to help the child and his family overcome the challenges, not to place blame.

Approaching a Treatment Program Realistically

Before beginning any kind of treatment plan—whether it is your own plan or that of professionals—keep these important points in mind:

1. No single theory of child development or behavior management has all of the explanations or answers.

2. No single treatment plan works for all children.

3. There are seldom simple solutions to complex problems. Things may initially get worse before they get better. Be patient, and be willing to modify goals and expectations according to the progress being made.

4. Beware of treatments or interventions that make you feel guilty or inadequate or that do not make sense to you.

5. Beware of becoming a clinical "expert" with your own child, particularly if you work in one of the helping professions. It is not necessary—and in fact may even be harmful—to analyze and discuss every detailed aspect of your child's behavior.

6. Be careful of statistics or dogma that claims to explain everything or create broad generalizations or truths.

7. Be wary of therapies that discourage parents from doing their own problem-solving or using informal, commonsense approaches. On the

other hand, don't try to do it all alone; keep in touch with the professional, even as you assume more responsibility yourself.

8. Ask your pediatrician for advice, or for a referral, in sorting out whether a treatment program is right for you and your child. If the program doesn't seem right, discuss it with the therapist. If you decide to stop treatment, talk it over in advance with both your child and the therapist so the last few sessions can be structured in a supportive way for your child.

PART V

· · · · · · · · · · · · ·

Family Matters

~ 18 ~

The Importance of Family

FAMILIES PROVIDE CHILDREN with a sense of belonging and a unique identity. Families are ideally a source of emotional support and comfort, warmth and nurturing, protection and security—a safe haven. Family relationships provide children with a sense of being valued and with a vital network of historical linkages and social support. Within every healthy family there is a sense of reciprocity—a giving and taking of love and empathy by every family member. Life continually evolves and changes; a cohesive yet adaptable family serves as a bedrock of support during times of transition.

Families are much more than groups of individuals, and together are worth more than the sum of their parts. Families have their own goals and aspirations. Within a family, every child and adult should feel that she contributes to the household, and her goals and plans should be respected and encouraged. The family should be a place where everyone's individuality is permitted to flourish. Although every family has conflicts, all the family members should feel as though they can express themselves openly, share their feelings, and have their opinions listened to with understanding. Conflicts and disagreements are a normal part of family life; in fact, they are important, as they permit people to communicate their differences and ventilate their feelings. Healthy communication between individual family members goes both ways.

The family instructs children and gives guidance about personal values and social behavior. It instills discipline and helps them learn and internalize codes of conduct that will serve them for the rest of their lives. It helps them develop positive interpersonal relationships, and it provides an environment that encourages learning both in the home and at school. It gives children a sense of history and a secure base from which to grow and develop. As life changes and transitions occur, adaptable families adjust and support each other.

Diversity Among Family Structures

The structure of the American family continues to evolve. Whether discussing dual-parent households, single-parent households, or homes in which the parent(s) work outside the home, the idea of family and the importance of communication within the family are important. If your own family is not like the one you grew up in, your situation is certainly not unusual. Families are diverse and include families headed by single parents (by divorce, being widowed, or never married), stepfamilies, LGBTQ families, or foster families, and most households have parents who work outside the home.

No matter your family structure, your children will have friends who live in households with different structures. From time to time you can expect your child to ask questions like "Why do people get divorced?" "How come Sophia's mother and father don't live together?" "Why does Connor's father live with another lady?" Because families are so important to children, parents need to be able to answer such questions and have a discussion with their child. As your children grow, their friends' households will evolve, and this also is important to discuss. By asking these questions, children are trying to understand two things about families: the different structures that families can take and the changes in structure, lifestyles, and relationships that can occur.

Any group of people living together in a household can create and call themselves a family. For example, to share expenses, a divorced mother with two children may live with another single woman with children; together, they may consider themselves a family. A grandparent who lives with her daughter, son-in-law, and grandchildren may become an integral part of their family. The variations of family structures and definition are endless, but they have certain qualities in common: family members share their lives emotionally and together fulfill the multiple responsibilities of family life.

A Vision of the Family

Your child's notion—as well as your own ideas—of the family and how it should work have largely been shaped by personal experiences. If you grew up as an only child, for example, and you have four children of your own who compete for attention, privacy, or possessions, you might feel concern with the way your family is functioning. Or if you grew up in a household where everyone was relatively calm and harmonious, and you have kids who are active and energetic, you may be concerned about relationships within the family because things are not in sync with your early experiences.

Other factors can help shape your vision of the family and how it actually works. Religious and moral beliefs, for example, help form your ideas of the way things "should" be. Your economic situation and living conditions will influence the functioning of your family, perhaps in ways that run counter to your preconceptions. Today's geographic mobility can put distance between extended families, with hundreds or thousands of miles separating grandparents and their grandchildren; if you grew up with your grandparents nearby, this is a different experience for you.

The prevailing cultural values as depicted and transmitted by the media may not coincide with your notion of family. Social networking, the internet, television, movies, and other media bombard us each day with images of the family. If your family doesn't measure up to these depictions—if your family isn't always as happy as families on the TV commercials, or doesn't settle arguments within a thirty-minute time slot—you might feel you aren't doing as good a job as you should. Some of the media more accurately portray the evolving roles that males and females can play today, with both fathers and mothers exercising more options in sharing the breadwinning and child-raising responsibilities.

The Family with School-Age Children

During the middle years of your child's childhood, many changes will occur within the family. Your child is more independent than before, better able to care for herself, and more capable of contributing to chores and other household responsibilities. Most families discover that routines can be established, and in many ways life seems more settled, yet children still need parental supervision and guidance.

During the middle childhood years, parents have two tasks that are especially important. The first is learning to allow and encourage your child to enter the new world of school and friends alone. The second is learning to be parents at a distance. Once children enter school, parents spend less than half as much time with them during waking hours as they did before. Parents' involvement in their children's lives must evolve in order to monitor, guide, and support them effectively.

Myths About the Family

Here are some commonly held beliefs about the family, all of which are more fiction than fact.

MYTH: THE "NUCLEAR FAMILY" IS A UNIVERSAL PHENOMENON

The nuclear family is generally defined as a family group made up of only parents and children. Although most people tend to think that this particular family structure has always been the dominant one, that is not the case. The nuclear family is a relatively recent phenomenon, becoming common only within the last century. Before then, the "traditional" family was multigenerational, with grandparents often living with their children on farms as well as in urban environments, typically with other relatives living nearby. The nuclear family has evolved in response to a number of factors: better health and longer lives, economic development, industrialization, urbanization, geographic mobility, and migration to the suburbs. These changes have resulted in the physical separation of extended families and in progressive fragmentation of the family.

MYTH: FAMILY HARMONY IS THE RULE, NOT THE EXCEPTION

Although family life is often romanticized, it has always been filled with conflicts and tension. Difficulties between partners are commonplace, with disagreements arising over issues ranging from how the children should be raised to how the family finances should be handled. Parents also must learn to maintain a relationship in which partnership and companionship may become more important than passionate love. Parent-children conflicts are commonplace as well. As parents assert their authority and children try to assert their autonomy appropriately, strife is inevitable.

While we often expect families to be above the chaos that exists in the rest of society, that outlook places unrealistic expectation upon the family. In the real world families are not always a haven, since they too can be filled with conflict. Although stress and disagreements are common, they can be destructive to families, especially when conflict gets out of hand. Families are under constant stress, being pushed and pulled from many directions, often without the support systems of extended families that may have existed in the past.

MYTH: THE STABILITY OF A FAMILY IS A MEASURE OF ITS SUCCESS

Change is a part of life. Death, illness, physical separation, financial strains, divorce … these are some of the events families must adjust to. Consequently, stability shouldn't be the only measure of a family's success. Many families function quite well despite frequent disruptions. In fact, one important measure of a family's success is its resilience, adaptability, and ability to adjust to changes and transitions. Daily life is full of stresses that constantly demand accommodation from family members.

MYTH: PARENTS CONTROL THEIR CHILDREN'S FATE

In reality, parents cannot determine how their children will turn out. Inevitably, children assert their autonomy, creating a niche for themselves separate from their parents. At the same time, many factors external to both the child and family can influence the way a child develops.

Even within the same family there can be tremendous individual variations among siblings in intelligence, temperament, mood, and sociability. Yet despite these differences, parents are responsible for imparting to each child a sense of being loved and accepted, for helping each child to succeed at various developmental tasks, for encouraging each child to be a contributing member of the household, and for socializing each child into respecting the rules and accepting the responsibilities society imposes.

Some parents perceive themselves as having total responsibility for their children's fate. This belief places a heavy and unrealistic emotional burden on them as well as their children. If the children are having problems, the parents often feel a sense of failure; likewise, the children feel as though they have let their family down if they do not live up to their parents' expectations. Parents can influence and shape but cannot control their children's lives.

At the same time, the role of a parent should not be that of a helicopter, to swoop in and solve all the child's problems for him. Nor should parents do what has been termed "lawnmower parenting": anticipating and solving all obstacles and challenges, paving a clear path for the child. Rather, the goal is to nurture self-empowerment skills and resilience to help our kids learn problem-solving skills, in an evolving, age-appropriate way as they grow.

During the school years your child will develop more self-confidence, overcome fears and self-doubts, test the limits of her autonomy, find role models, and learn and internalize moral and spiritual values. You and the rest of the family should pay particular attention to the following areas, which will become increasingly significant during this time of life.

School

School assumes a central role in your child's life when she reaches the age of 5 or 6, drawing much of her attention and energy away from the family unit. Her elementary school years can become a time of enormous satisfaction and excitement. As she learns to read and master other academic skills, she will develop a love of learning and a pride in her achievements. This can contribute to her self-esteem, not only because of her accomplishments in the classroom but also as she separates successfully from the home environment. In the process her teacher can become a source of support and an important role model in her life.

For some children, however, school may cause frustration and stress. Learning disabilities can interfere with the joy of learning. Poor study habits or a lack of motivation can create academic challenges. Sometimes children may have a poor relationship with their teachers, or they may experience separation anxiety that can interfere with their school attendance.

To make your own child's education as positive and productive as possible, monitor her academic progress and social adjustment, and get to know her teacher. Take advantage of opportunities to visit the school, whether it be Meet the Teacher Day, Parent Expectation Night, Mystery Reader, or other special occasions in which parents are invited to the school during or after school hours. Working parents may have a challenge adjusting their work schedules to visit the classroom; email the teacher to get advance notice about future dates and upcoming events. Parents can look at their child's school website or the school newsletters for helpful tips to stay updated on their child's school activities.

Discuss with your child what she is learning in the classroom and how she feels about school. Encourage her to demonstrate her newly learned skills and to practice them with you. Supervise your child's homework (but don't do it for her), and make sure she is preparing herself well for tests. Limit the amount of screen time and encourage her to read, write, and express herself creatively through hobbies and physical activities. If she or her teacher reports any problem areas, communicate openly with school personnel, and try to figure out how best to help your child overcome her challenges. Consult your pediatrician for suggestions to help solve these problems.

For more information about your child's education, see Part VI, "Children in School."

Friendships

As important as your child's family is to her, friends and acquaintances will become increasingly significant during middle childhood. She will spend more time with her peers, both in and out of school. These playmates will provide companionship, and your child will probably become preoccupied with being socially accepted by her friends. She will feel a strong need for both conformity (to be just like the others) and recognition (to be seen as unique).

Your family will also have to deal with the stresses associated with your child's peer relationships. From time to time she may have conflicts with friends, which can undermine her self-esteem. During these years, monitor your child's choice of friends and supervise, but do not interfere with, her play activities. Get to know her friends' parents and share with them any concerning observations about the children's activities. Offer support, understanding, and guidance to your child when problems arise in her peer relationships. When a conflict occurs, try to understand how your child feels about it and what she sees as the factors contributing to it, then discuss how the other child might view the problem. Ask, "What do you think?" and together work out ways to resolve the conflict. At the same time keep in mind that the family cannot, and should not, solve every peer-related difficulty—for example, you cannot run to the playground and intervene whenever a conflict arises. You can offer support and guidance, convey your own values and expectations, and help your child to navigate her own conflicts as they arise, all in an age-appropriate manner.

Older children who have been granted internet access or who have their own electronic devices will be interacting with their peers through texting and social media (for more on this, see page 315). Age-appropriate limits should be placed on such screen time, with the realization that it is easier to relax limits over time than set new limits in place after a child has been granted little to no restrictions. Texting and online interaction should *not* replace relationships IRL, "in real life." Promote device-free meals, and when friends come to your home encourage everyone to set aside electronic devices so that the kids can hold conversations, play board games, and experience other types of interaction.

Outside Activities

During middle childhood your child will develop a number of outside interests, from sports to Scouts, from music lessons to clubs. Many of these activities will require a commitment on the family's part, in terms of time, driving, and money. It may also require parental patience as children experiment with different programs before finding the ones they prefer. Many park districts offer classes that

Evolving Friendships Through the Years

Children ages 5–7 years: Children's view of friendship is simpler in these years. Classmates from school make for easy playdates. Screen time should be minimal to not present at all for these ages when socializing.

Children ages 8–10 years: At this age, kids have more relationships both within school and outside school with kids they meet through extracurricular activities. Friendships with kids who attend different schools are emotionally healthy for kids; it helps them to see there is a larger world out there, and helps "bully-proof" kids with this broader perspective.

Children ages 11–12 years: Older children have an increased focus on relationships outside the family. Encourage your preteen to invite friends to your home; this way you can get to know your child's friends and observe the dynamic. Ensure limits and supervision of use of electronic devices (for more on media, see page 315).

expose younger kids to a variety of sports, to help them decide which ones they prefer.

In general, the family should be willing to support the child with resources, encouragement, supervision, transportation, and, at times, direct participation as a parent volunteer. This sends a strong message to your child that she matters to you. At the same time, care should be taken to avoid overscheduling a child or the family as a whole. Many athletic team programs can be quite an investment of time and finances; make sure the needs of the child are being met, including relaxation and downtime as a family. Families should ensure family meals occur on a regular basis and maintain other important times to gather, connect, and simply be together. In most cases, quality sports coaches have the kids' best interests at heart—the goal should always be to have fun and get exercise. From time to time, parents should step back and look at the big picture. The developmental and emotional needs of the child should take precedence above the business pressures of twentieth-first-century youth athletics.

Is My Family Functioning Normally?

"Is my family functioning normally?" Parents may ask themselves this question, but there is no simple answer, since there is no such thing as normal. A better question to ask is "Is our family functioning well?"

There are several characteristics that are generally identified with a well-functioning family: support; love and caring for other family members; providing security and a sense of belonging; open communication; making each person within the family feel important, valued, respected, and esteemed; adaptability to help all family members navigate inevitable transitions and life changes.

Here are some other qualities to consider when evaluating how well your own family is functioning.

- Is there ample humor and fun within your family, despite the demands of daily life?

- Does your family have rules that have been clearly stated and are evenly applied, yet are flexible and respond to new situations and changes in the family?

- Are the family's expectations of each person reasonable, realistic, mutually agreed upon, and generally fulfilled?

- Do family members achieve most of their individual goals, and are their personal needs being met?

- Do parents and children have genuine respect for one another, demonstrating love, caring, trust, and concern, even when there are disagreements?

- Is your family able to mature and change without everyone getting upset or unhappy?

Family Leadership

Families are not democracies. Each family has its own ways of deciding who has the power and authority within the family unit, and which rights, privileges, obligations, and roles are assigned to each family member. In most families, parents are expected to be the leaders or executives of the family; children are expected to follow the leadership of their parents. As children in the middle years grow older, they will ask for, and certainly should be allowed, more autonomy, and their opinions should be considered when decisions are made; however, parents are the final authorities.

There will be disagreements among the generations. Your child may think he has too many chores to do; you may think he has just the right amount. Let him speak his mind, but the ultimate decision is yours. Explain why you've made the judgment you have, without becoming defensive or apologetic. Our primary job is to parent, not to be popular. It is a losing proposition to attempt to be your child's "friend." Kids may point out other families' rules; you can tell your child, "This is how our family operates."

Although generational hierarchies are the most obvious ones within families, other types of hierarchies exist as well. Sometimes they depend on gender. In the past, mothers and fathers often held different positions in the family hierarchy; now, the traditional gender-based structure is outdated. In many families one or both parents work outside the home. Thankfully, dads now assume greater roles in child-raising and household duties, which models excellent teamwork to our kids.

It is useful to consider what roles each family member takes within the family, and whether everyone is satisfied with the current arrangement. For example, the oldest children in the family may take on a caring role, helping to care for their younger siblings. Or grandparents may acquire an important place within the family by assuming a central child-rearing role while parents work.

Think about who is responsible for what within your own family and how the current arrangement is working. Some responsibilities may be open to negotiation, particularly if the family does not seem to be functioning optimally. For example, an older child may be resentful of having too much responsibility for watching over the younger children, while the younger children may also resent the older child playing a parental role. This will result in arguments whenever the oldest child is left in charge. Parents need to review what is going on, discuss how the children are feeling about it, and come up with some alternatives. Remember the advantages of chores and assigned household responsibilities: in the short run, a cleaner home; in the long run, the kids are learning important life skills and teamwork. (For more on chores, see page 309.)

Family Boundaries

As children grow through the school years, the boundaries that affect how family members relate to one another evolve. When your child was a newborn, for example, you were with or near her almost twenty-four hours a day, meeting her every demand for food, cuddling, clean diapers, and other basic needs. As your child matured, the situation changed, and greater emotional distance developed between the two of you. For instance, she may always have shared with you everything that happened at school, but at age 8 or 9 she may stop doing so. She may be trying to assert some independence and negotiate a new boundary that says, "This is my territory and not always yours to know."

When these situations come up, you need to learn to respect your child's wishes and allow her some privacy. If she is not having problems in the classroom, respect her wishes. Just as we adults will have days where we don't necessarily feel like rehashing all the events of our day, kids can have similar days as well. Do not pressure her to talk, but still provide opportunities for her to do so. For example, "If there's anything you'd like to tell me about school, I'd love to hear it, but if you don't feel like talking right now, that's okay too." (For more creative ideas on how to get a conversation started, see the box on page 188.)

Bear in mind that at some point early in middle childhood many kids may prefer to spend more time playing and talking with their friends than with their parents. This is an example of a child's renegotiating boundaries and relationships. That being said, your child should know that if he has been harmed by someone (either physical, sexual, or verbal abuse), if he has thoughts of harming himself, or if a friend is experiencing these situations, he should come to you for help. Certain secrets are *not* appropriate to keep.

Family boundaries are a two-way street. Everyone in the family needs some privacy, including you as a parent. Closed doors and shut dresser drawers must be respected. Teach your child about privacy by respecting her space and belongings.

Keep in mind that children are not adults. During the middle years of childhood, children are not emotionally or developmentally ready to understand or take on the stresses that adults face. Don't expect a child of this age to serve as your confidant or "best friend," burdening her with your problems and concerns. Your child will be sensitive to your moods and will recognize if something is troubling you; when this happens, be honest with her, explaining that you are experiencing some difficulties that may take some time to work through. However, a lengthy and complete disclosure of your problems is unwise; particularly if your sharing is intended to elicit emotional support for you, that can become a burden for your child and is not justified. The best approach is to acknowledge to your child that a problem exists. Discuss how it might affect the family's routines, but voice optimism that in time the difficulty will be resolved and things will be fine. Life's inevitable roadblocks are a good opportunity to model resilience and coping strategies to your child.

If you wish, discuss any concrete actions she can take that would be of help. If you have lost your job, for example, and there will be pressures upon the family finances, perhaps you and your child can together think of ways she could help save a little money—perhaps by taking a packed lunch to school rather than buying it, or postponing a planned activity or purchase until you become employed again. These actions by your child, however, should not become an emotional burden on her, nor should you present them in a way to make her feel responsible for "fixing" the problem.

Dealing with Family Conflicts

How does your family handle disagreements that occur in your household? Conflicts are basic to human relationships; they are inevitable and should not be avoided. Family members should know how to negotiate and resolve these conflicts. To negotiate, parents and children both need to make a genuine attempt to understand each other's attitudes, feelings, and desires. When disagreements are resolved successfully, family life is enhanced and relationships are strengthened.

Family members may deny that problems exist. Or they may draw a third person into the conflict, supposedly to mediate the difficulty, but who instead may take a position on one side or the other and thereby make the disagreement worse. Within every family, certain alliances, coalitions, and rivalries exist. At times, mother and daughter might form an alliance against father and son. Or the two parents might unite against the children on a particular issue. But within a healthy family these coalitions are not fixed—they change from situation to situation— and they do not disrupt the functioning of the family. If they become rigid and long-lasting, however, they can do damage to the family.

It is natural to be unaware that any alliances exist within your family. But to get a better sense of your family's dynamics, ask yourself questions like: "What family member do I tend to agree (or disagree) with most often? When my children are fighting, whose side do I generally take? With whom in the family do I usually spend my free time? Who in the family most easily angers me?"

The Adaptable Family

Family challenges come in all shapes and sizes; some are short-lived and easily managed, while others last longer and are difficult to handle. Stress points include transitions and events such as illness and injury, changing jobs, changing schools, moving, and financial difficulties. Adaptable families fare better navigating life's inevitable stresses.

There is no perfect family. Each family has its own strengths and weaknesses, assets and liabilities, challenges and problems. If your family is overwhelmed or there is a breakdown in relationships within your family, it may be helpful to discuss the situation with your pediatrician to see if family counseling or other forms of support are warranted. As a parent, your task is to meet the multiple demands of family life with energy, flexibility, and creativity, and nurture your children to take on age-appropriate, increasing responsibilities as the school years continue. Your kids will learn resilience by your example and develop the life skills they themselves will need as future adults.

Maintaining a Healthy Family

- **Do you treat each child as an individual?** Each child has his own temperament, his own way of viewing and interacting with the world around him. Parents may love their children equally, but naturally will have different relationships with each of them. Individualize your relationship with each of your children, reinforce their strengths and talents, and avoid comparing the child to siblings or friends. Make sure special one-on-one time with each child is the routine, not the exception.

- **Does your family have regular routines?** Children and parents benefit from having some predictable day-to-day routines. Morning schedules, mealtimes, and bedtimes are easier for everyone when they follow a pattern. Family rituals and traditions around birthdays and important holidays promote long-term bonding.

- **Is your family an active participant in your extended family and the community?** Families work better when they feel connected and supported by friends and relatives. Usually such relationships require that parents make an active effort to get together with others socially or for religious or civic projects.

- **Is your family adaptable to change?** The one constant of life is change; your family's situation will continue to evolve over the years. Job changes, house moves, and other situations pose challenges. Overly rigid and structured families have difficulty facing these challenges; a willingness to renegotiate roles within the family helps navigate life's inevitable transitions.

- **Are your expectations of yourself and other family members realistic?** Your child's self-awareness, knowledge, and skills are constantly changing. Observe, read, and talk to others to learn what can reasonably be expected of your child at each stage of development. Parents, too, have limitations on what they can accomplish, given their resources and the time available. There are no "superparents," just individuals doing their best given their current circumstances.

- **Does the time you spend with your family members contribute to good relationships among you?** Most of the time you and your child spend together should be fun, relaxed, meaningful, and relatively conflict-free.

- **As a parent, are you taking care of your own needs?** You should be leading a healthy personal life (including proper diet, exercise, and sleep habits). Set aside time, however brief, for things you enjoy. Your children will thrive when your own emotional needs are being met. On an airplane, we are asked to put our own oxygen mask on before helping others; we cannot help others if we are not taking care of ourselves as well.

- **Do you take moral and social responsibility for your own life?** You are the most important role model for your child. Demonstrate your value system through actions as well as words.

~ 19 ~

Your Family Routines and Dealing with Disruptions

FAMILY LIFE IS filled with everyday routines such as the kids getting ready for school in the morning, sharing the day's experiences at mealtimes, dealing with arguments and conflicts, and managing financial pressures. Families also face larger challenges such as a parent's deployment overseas, or moving to a new home. Families can use the following strategies to streamline their routines, bolster kids' growing confidence and life skills, and navigate transitions with resilience.

Family Routines

Maintaining schedules and routines helps to organize life. A schedule helps family members know what to expect, children and adults alike. Children in the middle years do best when routines are regular, predictable, and consistent. One of a family's challenges is to establish comfortable, effective routines, striving for a happy compromise between the disorder and confusion that can occur without them and the rigidity and boredom that can come with too much structure and regimentation. As a parent, review the routines in your household to ensure that they accomplish what you want.

It is also important for parents to take a step back from time to time and evaluate the big picture. All too often, especially as kids approach middle school, it is easy to fall into the overscheduling trap. Sports teams demand more time as the child develops her talent and skill. Music programs become more involved. Often your family is surrounded with other participating families who may be as overscheduled as you; this doesn't make it okay. Ensure that your child has downtime, and that the family has time to reconnect. School and religious education are often top priorities for families; after the nonnegotiables, prioritize top choices. It may be necessary to cut back on lower-priority extracurricular activities. Always remember that the individual needs of the child should take precedence over the pressures of the modern youth sports business.

Weekdays

Mornings. Most households are hectic on weekday mornings. The children are preparing for school. Parents are trying to get their kids out the door while making sure that they themselves get to work on time. To help the household function well in the morning, everyone should know what has to be done to get ready for the day. Many families get a head start on the morning by putting as many things in order as possible the night before. Prior to going to sleep, kids can pack up their books and papers for the next day. They also can help prep lunches and lay out clothes.

There can be obstacles that interfere with a smoothly running morning. Try to resolve any squabbles with a minimum of discussion or arguing. Kids should have some choice in the matter; for instance: "It's going to be chilly today, so you should wear a sweater. Would you like to wear the blue one or the red one?" At a certain point, though, especially for kids 10 to 12 years, you need to choose your battles. Within reason, kids should learn from natural consequences. If she doesn't wear a coat at the bus stop on a chilly day, the discomfort of the experience will help her remember the next time much better than any parental reminder would.

Keep the wake-up routine cheerful and positive. Kids can make use of an alarm clock by third grade. An affordable, simple alarm clock is preferable to an electronic device such as a tablet or smartphone, as such screens can interfere with good sleep habits. Keep tabs on the time to make sure your child is truly up and getting ready for the day. Persistent difficulty in awakening may indicate that she is getting to sleep too late or has some other sleep disturbance.

As a general guideline, limit your child's bathing or washing to ten minutes. Be sure she eats breakfast; even if she is not particularly hungry in the morning, have her get *some* food in her system to start the day. Some children regularly use the toilet after breakfast; allow these children adequate time so they do not feel rushed and omit this part of their routine.

Some parents realize that they are expecting their children to get everything done much faster than kids are actually capable of; for example, they may be giving their children only twenty-five minutes to accomplish tasks that actually take thirty-five minutes. Roughly determine the amount of time she needs to get dressed, wash herself, eat breakfast, brush her teeth, and get things ready for school (without an adult intervening). If necessary, schedule your child's wake-up time a little earlier so the morning will proceed more smoothly.

In order to keep kids on task with their morning responsibilities, many parents make a list of the tasks involved in getting ready. Charts and drawings about the morning routine can be fun to make as a family and can offer children a chance to discuss how they view the process and where they might be stuck. This strategy helps to pinpoint where problems are likely to arise and how to reshape the routines to reduce the chaos and confusion that can accompany morning time.

If you or your children just aren't "morning people," all of you might need a little extra assistance before getting going. For example, it might be nice to spend a few moments cuddling or talking about something pleasant before starting the morning routine. And don't underestimate the power of some upbeat music to get the household going. Music is a natural mood lifter. Avoid screen time, as this serves as a distraction from getting ready and out the door. Another benefit to no screen time during the morning hustle: if you have a daily newspaper subscription, kids of all ages will naturally start reading while they munch their morning cereal. Often this begins with the comic pages, but don't be surprised if your fourth-grader learns a bit of geography while scanning world news, or can recite sports stats thanks to the sports pages.

If mornings are stressful, you should monitor your own behavior to see if it might be contributing to the problem. Yelling, scolding, criticizing, and engaging in fruitless arguments will undermine your authority and diminish your child's respect for the rules. Even if things aren't going as planned, keep your emotional reactions under control, and handle any conflicts or mishaps with good humor.

Finally, round out each morning by saying goodbye to your children. A simple hug and a wave as she heads out the front door or slides out of the car are extremely important. They will give her a positive feeling with which to begin the day's activities.

After school. During middle childhood, children need adult supervision. After school the presence of an adult will provide them with safety, structure, support, and a sense of well-being. Many schools offer excellent after-care options for working parents, or transportation to reliable daycare organizations. For more on child care, see Chapter 23.

At times parents, due to their particular circumstances and their child's age and developmental stage, choose to have their children return home independently each afternoon; for more, see "Staying Safe While Home Alone," page 92. The American Academy of Pediatrics recommends that a child younger than 11 years of age come home to a parent, another adult, or a responsible adolescent. In general, 11 or 12 years of age is when parents can consider allowing their child to stay home alone for longer stretches of time. During daylight hours, and no more than three hours, is an appropriate place to start. Before settling on this decision, parents should consider neighborhood safety and whether there are adult neighbors available to help in case of an emergency. Each child has a different level of maturity and life skills even at the same numeric age, so it is important to determine if the particular child is ready for this next step of responsibility.

Particularly for younger children in the middle years, an after-school schedule is also useful, although every minute does not need to be planned. The routine should include a snack, exercise, relaxation, and study, in whatever order works best for your child. In general, after six to eight hours of school, children need time for active play—to invigorate themselves so they are better able to complete the tasks before them, to get their energy out, and to help them stay fit. Watching television, playing computer games, or other forms of screen time are not good substitutes for this active play.

Some kids try to complete as much of their homework as possible *before* dinner; TV watching and other pleasurable activities wait until later. Most children, however, go outside for some play and exercise after coming home, saving the homework until later, perhaps after sunset, when playing outdoors is impractical.

As an alternative to coming home after classes end, a variety of after-school programs and child care settings are available in most communities. Many are offered through the public schools, city agencies, or community organizations (YMCA, Boys and Girls Club) and are reasonably priced.

Before enrolling your child in one of these after-school programs, visit the site while kids are there. The staff should relate to children in a sensitive way, the child-to-adult ratio ideally should not exceed 10:1 or 12:1, and the size of the group should be no more than twenty-four. The facilities should be clean, safe, functional, and have convenient outdoor play areas. (See Chapter 23.)

Evenings. Dinner should be an important time for your family. As often as possible, all family members should eat together at the dinner table, without the distraction of electronic devices or television. For many families, this is the only time of day when the whole family is together. During dinner the family can share the day's activities and participate in enjoyable conversation. For more ideas on conversation starters, see page 188. Many families like to take turns going around the table for "Apples and Onions" (or "Highs and Lows"), sharing the "apples," or best parts of their day, and the "onions," not-so-great parts of the day.

It is important for children to participate in the preparation and cleanup of dinner. In middle childhood, they are capable of taking on a regular chore such as preparing part of the meal, setting the table, helping to serve, clearing the table, or rinsing the dishes. When they help in this way, it will help them develop good life skills, increase their awareness of the importance of dinnertime, and raise their level of investment in making dinner a good family experience.

If the entire family is unable to eat dinner at the same time—perhaps because Dad or Mom gets home late from work, or due to extracurricular activities—try to schedule another time of the day when the family can congregate for even twenty or thirty minutes of discussion, reading aloud, or playing games. Alternatively, parents can consider making breakfast the "family meal" of the day. Many parents have discovered that this is a wise investment of time during the middle years of childhood. Not only is this a period to enjoy your children, but if you have a strong history of sharing good times with your family, you will probably find it easier to make a difference in their lives during adolescence, when problems might arise and need resolving. At that time your relationship will already have become strong and important to both of you, and that strength can help carry you through tough experiences.

During the evening your children will need to finish their dinner-related tasks, perform their other chores such as emptying the garbage or putting things away, and complete their homework. Once these are done, they can relax by reading, having a conversation, playing games, or limited screen time. These should be seen as earned privileges and rewards rather than inalienable rights. If a child fails to finish her chores, she should forfeit some of her free-time leisure activities.

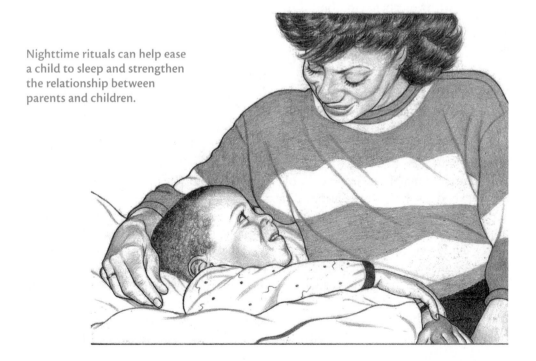

Nighttime rituals can help ease a child to sleep and strengthen the relationship between parents and children.

Bedtime. After some time for relaxation, most kids take a bath or shower and get ready for bed. On school nights, children need a regular bedtime to go to sleep. Lights can go out at different times for different children in the family, depending on how much sleep each child needs. In general, most of us, adults and kids alike, need more sleep. When deciding what time your child needs to go to bed, pay attention to how she functions the next day; if she is groggy and struggles through the morning and afternoon, then she needs an earlier bedtime.

Nighttime rituals can help ease a child to sleep, as well as promote intimacy between parents and children. These rituals can include storytelling, reading aloud, conversation, and songs. Try to avoid active play and energetic activities immediately before bedtime. Your child might enjoy reading in bed for thirty minutes before the lights are turned off.

The days can get quite hectic, and it is often at bedtime, especially when the child has their parent all to themselves, that he feels comfortable sharing something that has been on his mind or a situation that occurred earlier in the day. This is a fantastic opportunity to learn more about your child's world and connect. In addition, a few minutes of conversation at bedtime affords a good opportunity to resolve any persisting conflicts, putting them to rest so the child has a peaceful night and the conflicts don't continue into the following day. For instance, if you had an argument earlier in the evening, or there were some hassles related to homework, neither of you should take these conflicts to sleep. Say something like, "I know we had an argument. Let's put it to rest and start tomorrow fresh. I was unhappy with your behavior, but it's over now. I love you very much."

Weekends

Weekends are a good opportunity for family togetherness. Weekends are different for different families. Some families have work and school during weekdays. Other families may have a parent working weekends regularly, especially if parents work opposite each other so that one parent is home with the kids as much as possible. For these families, free time on weekends may be more limited.

Your child may have homework or long-term school projects to work on over the weekend, as well as obligations to a sports team, religious education, or other activities. In the middle years of childhood, since peers are becoming more important in your child's life, she may want to spend part of her weekends playing with friends too. Since knowing your child's friends is important, you might invite them to join your family in some activity. Find a balance between family time and your child's other priorities, while also allotting time for yourself for your own personal interests.

Many families carefully plan the weekend to avoid conflicts over time allocation. If one of your children is interested in tennis lessons and the other is deter-

Weekends and Free Time as a Family

Children ages 5–7 years: Special time as a family when kids are in kindergarten, first, and second grade does not have to be fancy or cost a lot of money. Think back to your own best childhood memories: often what really stays with a child are the simple times being together, such as raking leaves in the yard together and jumping into leaf piles, or piling in the car to drive an hour to a grandparent's house. The journey can be just as fun as the destination. Packing sandwiches for a local nature walk is budget friendly and arguably more relaxing for the family to enjoy together rather than an overcrowded, pricey theme park, for example. Often classmates will invite the whole class to birthday parties on weekends; while this is a great way to connect with other families in your school and community, if your family is overwhelmed with invitations it is okay to RSVP "no" from time to time in order to protect family time.

Children ages 8–10 years: Kids these ages have strengthening friendships. Invite these special friends to join your family—you can share some family time and also get to know your child's friends better. Simplicity is best— your child can invite a friend for dinner with your family followed by board games or a movie. Kids these ages can be helpers in the kitchen; have a weekend morning breakfast buffet and work together to flip pancakes and assemble a fruit kabob station.

Children ages 11–12 years: Preteens often have a hectic weekend schedule including sports team competitions, religious services and education, recitals, and more. Make sure you step back from time to time to look at the big picture. If you and your crew are exhausted by Sunday night, feeling stressed about not having enough time to make necessary preparations for the new week ahead, it is time to prioritize top commitments and let go of the less important things occupying your time. Your family needs protected time to simply be together, relaxing or engaging in something low-key and fun like a nature walk. This is especially important if you have multiple children in your family. There will be times of the year that will inevitably be more hectic than others (for example, August and September, when families are adjusting to a new school year, and December's holiday season), but a *balance* is a healthy choice for sanity and family connectedness.

mined to take ballet, work out a practical schedule for getting them to and from these activities. Morning routines will usually have to be altered so as to get the children ready in time, and carpooling arrangements may need to be made.

When one of your children has a special school assignment due, the weekend may be the best time for her to work on it. She should have all the materials she needs for the project, and thus trips to the library and stationery store may need to occur the previous week. Keep some time open in which you'll be available to help her if the need arises.

On weekends bedtimes may be a bit later than during the week, especially if you are gathering with extended family or friends. However, it is wise to not veer too much from the usual sleep/wake cycles. If a child spends weekend nights up too late and sleeps in the next morning, Monday morning and the "return to reality" will be a challenge. Sleep patterns are improved in the long run if attempts are made to keep weekend bedtimes as similar to weekdays as possible.

Family time on weekends is essential, and it is equally important for parents to set aside some time to reinforce their individual relationship. This strengthens the parents' bond with each other and sends a positive message to the children. Kids will enjoy their time with a trusted sitter while parents reconnect. (For more information, see page 303.)

From time to time, evaluate how your family allocates time. Are your family's weekends an opportunity to rejuvenate and reconnect? Or do you feel you are overscheduled, running from one activity to the next, scrambling on Sunday evenings to get the family ready for the new week? Be mindful of the big picture, prioritize your family's plans and activities, and don't be afraid to decline or say no to the items lower on the priority list. It's okay to RSVP regrets to a birthday party of a classmate that your child does not know very well in order to attend a family function. Be vigilant with your precious time, as it is all too easy to overextend yourself, resulting in frayed nerves and burnout.

Your Family Rituals

Every family should have activities that they enjoy together that become a regular, predictable, and integral part of their lives. Some can be serious pursuits, like attending community functions or religious services as a family; others can be more lighthearted, like going fishing or taking family bike rides. Whatever they are, they can help bond a family together.

Family meals. Connecting together over a meal, whether it is the evening dinner or a big breakfast on Sunday morning, is a great way for families to reconnect. Turn off phones and the TV, and put away other electronic devices.

Important conversations. Communication between parents and children should be a top priority in your family. Set aside time to talk, discussing the day's and the week's activities, sharing feelings, and really listening to one another.

Respect the privacy of each of your kids as they begin to assert their independence during these middle years; they may have certain problems and difficulties they may not want to divulge to their brothers and sisters. You should be able to have a one-on-one conversation with each child without all the other children listening in. If you honor his wishes for confidentiality, this can build trust between you.

Some families establish a weekly time for a family meeting. When everyone is present, family issues, relationships, plans, and experiences are discussed, and everyone from the youngest to the oldest gets a chance to be heard and to participate.

Recreation and cultural activities. Family recreation is an important way to strengthen the family. Sports (participation and spectator), games, movies, and walks in the park are good ways to increase cohesiveness and reduce stress.

Grocery shopping. Food shopping trips can provide regular opportunities for parents and children to spend time together. Let your children make lists, find items in the store, bag produce, carry the bags to the car, and unpack them once

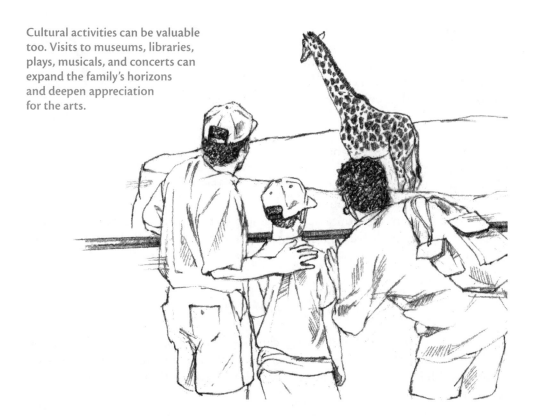

Cultural activities can be valuable too. Visits to museums, libraries, plays, musicals, and concerts can expand the family's horizons and deepen appreciation for the arts.

you return home. Allowing your child some choices and assigning some meaningful responsibilities can help build his self-confidence.

Reading time. Whether together or individually, reading time should be a scheduled part of the days and weeks. When kids see parents reading regularly, whether it be the daily newspaper, a book, or a magazine, it sends a positive message and establishes reading as part of the culture of a home. E-reader devices are okay also; however, because some have internet and gaming capabilities, ensure that reading time with an e-reader is truly reading. For younger kids, reading together is wonderful bonding time and boosts literacy. Reading together as part of a bedtime ritual is a wise move, and that idea can be extended to a quiet Saturday afternoon as well.

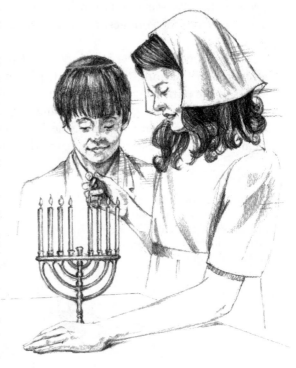

Holiday traditions. By learning about the history, significance, and rituals of a particular holiday, children will feel a greater sense of involvement in the holiday preparations and celebrations. As the years pass, these traditions become part of the family culture and history.

Spiritual pursuits. For many families, religion plays an important role in providing a moral tradition, a set of values, and a network of friends and neighbors who can provide support. Families can attend religious services together.

You do not necessarily need to go to a church, synagogue, or other place of worship regularly, however, to share moral values with your children and help them develop a sense of their history and the continuity of the family. Many families develop a strong spiritual life without the formal structure of organized religion.

Family Disruptions

When family disruptions occur, they can be stressful for every member of the family. Illness, conflicts, work-related travel, deployments, unexpected setbacks, mental health issues, or substance use can all interfere with the normal course of family life.

Illness and Injury

Whether it is a parent or a child who becomes ill or injured, the entire family is affected. While even a short-term illness like the flu can disrupt the normal activities of a family, a chronic disease (from cancer to epilepsy) can affect the way a family functions.

For a child in middle childhood, reactions to illness depend on a number of factors, including the nature of the illness (severity, course, and treatments), her previous experiences with medical problems, her resilience, and the support she receives from the family.

You may need to do some adjusting to the illness as well. With a short-term disease you might feel stress until the condition disappears. With a chronic illness you may experience feelings of guilt, fear, anger, or helplessness. You may need to set aside time for treatments as well as conferences with physicians and other healthcare professionals. You will need to learn as much as possible about the illness and its care.

With a chronic or long-lasting disease, you need to comfort your child. Explain the condition as honestly and fully as possible, and what she can expect by way of treatment and cure. Be realistic; do not make promises that can't be kept. Encourage your child to express her feelings too; not only should she feel free to talk with you about anything on her mind, but she should be able to trust the medical team. Discuss how to communicate about the illness with friends, classmates, and teachers. If it appears that your child is having strong emotional reactions or troubling behavior, she might also benefit from counseling. Remember that even younger kids usually know more than adults give them credit for. Ensure that your communication with your child is honest but simple.

(For additional information, see Part VII, "Chronic Health Problems.")

Arguments and Conflicts

Disputes between you and your children are inevitable in family life. If your family never has arguments, it probably means that issues are being avoided. To become productive adults, children need to be able to voice their opinions—even if they disagree with yours—and feel they are being taken seriously. That said, you can and should keep the negative impact of arguments to a minimum by adhering to the following guidelines:

- Prioritize and be selective about the issues you and your kids disagree on. When a potential problem arises, decide if it is really worth the battle; some issues probably are not. For example, if your child wants to wear an old

How to Have a Family Meeting

Weekly family meetings are an effective way to bring the family together, improve communication, set weekly goals, recognize and reward progress, and determine each member's needs and feelings.

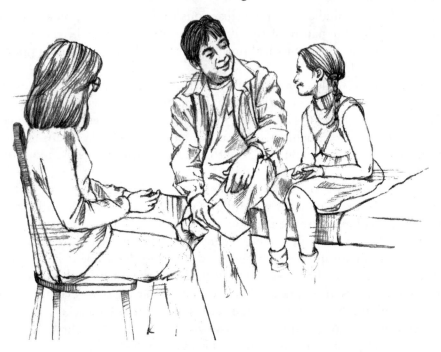

1. The meetings should occur at a regular, pleasant time—for instance, after dinner.

2. Parents can serve as discussion leaders and make sure that any ground rules are clearly explained and understood.

3. The meetings should emphasize both individual and family needs, goals, and accomplishments and discuss positive events and efforts. During the meeting parents can give allowances and praise and reward behavior progress and changes. They can also share other relevant family information, such as an upcoming school event to prepare for.

4. Each family member should be allowed to speak without criticism or interruption, to share his or her thoughts, feelings, achievements, and hopes.

5. The meeting is not a time or place to scold, punish, recall past mistakes, blow off steam, or single out a particular person. Those issues should be taken up separately and individually.

6. The meetings should last no more than twenty or thirty minutes unless the family wants to continue.

7. Everyone should understand and accept that parents have the final word in difficult decisions.

8. A record should be kept of the main points, rewards, progress toward goals, new goals, and agreements.

9. Before the meeting ends, anyone who wants to should have a chance to say how he or she thinks the meeting went, and what might be done to make the next meeting better.

pair of sneakers to school rather than the newer pair you recently bought her, or if she wants to wear her hair a little longer than you would prefer, you might decide to let her have her way, choosing to take a stand on more important matters instead. Pick your battles carefully.

As long as disagreements stay within certain boundaries, they are an acceptable and productive form of communication. They can continue as long as they are under control, remain respectful, and are moving toward a solution. Discontinue them if they degenerate into name-calling, if calm voices are replaced by shouting, or if you and your child are going around in circles without progressing toward a resolution. Never laugh at your child, no matter how ludicrous her arguments sound to you; by laughing you are essentially ridiculing her, minimizing her and what she is saying.

If you are unhappy with the essay your child wrote about the Civil War for school, for example, the two of you can discuss what you perceive to be its shortcomings. But remember, it is *her* school assignment and *her* responsibility. Her teacher is the ultimate judge. If the dialogue between you and your child starts to get personal ("You don't know what you're talking about!"), then it's time for a break. Tell your child: "This discussion isn't going anywhere. We need to stop, cool down, and come back to it later." Resume the dialogue later in the day, when one or both of you might have a new approach to the problem.

Some families actually schedule these follow-up discussions. A parent might say, "Come back with five points to support your argument, and I'll have five to support mine." Families can even create a format for these dialogues: the child speaks uninterrupted for five minutes, and then the parent responds during the next five minutes; after another round of five minutes each, you might find areas where you can agree or compromise.

- Let your child "win" sometimes. When you and your child argue, you need to do more than listen to her point of view; when she presents a persuasive case, be willing to say, "You convinced me. We'll do it your way." Let your child know that you value her point of view, that conflicts can be resolved through communication, and that sometimes her perspective on an issue has enlightened you.

- If conflicts about particular issues recur again and again, take a look at root causes and deeper issues that may be what is really at play. Think deeply about why you and your child are arguing about these matters, and try to take preventive action. For example, if your child rebels against going to bed each night, she may be using her outbursts as a way to stay up a little longer, or to get more attention. Or if she repeatedly argues about doing her homework, try to put an end to these conflicts by actually writing up a contract stipulating the expectations, responsibilities, rewards, and punishments for doing (and not doing) homework. Remember that the homework assignment is made by the teacher and is your child's responsibility. She may not do it your way, but if she is satisfying the school's requirements, you should not turn it into an issue at home. Both you and your child should sign the contract, agree to abide by it, and hopefully end the disagreements about the subject.

- Do not forget that children learn how to handle disagreements by watching their parents' example. How readily do you and your partner have "good" arguments, which end in successful reconciliation? Or do you stay angry, or avoid fights altogether? Your children model themselves by watching you.

Departures and Returns

Do you or your partner frequently travel for work? Are you or your partner serving in the military on an overseas deployment? These can be disruptive times for your child and for the family as a whole. To minimize problems, prepare your children for these extended separations. Spend as much time as it takes to explain where you are going and why.

Your child may be sad, anxious, angry, or all of these before and during your

Special Considerations for Military Families

A military deployment is challenging for all families, but especially if kids are involved. New stresses occur when a mom or dad has to take on the entire parenting role without a partner; kids not only absorb this stress but have their own issues. A school-age child will worry for his parent's safety. A 12-year-old has the usual preadolescent issues, but may also be angry with his parent's absence for a longer stretch of time.

What can families do to make deployments less stressful for the child? Beforehand, learn about programs and resources available to learn about what to expect. This includes feelings and reactions both at the beginning of deployment and when your partner returns home. Preparations will help you avoid surprises and handle issues as they arise. Open discussions help mitigate the stress; be sure to listen to your child and answer her questions in as straightforward and age-appropriate a way as possible. Let your child know that you are sad too, that it is okay and normal to have feelings, and that you love your child and will support her.

Monitor media use, as reports of bombings are stressful for kids. Older kids may have related school projects or hear people talking about it; parents should talk with kids about what they're reading in the paper or seeing on the news. Emails, letters, video chats, care packages, and journaling can help kids stay in touch with their parent. A stuffed animal, special necklace, or special photos of the deployed parent can help a child feel closer to that parent. Maintain the usual family schedule as much as possible to minimize disruptions that can add to the child's stress. If you feel your family needs additional help during the stress of deployment, discuss with your pediatrician what options are available.

Deployment stress symptoms can vary depending on the child's age. School-age children may have changes in eating or sleeping patterns, have physical complaints such as headaches or stomachaches, or display regressive behavior. Eleven- and 12-year-olds may be moodier than usual, may lose interest in normal activities, or may act out with risky behavior such as smoking or alcohol use. A child's stress may actually increase when the deployed parent returns home, either from fearing a future goodbye again or if the parent has her own physical or mental health issues. If your child's stress remains or increases after the deployed parent returns, counseling may help.

travels. You need to acknowledge and accept her feelings: "I know you're going to miss me. I understand that you feel this way. I'm going to miss you too." In addition to missing you, your child may also feel inconvenienced, insecure, unsafe, or worried about how you and she will fare during your absence. For those serving in the military, there is the added aspect of the parent's safety.

Remind your children that you will be back soon. And while you are away, maintain contact with phone calls, video chats, and texting, as well as written postcards or letters. Once you come home, make your return special; spend some extra time with your child and do something together that she enjoys.

Unexpected Setbacks

What happens if you lose your job? Or if the family has financial problems? These disruptions can be unsettling for your child. At times parents may try to shield kids from financial troubles, but keep in mind that children are smart and often know more than parents give them credit for. It is important to be honest and help your child deal with the situation directly.

If the family is having financial difficulties, your child does not need to know all the specific details; however, she deserves an explanation of why she may not be able to return to the same summer camp she attended last year, or why you may not be able to buy her the exact pair of sneakers she wants. Children need to know: "Mom lost her job, so we're going to have to reduce our spending until she finds a new one."

Children can be just as concerned about disruptions in the extended family—for example, the news that her uncle and aunt are getting a divorce. Don't be surprised if she asks what exactly is happening and how it might affect her relationship with her cousins. She may ask you: "Are you and Dad going to get a divorce too?"

It is unwise to protect your child from these kinds of family problems. Keep in mind that if she sees you becoming anxious, without an obvious reason, she may misinterpret it ("Is Mom upset with *me*?"). Keep the channels of communication open, encourage your child to express her feelings, and reaffirm the importance and the stability of your family: "Even though Dad has lost his job, we are all going to stay together as a family and we are all going to be okay." It is exactly this kind of challenge that can actually strengthen the family as they navigate the highs and lows of life together.

Parental Mental Health or Substance Use Problems

Depression or other mental illness in a parent affects all family members and colors their relationships with others. Depressed and anxious parents tend to create a less positive emotional tone in the way their family interacts. They do not respond as quickly or as appropriately to the emotional needs of their children. Many children of depressed parents may have problems relating to their peers or may have a lower self-esteem. These children can often benefit from close relationships with adults outside the family and from professional counseling to help them develop ways to handle the stresses within their families.

The children of alcoholics and other drug users may have similar problems; in fact, many adults struggling with depression turn to alcohol or substance use. Although family experiences vary, these kids often grow up with more negative life experiences, and a decreased sense of togetherness and open communication. Drinking is also tied to a greater incidence of parental depression, family violence, and marital problems. Active participation in school and extracurricular activities can go a long way toward helping these children achieve success and happiness. In the meantime, affected parents need to seek professional help.

Special Events in the Family

Holidays, birthdays, anniversaries, weddings, vacations—these are special times in a family's life and can create lasting memories. As treasured and important as these events are, some families try to make too much of them. Parents may try to turn each birthday party into the best one ever, or they feel they have to fulfill every wish on their children's gift lists. Inevitably, that kind of attitude creates anxiety and disappointment, since few events turn out perfectly.

Birthdays are a chance to celebrate a person's life; the experience of being together and sharing special times should be the focus, rather than on material presents. Many families are shifting the focus of these special events by celebrating with *experiences*, not *things*: for example, in lieu of hectic parties and excessive gifting, an alternative idea is to share a special experience with two or three close selected friends, such as an outing to a nearby city museum or a movie followed by a sleepover. Studies show that by producing pleasant memories, experiences boost long-term happiness—something that material items can't do. Some families with multiple children find a birthday to be a great opportunity to have a one-on-one meal with just the birthday kid alone; the year-round family schedule can be hectic, and this provides some terrific special time. Special events such as family gatherings, school recitals, and band concerts are other times to demonstrate the specialness of the people you care about.

In making decisions about vacations, think back to the summers of your own childhood. What did you like most about your family vacations? What do you wish you had done more often? The answers to these questions will help guide you toward what may be important to your own child. More than anything, children remember that their vacations took them to locations other than their home, that

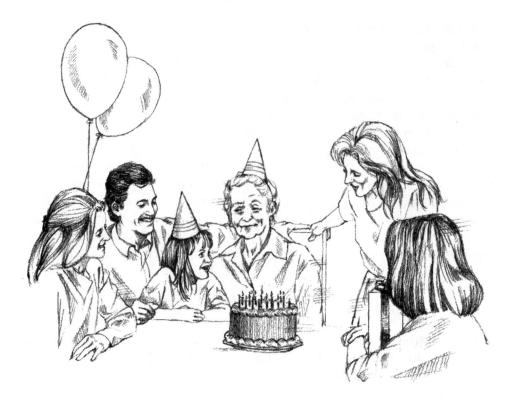

the family got to spend time together, and that there were long days and memorable experiences they did not get to enjoy the rest of the year. Often the car or plane ride itself is the most enjoyable aspect for kids! Do not fret if things go awry on your dream vacation; often these mishaps become the stuff of family legend.

Family Moves

In today's shrinking world, job transitions, job loss, and transfers are forcing some families to move frequently, across town, across the country, and even around the world. These moves can be quite difficult for the whole family but particularly for the children.

Most people think that, in general, moving is harder on an older child—middle school students, for instance, who are asserting their identities, forming meaningful friendships, and becoming achievement-oriented. Older children do benefit from permanence and stability. Nevertheless, younger school-age children have adjustments to make too, even if they seem more flexible. Children, of course, are different, and no two will handle a move quite the same. Stresses such as moving will tend to accentuate different aspects of your child's personality.

Positive Aspects of the Move

In helping your child prepare for a move, place as much emphasis as possible on the positive aspects of what awaits her. This is an opportunity for her to live in and learn about a new city, perhaps even a new country, and its people. She may be exposed to new cultural traditions and interesting and different ways of life. It also is a chance to meet new people and make new friends. Explain how the family will benefit from the move.

For some children the opportunity for a new beginning is an exciting prospect. It gives them a chance to be accepted in a new setting and to make friends free of their former reputations and self-images. Be cautious, however, of unreasonable expectations that a move will make things wonderful. Children take their likes and dislikes and personal strengths and weaknesses with them.

Children may worry about the negative side when a family moves. There is the loss of friends and, along with it, loss of a sense of belonging. In the new community the children will be newcomers and may need to learn some different social rules. In changing schools, they might have to leave behind extracurricular activities—a sports team, a school drama program—that were important to them. If they have been active soccer players, for example, signing up for a new team in your new community is a fantastic way to ease this transition. Upon arriving at their new school, they may find themselves either academically ahead of or behind their new classmates, depending on the curriculum in the previous school.

Making the Transition Easier

There are a number of ways in which you can make the move easier on your children. Keep these suggestions in mind during the planning stages and as you are adjusting to the new neighborhood:

Let your child express her feelings. Give your child adequate notice to get used to the idea of moving—even a year in advance may be appropriate. Acknowledge her sadness about leaving behind friends and familiar places. Let her know you are sympathetic and that you understand that she might feel nervous about what awaits her, whether it is the new people, the new school, or the new bus ride. At the same time, emphasize some of the positive aspects listed earlier.

If you are also experiencing stress about the move, be open with these feelings, keeping in mind that your own anxiety might rub off on your child. For that reason, try maintaining and communicating an optimistic attitude about what lies ahead. The stress of moving is greatest about two weeks before and after the move. Be sure to take breaks to relax and play.

Emphasize the excitement of moving. Remind your child that the move will be adventurous and interesting. Use the example of the pioneers (the Laura Ingalls Wilder Little House series) or the immigrants who overcame obstacles and traveled to new lands, where they encountered new and stimulating experiences. Give her some age-appropriate books that describe families moving from one city to another. Encourage your child to make plans for the move. Have her make lists of tasks and projects to do. Your child can research her new community online to teach the family about fun facts and interesting aspects of your future hometown.

Take your child to the community where you will be moving. She will probably discover that the new city is really not that different from the one she is leaving. Drive by her new school, and even contact school staff ahead of time for a potential visit and tour, so she can get a sense of what awaits her. Much of her fear of the unknown should dissipate with this trip.

Look for new things your child might enjoy. For example, if the family is moving to a larger house, maybe your child will get a room of her own for the first time. Perhaps the new city has a zoo or a science museum that she might find interesting. If you are moving to a different climate, there may be opportunities for new activities (skiing, sledding, ice skating; or, in warmer climates, the chance to play outdoors year-round). Plan in advance to enroll your child in sports, clubs, lessons, and the like so she has something to look forward to. Give your child the chance to participate in decisions that directly affect her.

Become involved in the new community. As you meet new people through local schools, groups, or organizations, you can open doors for your child to make new friends and connections. Reach out to people who have children about the same age as your own. Invite them over to make it easier for your child to meet other children. Investigate community sports activities, YMCAs, and Boys and Girls Clubs. As your child sees you finding your place in the new neighborhood, she will feel more comfortable and secure doing the same. If you are successful in finding a new friend for your child before school starts, they will have the security of knowing someone on the first day of school.

Maintain contact with the old community. If your child wants to keep her old friendships intact, help her do so. Host a farewell party with her friends, and take photographs as keepsakes. Encourage her to write letters, video chat, and make phone calls. If possible, visit the old neighborhood from time to time, and invite some of her old friends to spend time with you if possible. Let her know that even though you have moved, she does not have to break the ties that have been so important to her.

Make the move a family event. If you plan the move as a family and support one another as you adjust to the new community, it can bring your family closer together.

~ 20 ~

Your Development
as a Parent

AS THE SCHOOL years progress, children and parents alike evolve and develop, responding to the different challenges and situations that growing children experience. Your parenting style inevitably will evolve; how you parent your 5-year-old will (and should) be modified by the time your child reaches middle school. No single approach to parenting works for all families. Parenting is hard work and an extremely personal experience. Each family—and within that family, each parent-child relationship—is different. There is not a single way to raise a child. Rather, the goal should be a good fit between family values, family culture, and the child's temperament. You need to find out what works best for you and your family. Good parenting is often a matter of trial and error. A better understanding of your own parenting style, why you are drawn to the decisions you make, and the expectations you have will help you become the type of parent you wish to be. Parents should keep in mind that as a child grows through the school years, our job is not to solve every problem for the child; rather, we should nurture self-empowerment skills in our kids to promote resilience and life skills, in an age-appropriate way.

Parenting Influences

Many of the factors that influence the way you act within your family had their origins long before you became a mother or a father.

Your Childhood Experiences

Parents take into account their recollections of their own youth when setting their standards and expectations for parenting. As a first step toward understanding your own approach to parenting, and to use that information in a positive way, examine it through the prism of your own childhood. To begin, answer the following questions:

1. What do you remember about the family you grew up in, particularly your relationships with your parents? What do you appreciate most about their way of raising you?

2. What did you most enjoy doing with each of your parents? The answer to this question might give you a clue to the activities your own child might enjoy doing with you.

3. What were the greatest difficulties you had with your parents? This information might help you avoid problem areas with your own children, while understanding why you respond to certain parental situations the way you do. For instance, if you felt your parents were too strict, you might become too permissive with your own child; if you believe your mother and father were too withdrawn and quiet, you might insist upon talking with your child a lot.

4. What do you feel were their greatest shortcomings as parents? If your own father became abusive when he got angry, for example, you might feel anxious whenever tempers flare in your own household, and you might try to avoid angry confrontations.

Even though you may consciously try to avoid the actions of your parents that you thought were wrong, do not be surprised or upset if you find not only your parents' words but also their tone of voice coming out of your mouth. Pay attention to this experience and remember that children learn from what they see and hear.

You can also learn a lot from childhood relationships with your brothers and sisters. Ask yourself questions like: What were the best aspects of your relationship with your siblings? What did you enjoy doing most with them? What problems and conflicts did you have with them? How do you feel your parents handled these conflicts? If you were an only child, you might have difficulty adjusting to the way your own children relate to one another; you may find sibling fighting concerning, although sibling bickering is normal to some degree. Or if you were the oldest (or the youngest) child in your family, you might unconsciously identify more with your own oldest (or youngest) child.

As you reflect back on your childhood, think about the significant events that took place. What do you remember about moves to a new city? Starting school? Illnesses or injuries? Losses (the death of a pet, a friend moving away, a stolen bicycle)? These childhood memories can affect how you relate to your own children today. If you had a tough time moving to a new neighborhood when you were young, you might find it hard to put your own child through the same experience. If the first day at a new school was always difficult for you, you might feel especially anxious when your child changes schools.

Examine your own memories of teachers and classmates, your academic performance, what you liked and disliked about school, and important school events (tests, oral reports, class trips, science fairs). Think back upon your childhood friendships too: best friends, adversaries, activities with other children, and how you adjusted to changes in friendships, which are all normal situations in everyone's childhood. Keep in mind that technology has advanced and our kids have more access to the internet and its connectivity than most of us parents had growing up. Tackling media challenges is uncharted territory in this regard, and parental monitoring is a must. For more on media, see page 315.

As you reflect upon your childhood experiences, you might recognize how they have influenced your responses to your own child's interactions with others. For instance, your child may prefer coming home after school, playing a musical instrument, doing homework, and not spending much time in social activities. However, if you yearned to be more popular when you were young, you might push your child to participate more in sports or Scouting activities, although he might have no interest in them. These are issues you need to become more sensitive to.

As part of this self-examination, talk with your child about your own childhood recollections. He will love to hear stories about what life was like for you when you were his age. It will give him a sense of history and belonging. It will also help him through difficult times once he finds out that you too might not have been invited to a party you really wanted to go to, or that, like him, you had fears about giving an oral report in front of the class.

Your Personality Traits

You cannot change your personality, but by understanding your personal characteristics, you will get a better sense of how you approach others (including the members of your family) and what your strengths and weaknesses as a parent might be. Are you shy or outgoing? Are you intellectual or intuitive? Open-minded or opinionated? Self-assured or insecure? Rarely is anyone always one way or another, but we all have tendencies we should recognize as we approach child-rearing.

Although children are born with uniquely individual temperaments, certain personality traits develop through life experiences. For example, if your child has a tendency to be verbally expressive of his feelings, or if he is an affectionate child, he probably acquired these characteristics growing up in the family environment. Or if you or your partner complains a lot, he may tend to whine. Generally, children identify more with one parent than the other and unconsciously assume more of that parent's traits. If your own personality characteristics fit with or match those of your child, you may find living with him much easier than if your personalities conflict. (See "Temperament," page 131.) The more accepting you are of your own traits, the more you can relax and be a better partner and parent.

Keep in mind, however, that certain personal characteristics can have a negative impact on the family—for example, judgmental people tend to be critical of themselves as well as of others, which can interfere with the way they relate to their children; the offspring of judgmental parents often grow up feeling inferior or rejected. At the other extreme, however, some parents may accept *anything* their child does, even if he has adopted bad habits or negative values. You need to find a balance between these two extremes and communicate and model those personal traits you value.

Your Early Parenting Experiences

There is a whole history to your parent-child relationship that began at the moment your baby was born. To help you better understand the present, try to gain some insights into where you have been as a family. Think back on your experiences with your child when he was a baby, a toddler, and a preschooler. Ask yourself:

- How active a parent were you in those early years? Did you play a major child-raising role in the family, or were there other demands (such as long hours at work) that kept you from being as involved as you would have liked?

- What were your most enjoyable parenting and family experiences during those years?

Since those first years of your child's life, your parenting techniques may have changed. Perhaps you were quite anxious as a new parent but gained confidence as the months and years passed. Ask yourself questions like:

- What have you learned as a parent? What were the hardest skills to learn?

- What were your best traits as a parent of a young child? What were the areas in which you had the most problems? For example, did you find it difficult to relate to your child before he started to talk? Was it difficult for you to set limits when he entered toddlerhood? How did he respond to you in your parenting role?

- How did you develop yourself as a parent as your child grew? How successful have you been in making those changes? Keep in mind that as your child grows, you and the entire family need to change too.

Even if you made mistakes during those early years, you can amend them now. Children are understanding and forgive their parents for shortcomings. If you weren't there when your child took his first steps or rode his tricycle for the first time, you can be there for other special events to come, like your child's school play and his soccer games.

Your Current Parenting Experiences

Your child's school years are a time of transition, in which your child is seeking more independence and is questioning the family's rules. And, from time to time, you may have to help him with school-related issues. He will be developing more peer relationships too, and his interactions with siblings may change. While many parents are tempted to solve every problem that arises for their child, they should encourage their kids to tackle their own issues in an age-appropriate way, so that the children develop resilience and life skills.

When our children are babies and toddlers, they depend heavily on a parent for nurturing, food, and safety. As our children grow into the school years, parents need to be conscious of the fact that our role evolves. Our job is not to anticipate every roadblock ahead of time, or take care of every problem that comes our child's way. Often these tendencies are referred to as "helicopter parenting" (hovering nearby, ready to swoop in and resolve a situation) or "lawnmower parenting" (working ahead of the child, anticipating problems, smoothing out the path for the child). Life is full of inevitable bumps and roadblocks, and if a child does not get occasional practice developing these life skills, starting as early as second or third grade, they will not be emotionally or practically equipped to handle issues in the high school years and beyond.

Practically speaking, what does this mean? If your third-grader forgets a homework sheet at home, do not make a special delivery to the school. She can explain the situation to her teacher, experience the natural consequences, and from this early age learn better preparation skills than simply responding to parental reminders. If your fifth-grade competitive swimmer forgets to pack swim goggles for a swim meet, don't run home and grab them to "rescue" your child; she can brainstorm solutions and perhaps borrow a pair from a friend. These incremental steps of experiencing life's inevitable roadblocks will help develop resilience and life skills, and better prepare the child for the bigger challenges she will encounter in future years.

Your Child's Developmental Needs and Personality Traits

Your child, like all children, is unique, and thus there are differences in parenting each child. Some children are easier to manage than others. Each child's individual characteristics will affect your approach to parenting and the way your family functions. (See "Temperament" on page 131.)

As your middle-years child moves through particular stages of development, your own personality can influence just how well you adapt to these phases. For example, if you tend to be a parent who values routines and sets a lot of rules, you may experience challenges with a rebellious and controlling child. In the same way, if you are an energetic and sometimes impatient person, you might have trouble with a low-key and slow-moving child. These are the types of issues to reflect upon in order to better understand your relationship with your family.

Stages of Parenting

You had certain responses to your child when he was an infant and preschooler, and are now experiencing new issues as he enters school and negotiates new relationships outside the family. Children's entry into school and growing independence give parents an opportunity to consider what changes they would like to make in their relationships with their children. During these years separation becomes an issue for many parents: The child who once relied on them for almost everything has now become more independent. The trade-off is that the child may be more capable of new forms of companionship with his mother and father. As children approach adolescence, parents must learn again, as they did during their child's preschool years, to cope with challenges to parental authority.

Nagging Is Often Counterproductive

If you find yourself reminding your kids of the same tasks on a regular basis, it is time to take a step back and prioritize. Nagging sends a message to your child that you do not trust his ability to make the right choices on his own without reminders. Think of your own interactions with others; does the third, fourth, or fifth time hearing something help? Often the message is simply tuned out at that point. Nagging fosters resentment and sends a message that you, the parent, are in charge of the issue at hand, rather than handing over the reins of responsibility to the child.

Instead of nagging, listen to your child's concerns and perspective, and have an honest discussion about ideas he may have regarding the issue at hand. Prioritizing safety and education, you may decide to let certain issues slide for the sake of the big picture (approval of fashion choices in the third grade is an excellent example). At times, natural consequences may be the best option. Instead of constantly nagging a fifth-grader to bring an umbrella to the bus stop, recognize that getting caught in the rain isn't the end of the world and will serve as a better reminder than anything a parent can say. Within reason, natural consequences teach a lesson in a more memorable way than parental reminders.

Your Current Life Issues

For many men and women, the stress in their lives interferes with their ability to parent. If they are unhappy on the job, for instance, they might return home preoccupied and tense at the end of the day and be unable to handle the tasks of running a family as effectively.

Take a moment to assess how you feel about these and other important aspects of your life.

- Your career and occupation

- Your relationships at work

- Your living conditions, including your home and neighborhood

- Your lifestyle, including time for yourself and leisure activities

- Aging: growing older, slowing down, and experiencing changes in your body

- Your relationship with your partner

- Your relationship with your parents and siblings

- Your friendships

Evaluate problems in these areas, and how they might be influencing your family life. Whenever possible, find ways to deal with these difficulties in your life more effectively, so they will not interfere with your parent-child relationships.

If you are like many parents, your day is so filled with job and family responsibilities that you have little to no downtime, when you become a priority. Keep in mind, however, that most parents are happier people and better parents when they make time for things they find pleasurable, whether it be a book club, cooking or a craft, sports, or other hobbies. As your children move through their school years, they will develop interests and responsibilities (from friends to homework) that can provide you with more time for those activities that you find enriching. You do *not* need to devote every free moment to playing checkers or baseball with your children; in fact, as long as you are also setting aside some time for your child, they will probably feel good knowing that you are pursuing your own interests that you really enjoy. In addition, be wary of overscheduling your child; running from one activity to the next isn't doing anyone any favors. Everyone, both child and adult, needs downtime to refresh and rejuvenate.

Your Relationship with Your Child's Other Parent

To some degree, your own parenting style is affected by your adult relationships, most particularly the one with your child's other parent, whether you are married to that person, separated, or divorced. Think about how the two of you have divided up the tasks of parenting—from making sure your child gets up in the morning on time to tucking him in at night, and everything in between. How well is this arrangement working? Is the division of child-rearing labor equitable, which not only prevents burnout and resentment but, most importantly, models teamwork and cooperation to your child?

Ideally, both parents should work as a team, nurturing their children and family, showing consistency, and providing support for each other on issues like discipline. The two of you should communicate regularly about what is happening with your children. If there are particular issues that you regularly disagree on, you need to discuss and try to resolve them.

- Do you trust the other parent of your child—that is, how comfortable do you feel with his or her style of parenting? If you go away for an evening or a few days, leaving your child in the care of the other parent, are you confident that he or she will care for your child responsibly? How do you respond to his or her difficulties with your child? Keep in mind that often moms and dads can have a yin-yang approach and it can be healthy for kids to see that there is more than one way, or style, of parenting.

- Do you and the other parent have similar values and priorities regarding the family? Do you have similar expectations of your child's behavior?

- What kind of role models are the two of you providing for your child? Do you and the other parent apply the same standards of behavior for yourselves that you do for your children—that is, do the two of you expect your child to behave in a way that you yourself live up to?

Problems and Solutions of Co-Parenting

As you and your partner, or former partner, share the responsibilities of parenting and managing the family's day-to-day activities, problems will arise. Here are a few of the most common difficulties that today's parents encounter.

Inconsistency

Often parents differ in their rules and expectations for their child. Mom might say, "You can't have screen time until your homework is finished," but when she's away, Dad may say, "Go ahead and watch TV if you want to." Dad might insist that the child's bedtime is 8:30; Mom may say that stretching it until 9:00 is fine. Similar conflicts can develop over issues like approaches to discipline or a child's choice of friends. When these inconsistencies occur, one parent inevitably undermines the authority of the other.

To begin to resolve this problem, you and your spouse need to be explicit with each other about what your rules and expectations are. If necessary, write them down, review them, and be sure they are workable. In areas in which you differ, find a compromise that you both can live with—and stick by it.

Lack of Communication

If you and your spouse do not talk about the issues the family faces, one of you may be left out of important matters you should be informed about. To avoid this situation, you and your spouse need to commit yourselves to communicate about every significant issue in your family life. At least once a day the two of you need to check in with each other and discuss what happened that day that was important. At the same time, talk about long-term issues that may be confronting the family.

Confusion

Uncertainty about what stands to take and what rules to impose can create turmoil within the family. Too often, parents are perplexed about issues like the degree of supervision required for their children and the amount of freedom to give them. Parents frequently do not make decisions at all, and that can leave their children puzzled over what is expected of them. You and your partner need to resolve your own ambivalence on important family matters and agree on a position on these issues. Then you must clearly inform the entire family about your decisions and how their own lives will be affected by them.

Competition

Sometimes rivalry can develop between parents over their children's attention and love. If Dad wants his child to spend Saturday afternoon fishing with him but Mom wants her to go the library with her, they may struggle to get their way, putting the child in an unenviable position, right in the middle of the conflict. The two of you need to find ways to cooperate, not compete, with each other. You don't need to agree on everything, but you should be committed to working together toward a more harmonious relationship and family life; don't let differences undermine your common goals. Each of you needs to demonstrate some flexibility.

Overt Conflict

Parents will argue and openly challenge each other on family-related matters. Perhaps their child has gotten into trouble at school, and the parents disagree about how to handle it; the mother may think the child should be grounded, while the father believes it wasn't her fault. They start to argue—sometimes for hours or even over a period of days—and eventually, rather than resolving the problem amicably, one parent wins out because the other ultimately gives in, at least for the moment. The parental power struggle often begins all over again at a later time with a different issue, with some of the same anger from the previous conflict resurfacing. The wounds never fully heal and the animosity builds.

Parents need to learn the skills of conflict resolution. These include:

- Listening

- Clarifying points of difference

- Taking each other's feelings seriously

- Generating alternative solutions together

- Negotiating

Remember, the way you handle conflict in your family is how your child learns to manage disagreement. Many community colleges offer seminars and courses on conflict resolution. Partner therapy may be needed as well.

Parenting Principles

Parenting is one of life's biggest challenges. It requires loving, respecting, and empathizing with your children. It involves protecting, guiding, communicating, teaching, showing patience, setting limits, and resolving conflicts. If you feel you fall short in some of these areas, bear in mind that they can be acquired skills, learned and improved upon at any time.

Successful parenting begins with understanding and valuing yourself and your children. Without self-respect, you may have difficulty tolerating the inevitable trials of family life.

Too often, parents strive for perfection, but there is no such thing as the perfect family and the perfect parent. Every member of the family unit needs to work toward accepting the humanness of every other member, including faults and limitations. Rather than striving to be perfect, everyone should work toward doing your best, given your current circumstances.

A second key to successful parenting is understanding your child—reading his cues correctly, engaging in dialogue and listening carefully, and appreciating what makes your child unique.

When family difficulties arise, trust your gut and listen to your heart as well as your head. You have better parenting instincts than you think. There are few definitive "right" answers, so use your experience as a guide. Maintain connections with people you can talk to, share feelings with, and turn to for support and guidance, both inside and outside the family. Do not allow parenting to become a lonely experience, or you risk having frustration and fatigue get the best of you. In particular, parents of multiples or special-needs children benefit from connecting with other families dealing with similar circumstances. If you feel you need additional parenting support, discuss this with your child's pediatrician.

The Impact of Relationship Problems

Interpersonal relationships do not exist in a vacuum. If you and your partner are having relationship difficulties, they are likely to disrupt the entire family. When your relationship is not going well, your parenting skills and your children will suffer. Sometimes children are a convenient excuse for not dealing with serious relationship difficulties. Parents may think, "The kids require so much of our attention now; once they're grown, we'll have a lot of time to talk about the problems we have in our own relationship." Problems tend only to become worse with time, and once your children are grown, you may not have much of a foundation to build on.

The adults in the most successful families do not neglect relationship problems. They commit themselves to spending time together as a couple and working together to resolve any misunderstandings, jealousies, or conflicts. They make a commitment to communicate, praise, and forgive each other; they try to understand each other; and they routinely examine their relationship and how it can be improved.

~ 21 ~

Brothers and Sisters

AS CHILDREN GROW during the school years, parents can be surprised to discover how different each child is from his siblings, even though they have grown up in the same family. Differences among siblings are the rule, not the exception. A challenge for parents is to identify these differences and nurture each child as an individual.

The most obvious differences among siblings are in age and gender. Differences are also evident in temperament, interests, confidence, resilience, vulnerability, social style, sense of security, achievement in a variety of domains, physical and mental health, rate of physical and sexual maturation, and physical appearance. Even identical twins are two distinct individuals. While diversity and differences may be a source of pride for parents, they may also be a source of confusion and frustration, as well as uneven attention, praise, and other displays of affection.

Nature vs. Nurture

What are the factors that influence your child's personality and other attributes? Two major influences are at work: *nature* (genetic factors, heredity) and *nurture* (experience). These interact with each other in ways that are particular to each child. To better understand the similarities and differences among siblings, let's look at both of these factors more closely.

Nature

Because of heredity—the biological or genetic influences of the parents on each child—parents might expect their children to be alike. Overall, children have only about a fifty-fifty chance of expressing any particular inherited trait (physical appearance, personality, intelligence, aptitudes, health), and even when these traits are present, they can vary.

For instance, researchers have found that siblings tend to be more similar in their physical characteristics than in their likelihood of developing the same diseases. Also, while siblings may resemble one another in their intellectual aptitude and other psychological characteristics early in life, these similarities generally diminish by adulthood, while differences become more pronounced. Siblings with similar levels of intelligence may differ in their school achievement, since academic success can be strongly affected by the different life experiences of each child. Even identical twins can vary in personality and temperament.

Nurture

Nurture, or a collection of experiences, refers to the *non*-hereditary influences on your child's development. They include social factors such as relationships with siblings, peers, parents, and other adults, as well as environmental influences like illnesses, accidents, nutrition, and cultural experiences. Other forces come into play as well, including your child's perceptions of herself and others, past experiences, self-expectations, and the expectations others have of her.

Siblings share some experiences but have many others that are not shared. While shared experiences generally contribute toward similarities, even a shared experience may affect each child differently. And since most experiences are unshared, they contribute to differences between children too.

In the early school years, for instance, qualities such as intelligence and academic achievement are largely determined by heredity and shared experience. However, as children grow, they have more unshared experiences, which gradually help differentiate one sibling from another. Siblings even perceive and interpret shared events differently, and these different perceptions can be important in shaping a child's development and self-image.

Influence of Parents and Siblings

Do you treat all your children alike? Probably not. You *should* relate to and treat each child differently. Treating each child as an individual is part of what makes that child a unique person and is a way of appreciating his special characteristics. Remember that there will be stretches of time when one of your children "needs" more of you; this is normal and to be expected. The goal is to have balance over time with all of your children.

A first child "teaches" a parent how to parent, in a manner of speaking. As a result, the parent's relationship with that first child will be different from his or her relationships with subsequent children. Since parents develop and learn along with their children, parents' actions, conversational style, and displays of emotion will change with each new addition to your family. Younger siblings learn from their older siblings in addition to their parents.

Not only do parents change their style as they gain experience raising children, but each child has his or her own temperament and needs, initially because of birth order and inborn traits, and later because of experiences. Older children should be treated differently than younger ones. Sensitive children need different approaches than do easygoing ones. On every issue—rules, expectations, chores, responsibilities, rewards, and punishment—parents must individualize their parenting while striving to be fair to all. This last goal is nearly impossible to achieve. Even if parents interact with their children in a comparable manner, each child may perceive these actions differently.

Your behavior toward your children is determined in part by the age and developmental stage of each child. For example, you probably have tended to treat all your children in a somewhat similar way at the same age or level of development. A parent may be physically affectionate to her two children in their respective toddler years but less visibly affectionate when they reach school age. In a situation like this, the older child may perceive that the younger sibling is receiving more affection. Parents *should* treat children differently at different ages; problems occur when parents are not able to act appropriately for their child's developmental age and needs.

Birth order and family size also influence your children's development. The experience of an only child is different from that of a child in a larger family. An older child's experience is different from a younger one's: the older child has a younger sibling, while the younger child has an older sibling. A third child has two older siblings, and so on. Because of birth order and family size, no two children experience the same family the same way.

The birth order of your children also will affect the way you relate to them, the way they respond, the experiences they have, and thus the way they develop as individuals. For instance, firstborn children may feel neglected or unloved after the arrival of a new sibling. Though their parents may expect or at least hope for them to be more responsible and self-sufficient, firstborns may act younger or regress in order to attract parental attention. In turn, the parents may express frustration or anger with them because of their immature behavior.

The temperaments of parent and child influence the way each interacts with the other. A parent whose temperament fares best with order and predictability could find raising a disorganized, spontaneous, impulsive child a daily challenge. On the other hand, easygoing parents and children can readily make allowances for one another.

Each pair of family members has a unique relationship. A child relates in different ways to his father and to his mother. His sibling relates to each parent in his or her own way. Each sibling relates to each brother or sister in a particular way. Children are quite sensitive to these differences within family relationships; they monitor them, respond to them, and relate to one another in a manner based upon the nature of their experiences and how they perceive them. Some of the differences among siblings reflect how they perceive their roles and relationships within their families—how they have been loved, appreciated, respected, and understood. These factors can influence their self-confidence, sense of trust, and ability to cope with challenges and disappointments.

Over the years the relationships among siblings can contribute to increasing differences. Siblings compete for the affection and attention of their parents; they may compare themselves with one another, become aware of one another's strengths and weaknesses, and try to find the most comfortable and rewarding role for themselves within the family unit. In this dynamic interaction, differences develop and can become more pronounced with time, affecting everything from self-esteem and behavioral style to life goals and career choices.

Biological Differences

Age and gender are the most readily apparent differences and similarities among siblings. Older children earn certain privileges, in part due to the greater level of responsibility they are expected to assume in the household. Younger children may require special consideration because they are less independent.

Sometimes parents have difficulty treating children of similar ages differently, even though they realize that each child could benefit if they did not. All too often, boys and girls are treated differently in our society, which can lead to self-fulfilling prophecies in terms of academic success and other realms. Children have different physical, psychological, and social abilities. For example, a child with a learning disability may need extra time being read to or helped with homework. The special attention these children require can be a source of jealousy and conflict unless it is handled well.

Parents face a difficult juggling act in meeting the varying needs and expectations of their children. If you take time to listen to and observe your children, you will be more aware of their different perceptions and needs and can respond more successfully to each of your particular children and to the whole family.

Influences Outside the Family

The new people and experiences encountered by children in school, play, and other everyday events all contribute to sibling differences. Each encounter provides a unique opportunity for the child to test her innate personality and learned skills and wisdom with different people and new social situations. These interactions continually shape a child's perceptions, attitudes, beliefs, understanding, and behavior.

For instance, a child often has a particular relationship with friends. When a friend of one child is in the house, other siblings may join in their playing, but each will have a different way of relating to the visitor. These peer experiences can contribute significantly to the way a child views herself, and they magnify the differences between her and her siblings.

The way a child interacts with other people is strongly influenced by her relationships within her own family. Family experiences not only shape the personalities of individual children but also establish the patterns of interactions that will occur outside the family.

What Differences Mean for Parents

As you watch your children grow, remember that their similarities or differences are not as important as their overall development toward becoming positive, productive, healthy, and kind human beings. In order for your children to reach those goals, they need to feel loved, trusted, competent, and respected for who they are, not for who they are in comparison with their siblings. Children who are raised in this way will develop resilience, self-confidence, the capacity for risk-taking, the ability to set and achieve goals, and a sensitivity and respect for others. Parents should accept, appreciate, and respect the basic uniqueness of each of their children and nurture each child's individuality.

~ 22 ~

Sibling Rivalry

EVERY PARENT WITH more than one child has experienced the frustration of sibling rivalry. Despite best attempts at maintaining harmony in the family, brothers and sisters will fight over toys, argue, tease, or criticize each other. As upsetting as this rivalry can be, some jealousy and friction between siblings is a part of growing up.

Why does rivalry among your children occur? In part, it is a competition for your attention and love. You are very important in their lives, and they would rather not share you with anyone, particularly a brother or sister. That in itself is enough to cause dissension. Other factors contribute to this rivalry as well, including your children's personalities, their mutual or differing interests, their ages, the amount of time they spend with one another and with you, and even favoritism you may show toward one child, however unintentional. With so many factors at play, some squabbling is inevitable. (See Chapter 21, "Brothers and Sisters," for a discussion of sibling differences and similarities.) With patience, love, understanding, common sense, and humor, parents can handle sibling rivalry in a positive manner. The silver lining is that sibling rivalry will actually help your kids practice and develop social and interpersonal skills.

The Positive and Negative
Sides of Siblings

Brothers and sisters play very positive roles in each other's lives. They provide companionship and serve as ready playmates and confidants. They help one another learn to relate to the outside world. At times, they may find themselves protecting each other. As they grow, they have many of the same experiences and will share similar memories of family gatherings, holidays, vacations, and even family crises. They may have little secrets they share only with one another. These kinds of experiences can bond siblings for a lifetime.

Even the minor bickering is not all negative. Some squabbling is part of childhood and human nature. Kids develop social skills by interacting with their siblings. Children will try to dominate one another, to assert their authority, and to test different aspects of human relationships. Provoking responses from a brother or sister, whether that response is pleasant or conflicted, is part of children's normal and necessary learning. Through these interactions, siblings learn to be assertive, say what they are feeling, stand up for and defend themselves, and problem-solve to find solutions to their disputes. As they compete with one another, they can push themselves to excel.

However, when the rivalry becomes mean-spirited and creates stress and tension within the family, consuming a lot of a parent's time in breaking up and resolving arguments, then it has gone beyond the bounds of normal sibling competitiveness. If one of your children is aggressive or physical toward another, it has gone too far.

What to Expect

Although sibling rivalry can be present at any age, it tends to become more intense as children grow older, often peaking in the 8- to 12-year-old range. Siblings of the same sex are usually more competitive, as are siblings close in age or those who have similar interests.

In many cases, the oldest child in the family feels a greater sense of rivalry than the younger ones. The younger children may look up to and idolize the older brother or sister; by contrast, the oldest child may see his siblings as intrusions upon his privacy or the family unit and a threat to the special attention and status he is used to getting from his parents. Alternatively, younger kids can "gang up" on an older sibling. At its worst, sibling rivalry can take a serious emotional toll upon one or more children in the family. A child's self-esteem can suffer if he is being constantly harassed, belittled, or bullied by a brother or sister.

Brainstorm Different Ways to Strengthen Sibling Relationships

Sibling relationships teach children social skills as well as how to navigate long-term relationships. After all, the sibling connection is likely to be your child's longest-lasting relationship, lasting even longer than a parent-child relationship. Living together, sharing the same space, parents, and household, and possibly a bedroom, teaches kids give-and-take, how to share, and how to step away when needed, which are all great social skills for future relationships.

Just as it is important for a parent to spend one-on-one time with each child, it is nice for kids to spend time with only one sibling, separated from other siblings. For families with more than two kids, it can be healthy to break away from the crowd from time to time. For example, take just two kids with you for the weekend grocery shopping; this affords your 12-year-old and your 8-year-old some time together without the chaos of the rest of the crew.

On birthdays and holidays on which gifts are traditionally given, consider having each child brainstorm or craft a gift to give to each of their siblings. These gifts need not, and should not, be expensive—set a budget of less than $10. A special drawing, painting, or object created in art class costs next to nothing and means so much if it comes from the heart. The exercise of thinking about what the sibling enjoys or what hobbies she likes is a great way to help a child place himself in someone else's shoes and look at things from her perspective. Since younger kids often enjoy giving a gift that they *themselves* would enjoy, parents can help coach the child to think about what the *sibling* would truly enjoy. As an example, a 6-year-old could help select a desk organizer for $5 that would arrange his 9-year-old art-loving sibling's marker collection. You can help your child wrap the gift (a tricky skill and terrific to learn early on) and will enjoy the look on his face when his sibling opens her special gift. The gift of a small token or homemade craft, while a simple gesture, can allow the giver to feel a sense of pride and joy at having made someone else happy, and help the recipient realize that her sibling *does* notice her interests and hobbies. Families who have initiated this tradition enjoy seeing the creative ideas kids come up with, and how, through a simple gesture, kids can forge a stronger connection. The emphasis is not on the material item itself; rather, it's the thought that counts. This tradition is a simple way to help siblings think considerately of one another.

Stepsiblings

Stepfamilies have another variation of sibling rivalry. When two families become one, children adapt to a new marriage, stepparents, and perhaps a new home. When there are conflicts within the new family—for instance, disagreements over whom to visit during holidays—children may band together with their own parent, forming camps and aggravating any rivalries. (See Chapter 32, "Stepfamilies.")

What Parents Can Do

Sibling rivalry can change the dynamics of the entire family. Fortunately, there are ways to prevent or minimize problems.

Preparing for the Birth of a Sibling

Prior to the birth of a new baby, you can prepare your school-age child for the addition to the family. A child beyond the age of 5 is usually not as threatened by a newborn as a younger child is, particularly if the middle-years sibling has good self-esteem and feels loved and valued. Nevertheless, resentment may surface because of the attention the infant requires.

To prepare your child, be honest and straightforward about what is about to happen, using language he can understand. Explain the impending arrival of his new brother or sister, noting the changes that may affect him—both the good and the not-so-good. Have him help get the house ready for the arrival of his new sibling, fixing up the baby's bedroom, picking out a new crib, buying diapers. If your child is going to be moved to a different bedroom, make the move at least several weeks before the new baby is born, thereby spreading out the changes in his life over a longer period.

If possible, arrange for your older child to visit you at the hospital so that he feels included and part of the expanding family. Then, when you bring the baby home, make the newborn's sibling feel that he has a role to play in caring for the baby. Tell him he can hold the infant, although he must ask you first. Compliment him and use positive praise when he is gentle and loving toward the baby. When friends and relatives visit, ask them ahead of the visit to make a point to talk to your older child first, and then ask your older child to "introduce" them to the new baby. As challenging as this transition time is, don't make everything about the baby. Thankfully, newborns sleep a lot; use this as an opportunity to spend one-on-one time with your older child to talk about (or do) something unrelated to the baby.

During the first few busy weeks, respect the needs and activities of your older child. Give him permission to talk about any negative feelings he is having about the new sibling. Tell him: "A new baby means more work for the family, but if you ever feel that I'm not spending enough time with you, let me know so I can give you plenty of extra love." Make an effort to spend some time alone with him each day. Remember that babies grow quickly and within a few months everyone will be on a new, smoother routine.

Rivalry with Older Children

As your children grow and mature, treat each of them as an individual to minimize sibling rivalry. Every child should be recognized for her distinct achievements and strengths. Make sure you *listen* to each child, demonstrate your concern for her interests and needs, and ensure time alone with her. Show all your children that they are loved and valued.

To cut down on conflicts, clearly explain that there are different rules for each child based on age. Although you will do your best to be fair, things will not always be *equal* for the siblings. While a 12-year-old may stay up till 9:30 at night, an 8-year-old's bedtime might be 8:30. Electronic devices may be a privilege for older kids in the family, and your 9-year-old may wonder why she cannot have a tablet as well. (For more on media, see page 315.)

Teach your children that everyone in the family has his own personal space and belongings. Your middle-years child should ask his older sibling for permission to play with a board game that doesn't belong to him. He should respect the privacy of his brother or sister.

When it comes to chores in the family, make certain they are divided fairly. If there is a particular household job that none of the children enjoy—perhaps helping with the dinner dishes or carrying out the trash—be sure that everyone takes a turn with this responsibility. Many families simply rotate trash duty week to week among the children, writing down whose responsibility it is each week in the family calendar so it is clear and fair.

Cooperation and compassion are important family values to teach. As you spend time together as a family, children can learn the importance of supporting and caring for one another. They should be sensitive to any emotional distress that others in the family may feel from time to time, thinking beyond themselves and their own individual needs. Children learn a lot about relating to others by observing how their parents interact. Be conscious that the way you and your partner treat each other, respect each other, and resolve your differences presents a model that your children are likely to follow.

Avoid making comparisons between the children. For instance, one child may be a high achiever academically, while another struggles to get B's; or one child

Different-Age Siblings, Different Expectations

A challenge of having more than one child is that kids of different ages are at different developmental stages and are ready for different responsibilities and privileges. Younger children may not always understand why older siblings have certain privileges (allowed to see a certain movie they are not, for example), and older siblings may wonder why they are expected to perform more household chores than their younger siblings. As a parent, you will likely need to remind each child that privileges are *earned* with maturity and greater responsibilities.

Children ages 5–7 years: Younger kids may not understand why older kids are allowed to see certain films that they are not. Many superhero or action films are rated PG-13 due to violent scenes, yet manufacturers create toy sets based on these characters and market them to the younger children. It is an option for families to avoid toys based on films intended for older audiences to minimize misunderstanding and conflict; explain to your kids why the toys are not appropriate.

Children ages 8–10 years: These are the in-between ages, when children are maturing in some realms but not others. While ready for more independence navigating schoolwork and household chores, they still require limits on screen time and other privileges.

Children ages 11–12 years: Older children who wish to earn future privileges such as their own phone or increased screen time need household responsibilities, as well as self-initiative to complete their chores without frequent reminders. Education should be a top priority. Family decisions to increase certain privileges by age should be made hand-in-hand with frequent discussions with the child about the increased expectations that come with age. Older kids may wonder why 6-year-old siblings don't have to take out the trash; remind them of the difference in their privileges and expectations.

may be a star athlete, while another is more interested in creating art than participating in sports. One child may have a particular talent that is not appreciated by other family members, and as a result may feel sidelined and act out his feelings. Differences can be acknowledged in a positive way without negative judgments and comparisons being made. However, insensitive discussion of these differences can be very hurtful and may escalate hostility between siblings.

Rather than making comparisons, look for the strengths in each of your children and encourage their individuality. You might have to search out new interests and activities, nurturing them in each child. Also, find an activity each of your kids can do just with you, so they know you see them as special individuals. Children who might feel they are being "outshone" by a sibling may feel resentment toward that sibling. A child's own distinctive personal activities and interests can help him experience success and find a niche where he is not in competition with his sibling.

Resolving Problems

Siblings have a responsibility to solve their own conflicts reasonably and appropriately. The Golden Rule should be a theme in your home: treat others the way you wish to be treated yourself. Parents should set parameters for how siblings should resolve their disagreements—for example, physical violence is never acceptable. Act as an impartial judge, and help the children themselves negotiate their differences and solve their mutual problems.

Arrange regularly scheduled family meetings in which each child voices his concerns and desires. Additional meetings can be convened quickly for unforeseen incidents and issues that should be aired. In these discussions, allow each child to express his grievances toward the other, without interruption, name-calling, or other abusive language. Let them know that while these disagreements among siblings are normal, hurtful language and physical aggression are not permissible. After all sides are heard, restate the opposing viewpoints. Ask the children themselves to propose solutions to the conflict, and help them reach a middle ground. Initially, they will need help, reminders, practice, and rule enforcement from you. Eventually, they should be able to do this on their own.

Find out the reason for your children's resentment toward one another. It might be as simple as an argument over the choice of a TV program. However, it can go much deeper, perhaps with one child taking out on a sibling the hostility he feels toward *you*. It is much safer to lash out at a brother or sister than to shout or swing at a parent. Intense rivalry may reflect family tension or problems that are expressed through the children but don't originate between them. As you teach and discipline, be careful not to label one child as being the cause for all sibling conflicts, making him the scapegoat in the family. In some families, a timeout for both children involved in a conflict works well, letting tempers cool down before a solution is sought. (See page 204.)

At times, once the facts are on the table, it is clear that one child is at fault. In those instances, you may need to intervene with some consequences or guidelines to prevent the situation from recurring. Be fair and firm with your decision, making a statement such as "When your brother is doing homework in his room, you can't walk in and begin playing with his toys. He needs quiet. Knock on his door, but if he asks you not to come in, you have to respect his space."

As children grow older, sibling rivalries may decrease in intensity. An 11- or 12-year-old may develop more interests outside the home—perhaps youth sports or Scouts activities—and that can ease sibling conflicts. In the long run, efforts toward encouraging cooperation will be worthwhile.

~ 23 ~

Child Care

AN INTERESTING ASPECT of children's middle-years development is that at the beginning of this time of life, children require nearly continuous supervision, while at the end, they are much more autonomous. During the early years of middle childhood, they need reliable adult supervision, but as they approach adolescence, they may start to take on some limited child care responsibilities themselves.

Most families use a combination of child care arrangements to meet their specific needs. The arrangements may include parents only; care by a relative; before- and after-school programs; care by sitters, friends, or neighbors who are not relatives, either in the child's home or in an outside child care home; child care centers; and specialized child care for kids with special health needs.

Finding appropriate child care for your school-age children is a significant task. The first step is to determine what type of help you are looking for. Are you interested in someone who can watch the children on occasional evenings, or do you need a person to help out on a daily basis? Are you considering hiring someone to live in your home and to assume other duties such as housekeeping? How much can you afford to spend? What are your children like, and what kind of person do you think would be best suited to watch them? These questions need to be kept in mind when selecting child care.

Child Care Tips

How do you investigate local child care options and assess their quality?

- Ask neighbors and coworkers about the child care providers they use.

- Ask your pediatrician for recommendations.

- Look at quality online resources such as:

    - Child Care Aware of America (childcareaware.org)

    - The Child Care Resource Center (ccrcca.org)

    - National Association for the Education of Young Children (naeyc.org)

    - National Association for Family Child Care (nafcc.org)

Child Care Options

Before- and After-School Care

For school-age children, many communities have options for before- and after-school care. These may be offered by the school district itself, child care centers, home child care programs, youth programs such as the YMCA, or churches. Start by connecting with your child's school district to see if an on-site program is available, since a program offered by or contracted with the district can greatly simplify your family's transportation needs. Not all after-school care programs are regulated by the state; search on childcareaware.org by zip code to look into your local options. Such regulations set minimum health and safety standards and monitor regularly for compliance, but they are not the only markers of a quality program. Parents should also monitor online compliance reports on any program they select for their child.

When investigating before- and after-school care programs, ask the program's staff about caregiver-to-child ratios, the daily schedule including homework time and meals or snacks, and how staff are trained to administer first aid, CPR, medications if needed, and prevention strategies for child abuse. Once your child is enrolled, monitor his progress and proactively raise issues as they arise with the child care's staff.

Child Care by People Other than Relatives

If you are looking for an occasional sitter, you might decide to employ responsible adolescents from the neighborhood, typically teenagers who are looking to earn an income. There is an advantage to having young people as babysitters, since they can be energetic and entertaining for your children. The disadvantage is that they may be less strict than you are with discipline, and they may not be as experienced in handling problem situations. If your child is close to 12 years old, you will need someone considerably older to babysit; a teenager only one or two years older is not likely to have much authority. Be sure to speak with the parents of any teenager you are considering hiring, to get a sense of how he or she handles responsibility. It is also a good idea to check with other families who have used the teenager for sitting.

A good strategy is to develop a list of two or three sitters who know your child and can be called upon if your regular sitter is busy or ill. Make sure they all understand the rules that apply to sitting at your home regarding TV watching, internet usage, texting, visitors, smoking or drinking, telephone use, and taking your child outside.

If you need a sitter on a more regular basis, you may need to employ an older person. Word of mouth, online agencies (including background checks), and local colleges are a few ideas to recruit people. What qualities should you be looking for? In general, he or she needs to be mature, reliable, and friendly with children. He or she should be someone with whom your child enjoys spending time. As your child gets older, she should have some say in your selection of caretakers. Kids are very smart and have great intuition about people; respect their opinion.

Interview applicants thoroughly to get a sense of their reliability and competence. Ask them about other positions they have held, the ages of children they have cared for, and what their responsibilities included. Inquire about how they would handle various situations (such as your child not wanting to do homework). Ask about activities they enjoy doing with children. Explain your expectations clearly—for example, will the child care involve housecleaning? Ask for, and carefully check, references.

If one person stands out among those you've interviewed, have him or her come for a visit while you are home. Introduce him or her to your child, and pay him or her for an hour of child care while you are home as well. This first encounter will help you determine if the person is a good fit for your family. Later, ask your child about the sitter, and be receptive to her comments.

The hourly rate for sitting varies from community to community. In general, pay should increase with responsibility and with the competence of the babysitter. Caring for multiple children or adding household chores to child care merits a

Age-Appropriate Activities
with the Sitter

Give your sitter plenty of non-screen-time activity ideas with which to engage children:

Children ages 5–7 years: Children in this age group can read books, either picture books on their own, or a chapter book together with the sitter. Trips to the library are a great way to spend time on a rainy day, and best of all, the books are free. Play outside, weather permitting. Bike rides (always while wearing helmets), nature walks, and unstructured playground time are all good options. If there is inclement weather, look beyond building blocks' intended purpose; take a quieter part of the home and create a new "neighborhood" combining different random toy sets. Outer space action figures will enjoy having a tea party in a dollhouse.

Children ages 8–10 years: Like the younger kids, these children will benefit from library trips, reading time, and puzzles. Outdoor playtime can be unstructured at a playground or a more structured nature walk, weather permitting. In addition, kids this age can play more sophisticated board games. Don't forget about the classics such as chess. Don't know how to play chess yourself? No problem—many starter chess sets come with pieces that have the moves they are allowed to make printed right on the piece itself. Keep a spare side table ready to support a puzzle—the kids can work on it when able, and then safely set it to the side for a break, saving the partially completed puzzle for the next session.

Children ages 11–12 years: Being older and more mature, they won't need the degree of constant supervision that a 5-year-old needs. That being said, kids this age need to prioritize staying on top of school obligations, including homework and ongoing class projects. Kids should also remember their household chores (just because there is paid child care doesn't mean kids shouldn't have their own responsibilities; see the list of age-appropriate chores on page 310). After homework and chores, weather permitting, go outside and play.

higher hourly rate. In the weeks and months ahead, monitor your sitter and how he or she gets along with your child. Work with the sitter to improve his or her understanding of your child. Give advice and suggestions, and reinforce his or her positive qualities and strengths.

Some families prefer to hire an au pair. Typically, this is a college-age person from another country who agrees to live and work in the United States for a spec-

When Your Child Wants to Babysit

In the middle years, many children learn babysitting skills by being taken care of by an older sister or brother, or by helping their parents care for younger siblings. At some point, they may express an interest in becoming a sitter, and by the age of 13, they may be ready to do so.

Schools and organizations (YMCA, local hospitals, and fire departments) often provide courses in babysitting. However, nothing can compare to experience, preferably under the observation of an adult. Preteenagers, boys and girls, can seek some on-the-job training by working as a mother's helper, assisting in the care of young children when a parent is present in the home. This is particularly valuable if the family has expressed some interest in hiring your child as a sitter in the near future. She can observe how the parents interact with their children, while getting to know the children before taking full responsibility for them. She will also discover the tasks involved in babysitting, and how each child must be approached somewhat differently.

If your child has shown interest in becoming a sitter, emphasize to her the responsibility of taking care of someone else's children. When she is asked to sit, help her plan her schedule so other tasks such as homework do not conflict with the hours she has committed to child care. Also, assist her in formulating questions to ask the parents who are hiring her, such as what is expected of her and what she will be paid. Help her brainstorm activities she can do with the children.

The American Academy of Pediatrics publishes a training program called *BLAST! Babysitters Student Manual: Babysitter Lessons and Safety Training*. This program is designed for people ages 13 and older, their parents, and parents looking to hire a babysitter. The program can prepare children to begin babysitting safely and competently, with information on how to interview for a babysitting job, how to select safe and suitable games and activities, prevent accidents, and perform first aid.

ified period of time (usually one year). While an au pair can be expensive, he or she can bring cultural richness into your family. Recognize, however, that many of these individuals also need to be given support and assistance in adjusting to the United States. To find an au pair, use an agency that specializes in these placements.

Some families develop cooperative arrangements with neighbors or family friends who also have children; the families take turns providing child care for one another. Even in these cases, be sure you are clear about the rules you expect to be applied to your children. It is also helpful to keep track of how much child care each family is providing, so no family feels that the exchange of service is out of balance.

No matter what kind of sitter you select, make sure that the person with whom you leave your child has a list of all emergency phone numbers, including where you can be reached at all times, and the names and numbers of trusted neighbors, relatives, and your child's pediatrician. Make sure to have 911 and the national poison control center number, 800-222-1222, displayed on or near the phone at all times.

What should you do if your child challenges the sitter's authority? First, find out exactly what happened, talking to both the child and the sitter. In many circumstances, it will be appropriate to stand behind the sitter; a united front aids the sitter's role as an authority figure. However, if your child expresses a dislike for a sitter, or protests when hearing who is going to sit, take your child's concerns seriously. Explore what the problem is, and remember that with regard to child care, your child's safety and well-being are top priority.

Finally, be considerate of your sitter's time. Schedule and (if necessary) cancel well in advance. Respect the sitter's wishes to be with his or her family and friends on holidays and other special occasions. Remember, a good sitter is a valuable resource.

~ 24 ~

Responsibilities and Chores

AS CHILDREN GROW through their school years, they are increasingly able to manage homework and school projects on their own. Each year they should also take on more responsibilities in the classroom and at home. During the middle years kids can help clean their rooms, make their beds, pick up their toys, and help out in the kitchen or the yard. Kids can feed and care for pets. These daily chores and responsibilities are an important part of a child's development.

Parents should assign age-appropriate responsibilities to each child, as each child should be a contributing member of the family. Younger kids are naturally eager helpers—take advantage of these instincts and develop a teamwork spirit as a culture in your home. Pitching in with household tasks teaches life skills and cooperation with the group (in this case, your family). Self-esteem is boosted by contributing to the home running smoothly. Responsibility and initiative are learned through a gradual process of guidance and reward. Remember to keep expectations age-appropriate. Do not expect perfection in the early stages; praise the *effort* involved. Smaller steps taken now lead to further steps in the future.

Age-Appropriate Chores to Assist the Household

Kids who perform household chores develop life skills, boost self-esteem, and learn teamwork and responsibility from a young age. Start kids early; if you didn't already get your kids helping in preschool, now is the time! Don't insist on perfection; this is a learning process and children will develop their skills over time. Praise your child's effort in each task, not the outcome. Be consistent to make chores and household help the routine and the norm, rather than the exception. A specific chore chart or checklist can help as a visual reminder to keep all members of the family on task and provide each child with a sense of accomplishment with each completed task.

Children ages 5–7 years: Make their own beds, set and clear the table for mealtimes, weed and rake leaves, make and pack school lunches (for more on this, see page 412), dust, put toys away, neaten bookshelves, put dirty clothes in a hamper, fill pet's food dish, empty wastebaskets, sweep floors, sort laundry, bring in mail/newspaper, water flowers, and wash plastic dishes in the sink.

Children ages 8–10 years: All of the above, plus vacuum, help make dinner (for more on this, see page 32), make their own snacks, take a pet for walk, put away their own laundry, and put away groceries.

Children ages 11–12 years: All of the above, as well as clean the kitchen, change bedsheets, unload the dishwasher, do and fold laundry, scrub toilets and clean the bathroom, wash the car, cook a simple meal with supervision (see page 32), and watch younger sibling(s) with an adult present at home.

Staying on Task

As your child takes on more responsibilities, he will likely have periods of procrastination or needing reminders about expected chore fulfillment. Most kids do. During these times, encouragement, gentle guidance, and positive praise will point him in the right direction. Keep chores age-appropriate; most importantly, keep it fun. Especially for younger kids, if chores are fun, they won't even realize they are "working"! Sometimes parents may ask too much of their children, or criticize the outcome of the chore. They may assign too many responsibilities, resulting in children feeling overwhelmed and resisting taking on any responsibilities at all.

Parents need to avoid overloading, while still making sure that their children are assuming an appropriate level of responsibility. Children will inevitably differ in the personal traits and temperament they bring to tasks. Some are simply not very persistent and drift away in the middle of chores. Still others have trouble shifting from one activity to another. You should have a good sense of your child's style, and shape your expectations accordingly.

Children need to have obligations and duties within the family so that they learn to accept responsibility. Families whose kids are overscheduled in too many sports and extracurriculars may feel the child is too busy for chores and might not instill this basic life skill; this is a mistake. Ensure that kids develop skills to contribute to the household, with increased expectations as they mature. At times kids may point out different levels of responsibility their friends are assigned at their respective homes; as with many parenting situations, this is an opportunity to inform your child of what *your* family's rules and culture are.

What Parents Can Do

Keep chores fun and praise kids' effort, not necessarily the outcome. If your child procrastinates or needs frequent reminders of responsibilities and chores, here are some simple management techniques that are helpful:

1. Carefully spell out the tasks your child must perform. Make sure she understands what is expected of her on a daily and weekly basis. Star charts or chore lists posted in your child's room or on the refrigerator should clearly show what your expectations are. With a school-age child, particularly one who has not taken on responsibilities before, you should introduce one new task at a time; a long list can be overwhelming.

2. Honest praise from you can be the most effective way of motivating your child and guaranteeing her success. As your child completes a regular task, praise her and the effort she made. Initiating tasks on her own without a reminder, completing a special task, or doing an unusually good job with a regular one merits praise. You may also want to consider tangible rewards like allowances and stickers tied to completed chores.

3. Your child has a greater chance of remembering her chores if your family life has structure and routines. Encourage her to do her chores at the same

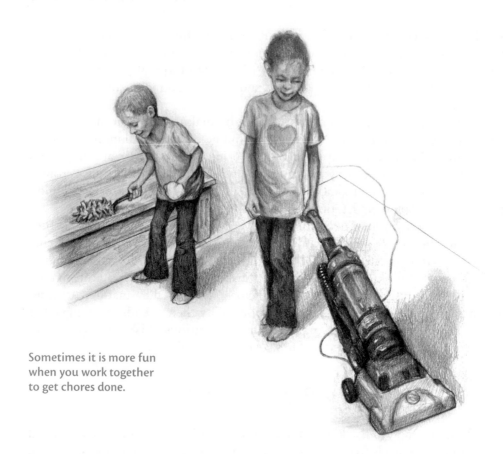

Sometimes it is more fun when you work together to get chores done.

time each day. Routines of other activities—including meals, homework, play, and bedtime—also can teach organization and help her develop responsibility.

4. Schedule family meetings at regular intervals to review your child's progress. Ask her for her ideas regarding chores and other responsibilities. Create new or modified "contracts" for the chores that are expected of her. Most important, supervise and support your child, which is the best way to ensure that she is being responsible.

5. When your child makes a choice not to complete her chores and other responsibilities, it may be necessary to implement consequences. For example, you might decide to revoke certain privileges or special activities. Badgering or scolding a child is not an effective method to get her to accept more responsibility. Rewarding successes and providing positive encouragement is always much more effective. Remember that electronic devices and screen time are privileges, not rights.

If you are concerned that your child is not taking on his household responsibilities appropriately despite various efforts, review your concerns with your pediatrician, who may reassure you that your child is behaving in an age-appropriate manner. The pediatrician may be concerned if your child *consistently* fails to complete everyday home responsibilities in addition to having similar issues in the school environment.

Allowance for the School-Age Child

While an allowance is certainly not mandatory, some families decide a weekly allowance is appropriate for their child. Some families tie the allowance to chores; other families see chores as part of the responsibility of being a member of the family and unrelated to the allowance. If you are considering starting an allowance for your child:

- An allowance for doing chores motivates children to assume responsibilities around the home. These tasks should contribute to the family's (and not just the child's) well-being. Yes, children need to learn to care for themselves (clean up their room), but they also need to contribute to the family.

- An allowance introduces children to the value of money—to saving, budgeting, and planning. These are life skills that are important to acquire. School-age children are not ready to assume the responsibility for purchasing necessary items, from clothing to school supplies, but their allowance can be used for discretionary purchases. For that reason, it should be only a modest amount (for more on money management, see Chapter 27).

Make sure your child clearly understands the purpose of an allowance. If you use it as a reward or payment for chores, then the rules should be clear about what your child needs to do to earn that money, and you need to abide by the agreement that you make. If the allowance is provided for discretionary spending and to teach money management, then a different set of rules applies. Spell out the amount, purpose, and expectations for the money in advance, and monitor the spending to teach important decision-making lessons.

~ 25 ~

Media

OUR CHILDREN AND our families are increasingly surrounded by media of all kinds. Every day children are inundated by endless messages intended to educate, entertain, or influence their behavior. Many of these sounds and images appear in media with the explicit intention of selling a product. Others, such as movies, computer games, and music, may be the product. Children in the elementary school years are frequent users of these products and important targets of advertisements. It takes commitment and effort on the part of parents to monitor, co-view, and help children interpret these external influences. Growing children also begin to delve into the internet, at first for school-related tasks and research, but in later years to play games, seek information, and text and interact with peers on social networking sites.

Your School-Age Child and the Internet

The internet, texting, social networking, television, online videogames, and email are a part of our daily lives, and are available twenty-four hours a day, seven days a week. As early as the toddler years, children learn how to watch and use screens and engage in the social aspects of digital connections from their parents and the adults in their world. Whether it's cuddling next to Mom as a toddler says hi to Grandma across the country or gathering with friends at a birthday party to smile and say "cheese" as Dad takes a smartphone photo or video to post on social media, young children have been interacting with media for most of their lives.

As with so many other aspects of parenting, it is key to remember that our children are learning lessons from us, their favorite role models, whether we are consciously aware of this or not. Parents can model good digital habits and citizenship for their children. How do *you* use technology in your everyday life? Do you check email on your smartphone frequently? Do you respond to text messages during family mealtimes? Are you able to enjoy a family function while having your smartphone stowed away, living in the moment as opposed to taking frequent photos throughout the activity? Respect for others means being attentive to them in the moment. Children are eager for their parents' attention, and, even at this age, face-to-face parent-child interactions are important for learning and social development.

Some parents might find evolving technology overwhelming. It is a challenge to keep up with the new apps and interactive games emerging on a continuous basis. Fads seem to come and go fast and furiously; a parent might finally understand a new online game using GPS location tags, only to be left in the dust with the latest and greatest must-have virtual reality program. Nevertheless, it's important for parents to educate themselves about the available digital options for their children; to test out a new app, game, or program before allowing its use; and to monitor how their children interact with the app and, in many cases, with other app users online. For the school-age child, interaction with peers historically was face-to-face during school hours, while playing in the neighborhood, during sports practice, or when spending time at each other's homes. With texting,

WHERE WE STAND

The American Academy of Pediatrics Family Media Use Plan can help parents and children develop a schedule for digital use that allows for unplugged mealtimes, physical activity, homework completion, and uninterrupted sleep, based on the requirements for each age group. The Family Media Use Plan is also available in Spanish. For more information visit healthychildren.org/mediauseplan.

email, and social networking apps, children can interact with peers twenty-four/seven. How can parents establish healthy, age-appropriate parameters?

Parents should remember that for children, electronic devices are a *privilege*, not a *right*. As a parent, you have the authority to determine and oversee your child's usage. All too often when a child obtains a new electronic device as a gift or a privilege, there is a family assumption that the child can access this device at all hours. However, doing so can increase the risk of negative health effects such as a sedentary lifestyle, obesity, and disrupted sleep. Therefore, for children of all ages, access to entertainment media should be limited and should not displace healthier activities.

While it is tempting to take your family offline and prohibit all devices and screen time, this is not realistic in today's era. As technology continues to march forward, we can nurture good media skills and habits in our kids, encourage them to use media wisely and obtain the benefits of such use, and help them navigate a world in which technology plays a major role. The goal as a parent in the twenty-first century is to introduce healthy online interactions to your child in an age-appropriate way.

Online Activity: Staying Safe on the World Wide Web

The internet, or World Wide Web, is a repository of a wealth of knowledge and experience. But it also is a portal to millions of users around the globe, not all of whom are good digital citizens or safe contacts for your child. Any internet user, whether via social media, email, or texting, can have their communication recorded, stored indefinitely, and shared with marketers and millions of viewers without their permission. A simple text, email, or comment on a social networking site can spread beyond the intended audience. Children should be aware that their texts, images, social media comments or photos, and any internet communication are the equivalent of standing up on a table shouting to the entire school cafeteria during lunchtime. Photos can be saved and shared. Text messages can be copied and forwarded. Even within social networking apps in which messages supposedly disappear, a user can take a screenshot of a message or photo and forward it on to third parties. A good guide: if you wouldn't announce a message in your school cafeteria during lunchtime, you shouldn't post it or text it. The same is true for sharing photos and videos that could be perceived as risqué or embarrassing if publicly viewed, such as with sexting, the sharing of sexually explicit messages or images. Additionally, sexting can also put children at risk of being cyberbullied, contacted by predators, or in violation of laws about underage sexual activity.

If there are missteps along the way, use them as a teaching opportunity. Communication online is not the same as face-to-face conversation. Without the benefit of visual cues, a seemingly innocent text observation can be misunderstood by a recipient, leading to hurt feelings. As your children grow, keep the doors of communication open and let them know you are available for advice if and when needed. As you experience your own online gaffes (we are all human, after all), let your kids be aware of your stumbles so they can see how you manage such an issue. For example, what do you do if a text message intended for a friend goes to your boss instead? We all make mistakes, and it is healthy for your kids to understand how to seek help, respond, and learn from your example. However, if you believe that a misstep may put your child or another child at risk, seek the advice of your pediatrician or school counselor. Teens whose communications and sexting have gone viral or who have been cyberbullied may be at risk of mental and physical health issues.

Internet Browsing and Searches

Age-appropriate blocks and filters on home devices and smartphones are a good start, but no app or technological childproofing device can replace one-on-one time using the internet together with your child. For example, if a conversation brings up a question about a favorite sports team, search the internet for your answer together. Point out how search engines often put paid advertiser results on the top of the results list; these are not necessarily the best sources of information, but rather come from companies who paid money to buy that position. Help your children be good consumers of information, helping them identify what is a quality website and avoid dangerous links. For example, websites that end in .org, .edu, or .gov may prove to be more reliable than those ending in .com.

An innocent online search may unfortunately pull up inappropriate content for your child. Again, childproofing blocks and filters are not perfect. Speak with your child about this possibility ahead of time. For younger children, let them know they should alert you if they see anything online that makes them uncomfortable. Older children have natural curiosity and may have been searching for such content intentionally. This is a great opportunity for you to share your family's values. Pornography, especially if viewed in excessive amounts, can unrealistically modify an individual's idea of what a healthy relationship is.

Email

Families may consider introducing the concept of email in a gradual process. One idea is to maintain a family account for which a parent has password access (e.g.,

Consider a Technology-Friendly Homework Zone for the Home

As an increased amount of homework is online, you'll want to create central spaces in your home so that technology needed for academics as well as entertainment is used under adult supervision. The kitchen table is a classic homework zone, especially if your children are using portable devices such as tablets and laptops. To keep tabs on your children's tech use, consider rearranging furniture and creating new tech-friendly zones in your home in family rooms or gathering areas. A central location near a parent or caregiver also allows children to ask questions and get help with homework assignments and online research. For example:

Children ages 5–7 years: As challenging words come up in conversation, you can search for more information together online. Model good online behavior, point out the inevitable pop-up advertisements, and show your child how to select quality information from among the large number of results that may be offered.

Children ages 8–10 years: Continue to be a presence in your children's online lives. Any initial forays into social networking or gaming should be done with an adult's participation after you have investigated the website, game, or app yourself. Adults should have passcode access. Playing a game with your child allows you to supervise your child's activity while educating and monitoring their play. For homework, research, and entertainment, continue to teach your child the difference between quality online results and less helpful options; websites that end in .gov, .org, and .edu are good bets. And remind them that you are available to help anytime they need assistance or feel uncomfortable online.

Children ages 11–12 years: Emphasize the Golden Rule when coaching your child's navigation of their online life: treat others the way you wish to be treated. Many parents "clock out" during this phase of your child's life, but do not mistake tech savviness with quality online digital citizenship. Now is an especially important time to educate your child about their digital footprint (for more on this, see page 321). Encourage your child to come to you for consultation or advice, especially if they are uncomfortable with their online experiences or have been contacted by strangers.

Email and Texting for a Growing School-Age Child

Children ages 5–7 years: Consider using a family account, to which a parent has full access, so that the child can email grandparents and other relatives with parental supervision.

Children ages 8–10 years: Use a family account that a parent has full access to and monitors regularly; children may email friends met at summer camp.

Children ages 11–12 years: Consider an individual email account that a parent has access/passwords for; children can email friends about spending time together and email classmates regarding group school projects.

SmithFamily@example.com). Younger children can learn to email grandparents, for example, using this account. Some families opt to record special memories by emailing special anecdotes and pictures to an email account restricted to the family, preserving memories online for posterity. Password-restricted and encrypted folders and albums on a server or the cloud can allow families to share photos and memorabilia as well. As a child grows, she can gain increasing experience using the account to keep up to date on classroom assignments and other school news, or perhaps maintain an electronic pen pal relationship with a friend she met at summer camp. Many children have moved from email to texting or social media to communicate with classmates, relatives, and friends around the world. Similar guidelines that protect children by allowing adequate supervision, coaching and mentoring, and privacy options can be implemented for these newer methods of communication. As with all digital media, these communications should fit into the Family Media Use Plan, and not displace face-to-face play and social activities, schoolwork, physical activity, and sleep.

Social Media and Interactive Videogames

Do you maintain social media accounts yourself? If not, you might want to consider signing up for one. You don't need to post frequently, or at all; the goal of enrolling is to be aware, as a parent, of what social media are and do. Social media offer users the opportunity to communicate and network with peers, friends, and family; to reach out to others with similar interests and experiences; and to learn about new information and opportunities. However, social media used by adults are often not popular with school-age children or teens. Therefore, it remains important to learn what media your child are using and continue to monitor your child's social media use.

Consider allowing your child to browse your social network with you as a learning tool. Show them the good points as well as the not-so-good observations. It is wonderful to see the evolution of an old college friend's life and family across the miles. It is not so wonderful to see a neighbor post rudely about his community and environment. Use online examples to discuss the dos and don'ts of online etiquette. And show your children how to block and avoid negative posts that may be hurtful, harmful, or illegal.

Both online games and social media may provide a venue for your child to interact with strangers. Children need to understand that others may present themselves online as different from who (or how old) they say they are. Teach your child to speak up and come to you if she encounters any online situation that makes her feel uncomfortable. Your child should "friend" people on social networks only if they are people she knows in real life, and whose identity can be verified.

It is important to note research that has shown overuse of the internet and social media for *any* age group (including adults) to be linked with depressive symptoms. Individuals of all ages who utilize social networks need to remember that users tend to post their lives' highlights, not the entire balanced picture of life's ups and down, or the mundane day-to-day activities and problems that everyone encounters. Users may get the impression that everyone else is having a fantastic life, and may not realize they are only seeing the top 2 percent of others' experiences.

The Data Trail, or Digital Footprint: The Internet Lasts Forever

Have you taken a photo of your 8-year-old building a snowman and posted the image to social media? If so, have you considered asking your child if he would permit you to do so? It's important for both children and parents to understand the concept of a data trail. A great way to introduce this concept is to type your child's name into an internet search engine. You may both be surprised to see that there may already be results listing your child's name and information, perhaps from a sporting event your child participated in or a relative's personal blog post that may include photographs.

The internet is "forever," meaning that even a silly online comment posted as a 9-year-old, if labeled with a child's name, can be searchable for years to come. Even sending a photo using an app that promises to delete the image after only a short time cannot prevent a recipient from taking a screenshot and storing or sharing the photo with other individuals outside the intended audience. Therefore, everyone should be careful about what they do, say, and post online.

GPS location apps can help parents and children locate each other, especially in an emergency; they can also be used by parents to supervise and monitor children to promote safety. However, GPS can also identify a child's location to others when he or she sends a selfie or other photo. Most smartphones and tablets have a default setting that tags the GPS location where the photo was taken, identifying your child's whereabouts. Certain social networks and online games use GPS location for marketing purposes, but there is no reason strangers (or even friends) need to identify your child's location. Before using a digital media device to transmit communications, make sure these GPS default settings are turned off, and, as you coach their media use, remind your child about this important safety issue.

Cyberbullying

The Golden Rule is a valuable ideal for both children and adults: treat others as you wish to be treated. This guideline applies to online activities as well. Unfortunately, individuals who in olden days might have bullied a classmate in the schoolyard have found a new medium to harass others: the internet. The impact of cyberbullying can be devastating—not only is the bullying hurtful, but the cyberbully has the potential to reach thousands of viewers and engage in attacks twenty-four/seven online. Being online removes the empathy that face-to-face contact creates, and may allow mean behavior that would be held in check in real life. Even mildly negative words about others can be easily spread with the openness of internet communications. Teach your kids that if they observe or experience a situation that makes them feel uncomfortable, they should reach out to a parent or trusted adult, such as a school counselor, right away. Teens bullied online have experienced depression, and a few, sadly, have committed suicide.

Studies show that the child being bullied often knows the bully, and children are often hesitant to report online bullying to adults. Underresourced schools may not always be quick to intervene either. Parents should monitor their children for subtle signs or changes in behavior such as not wanting to go to school or participate in a favorite activity; becoming upset after using the computer or smartphone; seeming more withdrawn or moodier than usual; or avoiding questions from you about what is happening. Surprisingly, children who bully may display similar behavior, but you may also notice unusual computer activity such as switching screens when you walk in or multiple log-ins on a website or phone history that you do not recognize.

Any behavior that is a significant change for a child, especially if it is extreme and interferes with home, school, and friends, warrants further review. Call the school to see if grades are slipping, and call your pediatrician to arrange an evaluation, including a discussion of whether resources such as counseling might be of help.

If you are concerned that your child is being bullied, save all emails, screenshots, and texts, and talk to school administrators to encourage an investigation; other parents may have similar experiences with their children, and many school districts have rigorous policies against online bullying. However, if the bullying seems to place your child in serious danger, or if there is a significant threat, call the police. The police can track the IP address (internet protocol address, which identifies the specific computer being used) to find the bully, intervene with the family, and keep your child safe. Do not attempt to contact the bully's family; that is better left to school officials or the police.

Any child spending time online is at risk for being bullied. Parental instincts for detecting that something is off with your child will help you pick up that something negative may have occurred and spur you to ask your child about her online experiences. Because children may find these conversations very difficult, parents may also consider using special software monitoring programs that help uncover situations that your child may not know how to talk to you about. However, no technology can replace a parent's close involvement in his or her child's online life.

Online Homework and School Projects

Assignments become more complex with each grade, and internet research becomes a more prominent tool. Parents should coach their children how to appropriately search for and use the information they find online. For example, if children, even at younger ages, are gathering information for a school project, they should record and cite their sources. It's not too early to educate children about plagiarism and how to avoid it.

Strategies to Protect Dedicated Screen-Free Time

As parents, we may find it all too easy to fall into the trap of being available via our professional emails twenty-four/seven. We may occasionally have unavoidable work obligations and special projects, but, as a general rule, it is wise to put away

Techniques to Find Quality Parenting and Medical Information in the Internet Era

We live in a time in which a wealth of information is more readily at our fingertips than ever before, yet the irony of this situation is that it is a challenge to distinguish quality information from false claims or less reputable sources. Parents, now more than ever, need to be wise consumers of the searchable information available.

The internet can be a helpful source of information and advice, but you and your children can't trust everything you read online. *Anyone* can put information on the internet, and not all of it is reliable. Some people and organizations are very careful about the accuracy of the information they post, and others are not. Some even give false information on purpose.

HealthyChildren.org is the official American Academy of Pediatrics website for parents where you can search for reliable, pediatrician-approved children's health and safety information. Websites that end in .gov and .org are safe bets for quality information as well. If an article mentions research findings, the authors should give the source information so readers can tell where the information comes from. And ultimately, if your instincts tell you the information you're reading online is not reliable, share your questions with your pediatrician, who can help guide you to quality, trusted information.

devices and smartphones during dedicated, regular family time—for example 6:00 to 8:00 on weeknights. Your Family Media Plan can help designate the duration of this unplugged period, but mealtimes are an excellent time to go device-free. A no-phone zone can be a special time for a parent and a child to reconnect face-to-face without the distraction of glowing screens. Your attention and conversation are what a child craves and needs during his formative school years, and you lead by example by showing your child it is okay, as well as emotionally healthy, to put devices away from time to time. Save checking new emails until after your kids go to bed for the evening, or until the next day.

Consider instituting a family ritual of device-free meals every day, even on weekends. If devices are not needed for schoolwork, some families opt to go screen-free for summer vacation, for example, giving parents and children an excellent opportunity to reconnect. Timers to keep families on track with their Family Media Plan are an excellent idea; you can set timers either on the device itself or use handy kitchen and egg timers if available.

Reading Time: E-Readers vs. Paper Books

E-readers or tablets are a convenient way to download books; however, parents should continue to incorporate paper books into your family's reading repertoire. All too often tablets and e-readers have many functions beyond simple book reading, including internet capabilities and gaming, that might be more tempting to a child than the e-book. Reading out loud with your family and acting out parts can be a fun activity. Another option is to choose a dedicated e-reader for your child that loads only books, not games. That said, if your child is snuggled up at bedtime curled up with a good paper book, you won't need to wonder if they're actually playing Minecraft.

Is There a Right Age to Own a Phone?

As with so many other parenting decisions, there is no one-size-fits-all approach to the question of if or when your child should have his own phone. Just because classmates and same-age peers are starting to get their own phones does not mean your child should, even if your family can afford the expense.

Ask yourself why your child might need a phone. Does your child spend time between two parents' households, thereby needing a way to stay in touch with the non-hosting parent? Are there child care arrangements that require that you monitor your child's location? Is your family living in an area at high risk for natural disasters or emergencies that might require calling 911 or a trusted adult?

If the need isn't strong to purchase a phone, there are alternatives for younger children. Smartwatches are available with GPS tracking that can identify a child's location and send simple text messages; this is a viable alternative if your main need is communication during extracurricular activities at which a parent is not present.

Any smartphone purchase must be made only after good communication between child and parent outlining basic rules and expectations for the device's use. Children should know that the parent can and will check the phone at any time (including unannounced), and that the privilege of the phone may be taken away for a specific amount of time if the child is not following family rules regarding phone and digital media usage. Some families choose to draw up a "contract" with agreed-upon rules for both parties to sign. Again, parents need to remind kids that a smartphone is a privilege, not a right.

Internet purchases can be a potential trouble spot for a kid new to her smartphone. An assigned credit card on the phone can rack up a surprisingly expensive app bill in a short amount of time. Instead, consider designating a preset amount on a gift card that allows a child to make limited app or music purchases.

Television and Streaming

Almost every American household has a TV set, and in about half of these homes there are two or more sets. Although viewer habits vary, the average child in the middle years views two to four hours of TV each day. Many children watch TV for more hours than they devote to any other waking activity. With the availability of various online streaming choices, there is the potential for a large amount of TV viewing. Over the course of a year most children spend more time with television programs than they do at school, playing sports, or with family and friends. Not surprisingly, during the formative school years, TV programs impact children's lifestyles, values, health, eating habits, family interactions, sleeping habits, cultural perceptions, and selections of role models. Despite ongoing debate about whether TV viewing is harmful, one thing is certain—when a child is watching TV, he is not doing something else that could be better for his health.

Families and Television

Families lose important opportunities to communicate and bond when media viewing replaces time parents and children could have spent together. Children lose out when TV serves as a babysitter or is used as an alternative for healthy after-school activities. TV viewing displaces many family activities—active play, conversations, and even shared mealtimes.

> Media (including television, movies, videogames, virtual reality, apps, online streaming, and social media) present advertisements to sell products and content that can influence child development and behavior in our society. Media can impact and affect what children learn, how they view their world, and how they interact with others. Research has shown that some media can be a public health risk factor to children and adolescents, leading to risk-taking behaviors, aggression, or negative attitudes about nutrition, sexuality, and self-image. Parents must understand the influence media can have on child wellness and health and monitor children's media exposure and use in terms of both quantity and quality.

Many children today are busier than ever with scheduled activities—soccer, Scouts, music lessons, tutoring—and have less free time. Yet media, not the family, dominate whatever free time remains. Video programs on TV or online also draw attention away from children's homework, often creating conflict and tension within the family. As a rule, homework and TV don't mix; if your child needs to study, the television set or streaming service should be off-limits.

Physical Health and Screen Time

Unfortunately, overuse of media, including TV, can have a negative impact on physical health. Glued to media products and apps, children spend less time outdoors playing or exercising and increased time sitting; their fitness suffers. With the availability of online streaming of tens of thousands of movies and shows, adults and kids alike can favor binge-watching over exercise, healthy activity, and conversation. Overuse of media also increases the risk of obesity for many children—and adults.

Learning and TV

Children who have learned critical viewing skills and who belong to families that actively select high-quality programs and apps can learn from television viewing and app use. However, real-life parent or caregiver teaching tends to result in greater learning and longer retention of learned material than the knowledge gained from educational apps.

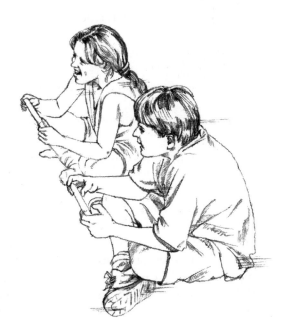

Parents should endeavor to ensure that screen time does not replace family time. The next time your child watches TV, look at her instead of the screen and ask yourself, "What is she doing?" or, perhaps more appropriately, "What is she *not* doing?" Sitting in front of the television set, children are giving up opportunities for more active intellectual, emotional, artistic, and physical growth. Instead of playing outdoors, reading a book, conversing, exercising, or doing homework, they spend hours sitting. Children learn best in the context of relationships and meaningful interaction with people they respect in the real world, not the virtual one. In most cases, even in a group, television viewing is a passive, solitary activity. More evolved media that allow for social interactions and creative opportunities provide some benefits, as noted above, if the engagement is time-limited and of high quality. However, the critical factor in promoting child development is avoiding overuse of all media and the displacement of healthier activities by media use.

If your child is watching TV, he is probably not doing any of the following:

- Solving problems

- Being creative

- Asking questions

- Exercising initiative

- Practicing eye-hand coordination

- Playing outdoors (some experts have discussed the concept of "nature deficit disorder," in which kids, as a result of spending less time outdoors, develop a wide range of behavioral problems)

- Scanning (useful in reading)

- Practicing motor skills

- Thinking critically, logically, and analytically

- Practicing communication skills

- Playing interactive games with other children or adults (helpful for developing patience, self-control, cooperation, sportsmanship)

Though parents often worry about media's negative influences, media can play a positive role in children's lives. If the programs and apps a child uses are carefully selected, they can provide fun learning through entertainment, exposure to other cultures, and positive social values. News sources, filtered for age-appropriateness, can inform children about current events, especially if co-viewed and discussed with parents. Through special programs she can learn about the wonders of nature and the fascinations of history. When a family watches, uses, or plays together, media can provide an opportunity for them to share time with one another, talk to each other, and grow closer bonds.

Although there are some worthwhile media options, parents need to research the options carefully. Apps and programs for children may make promises about quality that are not supported by research. Nonprofit organizations such as Common Sense Media at CommonSenseMedia.org have tools to help parents identify age-appropriate media for children. Unfortunately, too many TV shows,

WHERE WE STAND

Media often glamorize harmful and dangerous behavior for older children and teens. TV and films may promote the use of alcohol, tobacco, and other drugs. Music videos contain references to or graphic displays of sexual behavior, drug and alcohol overuse, and suicide. Parents should research the media their children will access, and pay close attention to ratings for TV, movies, and videogames to guide them in selecting media with high-quality content.

Pediatricians, parents, and teachers should help children develop critical thinking and viewing skills about what is portrayed in the media and how it is presented. When children understand that media are constructed to elicit a specific opinion or response, they become more critical of the messages they see and hear. Children who are educated about media are less likely to be influenced by media messages and more likely to withstand potentially harmful effects.

Children are exposed to violence in television, movies, videogames, and music. Media glamorize the use of guns and wrongly teach children that it is acceptable to use violence to resolve problems. Children need to know that violence on TV, in the movies, online, and in videogames is not real. By watching television or other media with their children, and discussing the content, parents can address objectionable content and use the medium as a springboard for family discussion.

Quality programming can both entertain and educate children, but too much media use detracts from time spent reading or using other active learning skills. It also has been associated with obesity. The AAP recommends that families develop a Family Media Plan (healthychildren.org /English/media/Pages/default.aspx) that ensures that healthy activities such as uninterrupted sleep, device-free meals, and physical activity have priority each day over entertainment media use.

videogames, online games, virtual reality games, and apps depict violence and aggression or promote family-role stereotypes that may not reinforce the values you hold. Others can be venues for targeted advertising. Commercials and other advertising expose children to products that parents often do not approve of and cannot afford. They normalize and promote the adoption of unhealthy behaviors by children and adolescents. Additionally, younger children may have difficulty distinguishing between fantasy and reality, and may be disturbed by the animated violence in cartoons. Studies suggest that violence in TV programs, music videos, and motion pictures can cause antisocial behavior in children and make them more likely to hurt others, behave more aggressively on the playground, and display callousness toward other people's pain. They can also create fear and suspicion in young viewers. Parents should make a conscientious effort to minimize or eliminate your child's viewing of violent media; see the suggestions in the box on page 329.

Media Education: What Parents Can Do

Here are some suggestions to help you keep your child's screen usage in balance:

- Develop a Family Media Plan (healthychildren.org/English/media/Pages /default.aspx). Ensure that healthy activities, homework assignments, and household chores have priority before entertainment digital media use. Provide alternatives to screens—such as after-school sports, hobbies, chores, and family activities—to engage children and make the transition easier.

- Review the media that your child uses. Sit down and watch the programs or use the apps with them, and, if any depictions of sex, alcohol or drug overuse, violence, or negative stereotypes should appear, use them as springboards for family discussions, helping your child put them in context. Use these opportunities to promote dialogue that can reinforce your family's values.

- Guide your children toward becoming more critical viewers by discussing the behavior and attitudes of characters, as well as the sales pitches in commercials. Children may want the toys and junk foods advertised on TV, but you can explain how commercials are aimed at persuading people to buy items they may not need or which may not be good for them.

- When good programs air at inconvenient times—perhaps educational programs telecast during school hours, or programs that conflict with family activities—record them so your child can watch them at a later date, preferably with you.

WHERE WE STAND

The primary goal of commercial children's television is to sell products, from toys to junk food. Young children in particular may not be able to distinguish between programs and their commercials, nor fully understand that commercials have been designed to sell them (and their parents) something and make money. Additionally, most digital media are in the for-profit business. General advertisements in apps, in games, and on websites are now accompanied by targeted advertisements that are aimed at a specific user. Advertisers are now able to track users' choices and purchases online, and design ads that can appeal to specific populations, including children and teens. Unless legislation limits the extent and type of such advertising, it's important for parents to educate their children about how to interpret and understand advertising using media literacy skills.

Media remain profoundly influential, especially for younger children and teens. Images presented in media (including television, movies, and online) can affect children's perceptions and self-esteem. Programs and shows may not reflect reality in areas such as culture, diversity, and mental and physical health and wellness, and may promote negative themes such as drug use, alcohol use, smoking, vaping, or unsafe sex in the interests of marketing and sales. Therefore, parents should advocate for high-quality educational-content media, and select their families' media options carefully. Co-viewing media with children and teens can also help to encourage discussions about media and what they have viewed, as well as hone media literacy skills.

The American Academy of Pediatrics strongly supports legislative efforts to improve the quality of children's programming and media. The AAP also advocates for content-based TV, film, videogame, and virtual reality ratings systems.

■ Keep books and other reading material readily available in your home. Make regular trips to the library with your child and help him select books to read. Board games that the whole family can play are a wonderful family activity.

■ Set an example of behavior you wish to instill. Parents are powerful role models. If you want your child to read more, that is what you should do too. If you would like him to go outdoors for some physical activity, go on a family bike ride or take part in a group outdoor activity.

- Do not permit electronic devices or TV watching during dinner. The evening meal is often the only time that families are able to be together for any sustained period. Screens will interfere with or terminate conversation. In addition, turn off digital media devices at least one hour before bedtime.

- Do not allow your child to have screens in his bedroom. When a child uses media in his bedroom, his sleep may be disturbed, causing problems with fatigue the following day at school. A good option is to have a central device charging area in the living room or kitchen where all the family devices can charge overnight.

- If media become a source of tension and conflict, simply unplug for a while. Some families institute TV-free days or weeks, or even go without TV all summer long. Children become very creative and are certainly more available when TV is not dominating their attention and time. Your pediatrician can help your family with challenges in developing and implementing a Family Media Plan to help kids balance their media use.

~ 26 ~

Pets

WHETHER THEY ARE dogs, cats, hamsters, fish, or parakeets, pets are found in millions of American households. Most families at least consider acquiring a pet, and for children an animal to love and care for can provide one of their most memorable experiences growing up. The attachment to animals developed in childhood can last a lifetime.

By the middle years, most children are capable of caring for their own pet. Not only can they fully enjoy the animal, but they are old enough to assume some or all of the responsibility for its care. At the same time, the presence of a pet can teach important lessons about love, respect, empathy, and sensitivity toward other living creatures. Children with special needs especially benefit from the comfort and companionship of a pet. A child's self-esteem can be boosted by caring for a pet, as she recognizes that she is capable of handling the caretaking duties. She might also feel particularly good about herself if she becomes an "expert" on the type of pet she has. Pets can help children connect with their peers too.

The decision to adopt a pet should not be taken lightly. Make sure you and your child understand that the responsibilities associated with a pet are continuous—and if she commits herself to bathing the dog or cleaning the litter box, it is a long-term obligation, one that will likely last for years.

Choosing a Pet

When selecting a pet, keep your child's developmental stage in mind. If this is going to be *his* pet—and thus he agrees to care for it—choose an animal whose needs can be met by your child. Some pets, like dogs or cats, require daily attention; they must be fed, groomed, cleaned up after, and exercised. Others—like fish, turtles, birds, guinea pigs, and hamsters—demand minimal care and may be a good choice for a younger child who is just beginning to learn about what is involved in having a pet. A goldfish, for example, requires feeding only every two to three days, with its water changed periodically; by contrast, a dog cannot be neglected for a single day.

Some pets have easygoing temperaments conducive to being around children. For instance, dogs such as retrievers and beagles tend to be gentle with kids, while other breeds, such as boxers, German shepherds, pit bulls, Doberman pinschers, and miniature French poodles, may be more unpredictable. Keep the animal's characteristics in mind when selecting a pet.

The dander (shed skin cells, hairs, and feathers) of some animals can evoke allergic symptoms in certain children. If your child has asthma, allergies, or eczema, or your family has a strong history of allergic disorders, discuss your options with your pediatrician.

Almost every type of pet is a potential source of disease that can infect your child. All reptiles, for example, can carry and transmit salmonella bacteria, which

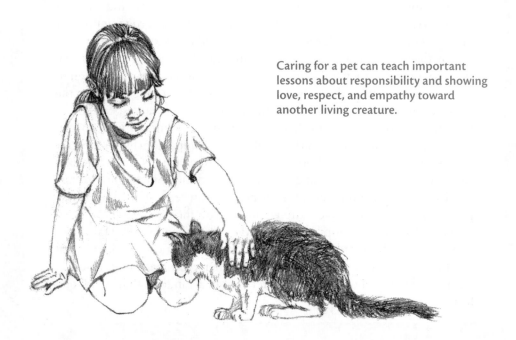

Caring for a pet can teach important lessons about responsibility and showing love, respect, and empathy toward another living creature.

can cause serious diarrhea. However, as long as your child practices reasonable hygiene, especially handwashing after playing with a pet and before eating, he should be safe. Children whose immune systems are suppressed, however, need to be especially careful, and generally should avoid most pets. Buy pets only from reputable breeders and shelters; otherwise you increase the risk of purchasing an ill or diseased animal and endangering your child and yourself.

Before bringing the pet home, discuss with your child the needs of the animal and everything that is involved in caring for it. Books on pet care from the library or the pet store can help him understand what is expected of him. Also helpful is a visit to the home of a friend who has a pet. This way you can see firsthand what care of a pet involves.

How should you react if your child loses interest in caring for the pet several weeks or months after the family adopts it? If he has made a commitment to be the primary caretaker but does not live up to that agreement, perhaps someone else in the family would be willing to take over the responsibility. If not, let your child know that you are unwilling to jeopardize the well-being of the pet because of his neglect, and unless his interest in the animal changes, you will need to find another home for it. During this discussion, do not accuse your child of any personal inadequacy. Instead, be as logical as possible, saying something like "The

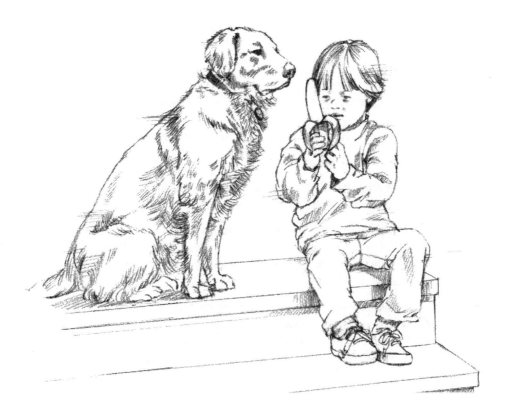

dog needs a dependable caretaker, and you haven't followed through on your promise. We need to find another family who can care for him."

Safety Around a Pet

Although most animals are friendly, some can be dangerous. More than any other age group, children between the ages of 5 and 9 are the victims of animal bites. Children 9 to 14 are next in line as the most frequent victims of bites.

When a new pet comes into the home—or if your child is sometimes exposed to dogs or cats in the neighborhood—make sure he knows how to minimize his chances of being bitten or scratched. Most often, a child is at risk if he teases, hurts, or plays too roughly with an animal. A dog might lash out to defend itself or to protect what it considers its territory or food. Incidents are rare in which a dog aggressively attacks when unprovoked. The box below offers some guidelines on how to reduce the chance of bites.

Teaching Kids to Properly Interact with Animals

How can your child protect himself from attacks from his own or other pets? Here are some suggestions to talk over with your son or daughter:

- Do not pet or otherwise disturb a dog or cat that is sleeping or eating.

- Do not tease or abuse an animal.

- Never pet an unfamiliar dog or cat. Also, be cautious about touching puppies or kittens within view of their mother.

- When a child is approached by an unfamiliar dog, he should not run; that can often make the dog aggressive. Instead, he should refrain from making direct eye contact, slowly back away, and avoid sudden movements while still keeping the dog within view.

- If your child is riding his bike and is being chased by a dog, he should not try to pedal quickly away from it. Rather, he should stop the bike and dismount from it so that the bike is between him and the dog. Before long, the animal may lose interest in a nonmoving "target."

If your child is bitten by a pet or other animal, know that infections can occur—more often from cat bites than dog bites. (For care of these wounds, see "Animal Bites," page 598.) Be sure any dogs or cats you own are fully immunized to protect both your pet and your family. The bites of wild animals such as raccoons, bats, or squirrels pose a special risk of rabies, particularly in some locales. Bites by wild animals should be examined promptly by your pediatrician, and public health recommendations about treatment to prevent rabies should be followed.

Teasing or maltreating animals not only is dangerous but may be a symptom that your child is having some emotional problems. Purposeful maltreatment of an animal is a cause for concern and should be discussed with your child's pediatrician. If your child continues to tease animals after you have talked about it with her and made it clear to her that this is unkind as well as dangerous, your child may benefit from the counseling of your pediatrician or a mental health professional. (See Chapter 17, "Seeking Professional Help.")

A Pet's Affection

A pet's love is unconditional, and the bond that develops between child and animal can become important to both of them. Even when children are rejected by friends and are feeling lonely, they can still depend on their pet for acceptance. Kids who come home from school to an empty house because of working parents often rely on a pet for companionship and sometimes protection (for more on after-school issues with kids, see page 304). Pets are also often recommended for children with chronic medical conditions or special needs, as they can serve as good companions. Some psychotherapists use specially trained therapy animals as part of their treatment programs, employing dogs or cats as a way to teach love, friendship, and responsibility.

When a Pet Dies

The loss of a pet—either through death or because it has run away—can be emotionally traumatic for a child. If your family loses a pet, spend time with your kids to help them understand their feelings and come to terms with the sadness. Share with your children any sorrow over the pet that you may be experiencing. Children learn important lifelong lessons about loss and death through their relationships with pets.

If harm, or worse, comes to the pet as a direct result of the child's actions, such as not properly tying up the pet, the child will understandably have a strong reaction. In cases like this be especially sensitive to what your child is experiencing. The natural consequences are punishment enough in this situation.

At times acquiring a new pet can help the child get over the loss of the old one. Explain to your child that while another animal cannot replace the pet that has died, it can become a new companion and someone he can love. Let him help decide if and when the family should get a new pet, and let him participate in the choice.

~ 27 ~

Money Skills

Money Management Skills for Kids Ages 5 to 12 Years

Boxes arrive on a doorstep, seemingly by magic, filled with toilet paper and other essentials. Between two jobs and hectic school and activity schedules, many families opt to order household necessities online for convenient delivery. How does the first-grade child interpret the purchase and arrival of these items? How can an understanding of the value of money be passed on to the child?

A trip to the grocery store: ingredients for school lunches and weeknight dinners are purchased. A third-grader helps his dad load up the cart. When all has been rung up at the register, Dad produces a debit card from his wallet to swipe before they are on their way to load up the car. Again, how can the child understand the concepts of budgeting and the value of money from this deceptively simple transaction?

In the twenty-first century, financial lessons should continue to evolve to coach our kids how to understand how money works. From kindergarten through middle school, children begin to take steps to learn about simple finances, the value of money, how household essentials are paid for, and the concept of saving and "waiting" for a planned purchase.

This chapter is meant to inspire parents and caregivers to consider how to introduce money skills in an age-appropriate way as children grow.

Allowance or Weekly Stipend

Some families use the concept of a weekly allowance for their children, with an understanding and expectation of what specific household chores the child should be completing on a regular basis. Other families consider household chores as part and parcel of being a family member contributing to the team effort, and prefer not to attach a financial amount to daily and weekly tasks performed by the child. Yet other families use the idea of a chore jar, where specific tasks are assigned a particular financial amount to be rewarded upon completion of the assigned task.

Whatever model you choose, be consistent so kids know what to expect. An early introduction to saving money (for example, even a first-grader can learn how to save special coins from the Tooth Fairy) serves as a stepping-stone to build on financial concepts as the child grows. You may find that as your children grow you may need to tweak the system with some trial and error; however, you'll want to avoid making modifications on a weekly basis to avoid confusion.

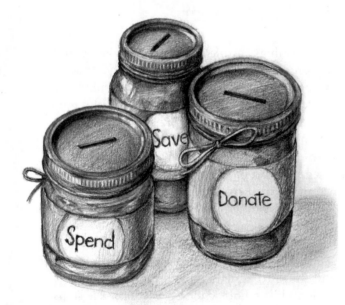

Sometimes it is easier for kids to understand money when they can see a visual. It makes them feel good to know how much they saved, donated, and have to spend.

Bank Accounts

Consider setting up a savings account for your child at a financial institution. Many banks will allow minors to set up a separate savings account, connected to the parents' accounts, that conveniently has no minimum balance requirement (handy if the child is saving Tooth Fairy money). If a family member gives your child money for a birthday, for example, the child can gain experience depositing it in her bank account. As time passes she can see the dollar value slowly grow with time, and parents can discuss with her the benefits of saving as opposed to using the money to buy gum that will soon be gone.

Let your kids know that money doesn't magically come out of an ATM; your family has earned it through work, you keep it safe in the bank, and the machine is used for convenience to retrieve your money when you need it.

Many families encourage smart finances by teaching their kids about the idea of thinking of your finances in thirds: save a third for the future, spend a third, and donate a third. In our current age of instant gratification (ordering items online that arrive quickly, within days) the idea of planning for a purchase, patiently saving money over time, and perhaps brainstorming ways to raise more money (e.g., by performing extra work around the house) is a concept you may wish to employ to encourage your child to learn these important life skills.

Cash or Credit?

Our kids are always watching the adults in their lives. More and more frequently we purchase items with credit or debit cards, and even built-in smartphone readers. From time to time use cash (yes, actual dollars and coins) and allow your kids to help you count coins for practice—excellent for building mental math skills (working with numbers in your head without need for pencil or paper). Even better, as kids get older, give them experience buying apples themselves with cash at the grocery store, for example, by coaching them through a cash payment at the cashier together, fostering these life skills further as the child grows. A 12-year-old should be able to independently handle a simple cash transaction at a store for a straightforward purchase.

Family schedules can be hectic, but ensure that as your kids help you with errands, for example, you are mindful to use these interactions as teachable moments to foster age-appropriate money skills for the future.

~ 28 ~

If You Choose
a Summer Camp

A SUMMER CAMP experience, while certainly not a requirement of childhood, can broaden a child's horizons. If financially and logistically an option for a family, camp offers a time for children to learn about themselves and other people, to explore aspects of the world to which they might not normally be exposed, and hopefully to spend a lot more time outdoors than during the usual school year. The best camps are free of electronic devices. There children meet and interact with new children, often from different parts of the city and state, and with different backgrounds. An overnight camp may also be a child's first experience being away from her family for more than just an overnight visit with a friend or a grandparent. Camp is a place to learn new skills and proficiencies. Some camps are designed to offer special and therapeutic experiences for children, helping them mature and learn to be more responsible for themselves. Specialized camps exist for children with food allergies, type 1 diabetes, leukemia, and other medical conditions; these allow a child to meet new friends with similar experiences, as well as develop self-responsibility toward her care in an encouraging, safe environment.

A sleepaway overnight camp is not financially or logistically possible for many families. Local day camps can provide a child with summer adventures not possible during the school year, and provide quality child care and ease the family schedule if parents work outside the home. For more on child care, see page 303.

Middle childhood is a time when kids may have their first overnight camp experience; however, as a parent you need to determine whether and when your child is ready. She needs to have the physical and emotional maturity to live away from home for a week or two. A key indicator of readiness is whether she is excited and enthusiastic about the idea of attending camp. Some camps are designed especially for younger children (ages 6 through 9) and are accustomed to giving extra support to kids who may be uneasy about being away from home for the first time.

Before your child decides to attend an overnight or resident camp, see how she does at a day camp first. If that turns out to be a positive experience, then you might start thinking more about an overnight camp.

Matching Your Child to a Camp

The financial cost of a camp is an important consideration; a more expensive camp is not necessarily a better camp. Your family budget will direct your choice of camps. Great camping experiences are available at reasonable prices through the YMCA, Scouts, and religious groups. Look at camp brochures and websites with your child. If he has a particular interest—for example, if you think that he would have a special attraction to a camp specializing in sports or music—be sure to look into these facilities. Or if he has certain health conditions, such as type 1 diabetes, asthma, or cancer, there are camps devoted exclusively to these children, which have medical personnel and facilities on-site to ensure that the children's needs are met. Your pediatrician can help you identify such specialized programs. Keep in mind that some camps "mainstream" children with health issues, mixing them with other children. It's not surprising that kids do very well in these settings; this approach provides valuable learning experiences for all campers, whether they have health issues or not.

As a parent, you are the best judge of where your child will be happiest and have the most valuable experience. Ideally, visit the camp and meet the camp director and counselors ahead of time, and observe the activities that are available. Ask the camp director for the names of parents of past campers whom you can contact to get their impressions and advice.

When you visit the camp ahead of time, look to see if the children attending the camp represent a mix of social classes and cultures. How structured is the schedule of daily activities, and how much freedom in choosing activities is best for your child? Ask whether the camp is accredited by the American Camping Association (ACA), indicating that it has met or exceeded a set of standards that include staff qualifications, first-aid and other healthcare facilities, and transportation. Inquire about the staff's background and training, and the staff-to-camper ratio. When investigating costs, be sure to inquire as to whether the camp fees are all-inclusive or whether there are additional charges for laundry, accident insurance, special lessons, and so on.

Getting Ready for Camp

Once the choice of a camp has been made, it is time to prepare your child for her camp experience. The director of the camp you've selected should tell you well in advance what your child should bring with her, and what you will need to take care of in advance—for instance, a physical examination, an updating of immunizations, and health insurance.

As the time for camp gets closer, encourage your child to talk about what she expects camp to be like, and what she will miss while away from home. Let her air any anxieties, and reassure her that the camp's staff is there to make her comfortable and create an "at home" feeling. Remind her of the fun she will have, and tell her that because of your love for her, you want her to have this enjoyable experience. Also, promise to write her frequently while she's away, and let her know that you want to receive letters from her too, so you can hear about all her experiences. Remember that many camps do not have internet access, or will limit or prohibit access to electronic devices, texting, and the internet. Prepare your child if this will be the case for her camp. You can follow along on your child's adventures through their written letters and by checking the camp's social media pages, where they will often post updates.

Among the things to discuss with your child before she leaves for camp is your confidence in her judgment about people and new situations. Although she is there to learn and have more experiences, encourage her to trust her feelings and to resist joining in activities with other campers and counselors with whom she feels uncomfortable. If the opportunity is available prior to camp, or at the time you take your child to camp, take a while to get to know the people who will be caring for your child. Once your child has left for camp, be sure to stay in touch. In fact, it is a good idea to send your first letter to her *before* she leaves for camp, so she receives it on the first day or two that she is there.

If you are feeling guilty about sending her away for a week or two, keep in mind that homesickness is usually short-lived. Once she makes her first new friend and becomes involved in camp activities, her time away from home will probably pass very quickly. Most children adjust rapidly to their new surroundings and enjoy their camping experience immensely.

Home Again

Encourage your child to talk about his camp experiences, what a typical day was like, who his friends were, and how he got along with the staff. Find out what experiences were new, which were most rewarding, and which were challenging. Were there especially good moments? Were there bad ones? Most kids return home from a camp experience with more confidence, a boosted self-esteem, and an appreciation for home sweet home.

~ 29 ~

When Both Parents Work

MOST SCHOOL-AGE CHILDREN live in homes in which both parents work. In the hours after school ends but before parents come home, kids may be cared for by another adult—either in after-school care, in a designated child care facility, or by a relative, neighbor, or employed sitter. Families in which both parents work benefit from a teamwork approach to running the household. Children of working parents learn the value of work as parents role-model setting and working toward their career goals.

The Impact of Working

There are advantages to a household in which the parents work outside the home, aside from the financial benefits. When both parents work, there is potential for greater equality and teamwork in the roles of partners. Depending on the nature of the parents' work, as well as the family's values, fathers may assume more responsibility for child care and housework. Sharing child-raising roles is particularly evident when parents have staggered work schedules—for instance, if one parent works daytime hours and is home after school and in the evening, while the other parent works a shift such as 4:00 p.m. to midnight. Dad may then be responsible for preparing dinner, cleaning up the kitchen, and helping the children with their homework.

Considerations of Shift Work

Many families feel the stress of overscheduled lives, especially families in which parents work at different times of the day. When parents work different shifts and are not home together often, a strain is put on their relationship and the family. Even more difficult are jobs that have rotating shifts—firefighting and nursing, for instance—in which parents work different hours each week; those schedules can prevent families from establishing routines and rhythms.

In these families, partners often have little or no time together. If they are lucky, they have a day or two during the week when they are both off, but their sleep schedules may be so different that they still spend little time with each other. These parents need to pass messages to each other, like ships passing in the night. Parents in these situations work especially hard at giving their children the feeling that their family is a unit, despite the difficult schedules. They need to make the most of weekends and vacations and support each other in areas like household responsibilities and discipline.

For some families, shift work is a solution to provide good child care and supervision for children who would otherwise be left in the care of another adult or on their own. Such arrangements may provide a financial benefit to the family and a sense of comfort to the child.

Parent Roles

In two-income families, do men assume an equal share of everyday responsibilities at home? Surveys have shown that while many men are willing to help with the grocery shopping and cleaning up in the kitchen after dinner, for example, the overall balance of the chores and planning involved in running a household is not yet even. The hope is that more households will have less gender-based divisions of chores and responsibilities. Not only does this make for a more equitable partnership with less-stressed partners, but it sends a strong positive message to kids about teamwork.

Women who work outside the home report significant benefits associated with their jobs and careers, including higher self-esteem and a greater sense of autonomy. When a mother enjoys her work and gains a sense of satisfaction from it, her children benefit. When women bring home a paycheck, they often have more leverage in the family and have a greater sense of independence in the relationship.

Working parents should consciously schedule time for each other and for their individual pursuits, as these activities may get lost in the hectic pace of balancing work and family life. Each day should have time dedicated to each of your kids. Let them know just how important they are to you, not only through words but through your presence and listening. The financial benefits of two-parent working families are no substitute for a parent's *time*.

Some parents awaken their families a few minutes earlier each morning so that everyone can eat breakfast together and share a few minutes as the day begins. In the evenings they turn off the television, put away the electronic devices, and participate in family activities like games, sports, music, and conversation. Email and work texts can easily consume twenty-four hours of the day, and working parents should make a deliberate decision to put away their devices at designated times each day. This not only models good life skills for kids but will reduce the working parent's stress.

A family with two wage-earners can be a positive influence on children. Everyone—both children and adults—will enjoy some of the benefits. Both boys and girls perceive themselves as having greater career options if they have a mother who works. Children also feel proud that their parents have careers. Depending on their after-school child care setting, middle-years children also have greater exposure to other kids and new social experiences, which can contribute to their development. It is healthy for kids to pitch in with household tasks and become more independent and self-sufficient each year.

Avoiding Burnout

If you are starting to feel burned out from your many responsibilities at home and at work, here are some ideas to help you ease the pressure.

- Throughout your workday, fit some relaxing moments into your routine. If possible, close your office door for ten minutes, shut your eyes, and perform a relaxation exercise. Or during breaks take a short walk in the fresh outdoor air, if possible. Diversions like these can reduce stress, improve efficiency on the job, and make you feel more vitalized when you return home in the evening, creating a more amicable family life.

- If you regularly come home tired, try to develop rituals that improve your frame of mind when you arrive home. This may mean spending some time by yourself in order to put a distance between you and the day's stresses. Coming home is an important moment; your children are eager to be with you and to share their day's experiences.

- Assess how you are spending your time during the day. Look for areas in which you can reduce stress. For instance, can you bring in dinner two or three nights a week? Can you hire a high school or college student to help for an hour or two in the evenings, perhaps doing the laundry or cleaning up the kitchen? If you can save a couple of hours a night this way, you will have more time to spend with your children or to relax or sleep.

■ Look at the big picture and make sure your kids are not overscheduled with too many extracurricular activities, adding to family chaos. In lieu of a travel sports team, would a more casual park district program be just as fun with less expense and travel time? Prioritize the activities that your kids are truly enjoying and are passionate about.

■ Involve the entire family in the evening responsibilities that are a drain on your time and energy. For example, the family can work together to clean up the kitchen after dinner; with everyone's help it will get done much quicker and free up some time for you in the evening. Do the same on the weekends too: if the house needs cleaning, have everyone pitch in on Saturday morning. This will help build family cohesiveness while finishing the job faster, leaving more time for enjoyable family activities.

■ Keep your expectations realistic. On certain evenings you might have to choose between going to the grocery store and doing the laundry. Some tasks just may have to wait until the weekend.

■ On the weekends, schedule some relaxation time for yourself. Go for a walk or go to the gym. Do some recreational reading. While family time is important and certain chores need to be done, time to unwind and recharge your own batteries is essential too.

Finding Child Care

During middle childhood, kids need supervision. A responsible adult should be available to get them ready and off to school in the morning and watch over them after school until you return from work. Even children approaching adolescence—11- and 12-year-olds—should not come home to an empty house in the afternoon unless they show unusual maturity for their age. For more on child care, see Chapter 23. Maturity is the key here and is a much more important criterion than age. Some 14-year-olds still require supervision; some 12-year-olds can be trusted to come home, do their homework, and care for themselves responsibly.

Although being physically present is the best way to supervise a child, sometimes that is not possible. If alternative adult supervision is not available, parents should make special efforts to supervise their children from a distance. Children should have a set time when they are expected to arrive at home and should check in with a neighbor or with a parent by text, telephone, or video chat. Parents and children should agree upon a regular routine for the child that is written down and posted in a conspicuous place alongside emergency telephone numbers. Such a schedule might consist of having a snack, doing homework, feeding a pet, and setting the dinner table. On some days the child may have an after-school activity or go to a friend's house to play. Parents should always know where their unsupervised children are and what they are doing.

When evaluating child care options, determine whether other family members can handle these responsibilities. For example, does a grandparent or other relative live nearby, and is he or she available and willing to help? Is there a responsible teenager—perhaps an older sibling—who can supervise your child for a couple of hours in the afternoon until you arrive home?

If you choose a formal after-school program, inquire about the training of the staff. There should be a high child-to-staff ratio, and the rooms and the playground should be safe. Many school districts and YMCAs hold after-care or after-school programs. Talk to personnel at your child's school and at the local YMCA about after-school programs, which are growing in number in many parts of the country. These programs tend to be structured, offer a variety of activities, and include time for homework. Many are reasonably priced. For more on this option, see Chapter 23, "Child Care."

If cost is an important factor, consider pooling resources with neighbors and hiring one parent to watch the children of a number of families. Or set up a co-op of several families in which each parent shares after-school child care on a rotating basis.

Some companies now offer their employees flexible time schedules—perhaps allowing parents to start work early so they can be home earlier in the afternoon, when the kids return from school. Some employees take work home with them, spending their last two job hours at home. Twelve-hour shifts, with four days off each week, and part-time employment are other alternative patterns of work that some parents find helps the family schedule. These options can be effective solutions to the child care problem for school-age children. Each family has its own needs and each must look for its own best circumstances.

Managing School Holidays and Vacations

School vacations, legal holidays (like Martin Luther King Jr. Day and Presidents' Day), and teacher in-service days can be challenges for working parents. These are days when the child is out of school but parents usually have to be at work. Advance planning is helpful for these situations. To help in that process, get copies of your child's school schedule as early as possible so you are aware of vacations and days off school several months in advance. Children's school schedules often dictate family vacation plans. With sufficient advance notice, you may be able to block out your own vacation time to coincide with that of your child.

Few parents have as much vacation time available as do their children, so arrangements need to be made for child care and supervision within the framework of the demands of the parents' jobs. Many school district after-care programs also run special all-day camps on school holidays, similar to how summer camps are run, recognizing the needs of families with working parents. If your spouse has some flexibility in his or her work schedule, divide the home responsibilities so one of you takes time off during different parts of the children's vacation. Some couples are able to work out a plan where Mom is home in the morning and Dad replaces her in the afternoon; perhaps one or both can work flexible schedules (6:00 a.m. to 2:00 p.m. for one, 2:30 p.m. to 10:30 p.m. for the other) so that at least one parent is home at all times.

Sometimes neither you nor your spouse will be able to get off work, or you will need a backup or alternative strategy for unexpected job demands or the sudden loss of a caretaker, both of which require some last-minute juggling of schedules. It is important that school-age children are always supervised, directly if possible and indirectly if not. Indirect supervision means providing a safe environment and a structured schedule of activities, including regular times to check in, even by phone, with a responsible adult. This latter option should be considered only for mature preteenagers and is never the preferred alternative.

When you can't break away from the office, see if extended family members are available and willing to help. Some parents are able to work out a timetable with several families, where each assumes the caretaking responsibilities for all the children one day a week, or they trade hours of babysitting with each other. Some high school and college students, or after-school child care employees, are willing to work on holidays, perhaps coming to your home to assume the care of children from several families. Many high schools and colleges have job placement offices to find employment for students on vacation; ask for and check references before hiring these young adults for child care. (For more on finding good child care, see Chapter 23.) You may also inquire about special holiday programs and camps that might be planned by local YMCAs, Boys and Girls Clubs, and other community organizations.

For some parents of school-age children, the best long-term solution is to work at home all the time, often in a small home-based business of their own. However, while this can be a good option, it is not available to everyone, and working at home poses problems of its own.

Making the Most of Time off School and Work

Before your child's school break, planning can make time off memorable.

1. A great deal of the enjoyment of time off school and work together is the *anticipation* of the time. You and your child can work together to plan activities with internet research, whether staying at home for a "staycation," enjoying parts of your local area your family is usually too busy to explore, or traveling elsewhere. Build on previous interests and offer some opportunities to learn something new.

2. Make ordinary activities fun. Maintain a relaxed mood and try not to do too much in too little time. Everyone enjoys some downtime together, perhaps just taking a walk as a family. Many families report that even after a trip visiting a different area, the kids' favorite part was the drive to get there, or some other aspect that we adults may not expect to be most memorable. Kids can see the joy in the simple, mundane aspects of a trip. Avoid peer pressure from other families and remember you don't need to plan elaborate, expensive, or exhausting events and trips. The most valuable gift you can give your child is time together, whether you are riding bikes, enjoying an ice cream cone on a park bench, or putting together a photo album and telling stories about when your child was younger. Your child wants attention from you, and even one fun activity a day together can be very satisfying for both of you.

3. A short, easy, and inexpensive vacation can be just a day and a night away. For example, if you feel the need to get away from familiar surroundings, try an overnight stay at a nearby hotel, where the pool, room service, in-room movies, or nearby miniature golf course can make it into a special vacation. Enjoy the moment rather than comparing your activities with what other families are doing. Sometimes divorced parents try to outdo each other, often with the weekend parent feeling obligated to plan something special and expensive; this usually puts a strain on everyone.

Some families find that spending work and school time off doing the same activities each year becomes a valued ritual. These traditions become part of a family's history and are saved in a child's memory bank, boosting togetherness and bonding.

~ 30 ~

Separation, Divorce, and the School-Age Child

WHEN PARENTS DECIDE to separate, whether temporarily or permanently, there is an inevitable emotional impact on their children. Children respond to divorce differently, depending on their age, sex, temperament, development, and life experience. Kids may be confused as to why these family changes are happening, and even blame themselves for it. Parents undergoing separation or divorce should remember to prioritize their child's understanding of and emotions regarding the transition.

When discussing your separation or divorce with your child, keep the discussions honest, simple, and age-appropriate. Children typically understand adult situations much more than adults may give them credit for, and if the household has had disagreements and conflict up to the point of separation, it is likely that the child is not going to be surprised. Keep the door of communication open with your child as your family navigates this transition, allowing the child to ask questions as they need to. Maintain regular routines at both households as much as possible, avoid criticizing the other parent in front of your child or involving your child in arguments, and respect the child's relationship with his other parent.

The Significance of Divorce

Regardless of the circumstances that lead to the decision of parents to divorce, it is a disruption in the lives of children. A child's initial emotional response may vary: younger children often describe sadness as their main reaction, while older children say they are angry. Almost all have experienced a breach of faith and have a fear of what the future will hold. At the same time, most child-health professionals believe that divorce is preferable to a conflict-ridden marriage, which can take an emotional toll on children.

Separated and divorced parents can take steps to minimize the trauma their children experience, assist them in adapting to their new circumstances, and model appropriate behaviors to help them achieve healthy relationships throughout their lives. If you are divorced, despite the difficulties you and your former partner are going through, remember that though you no longer share a marriage, you continue to share parenthood. If the two of you, alone or with professional help, can put aside your marital conflicts and get on with your lives, your children will benefit over the long term. The most important predictor of a child's long-term adjustment to divorce is the way his parents adapt to their separation—specifically that the divorce ends the discord the child was experiencing.

What Should You Tell the Children?

Children have a right to know about an impending change in the family, particularly how it is going to affect them. This information should be saved until you and your partner have made some final decisions and are able to provide the children with a structured plan and answers to most of their questions. Avoid statements such as "Your father and I are thinking about getting a divorce; we'll let you know what we decide."

If you and your partner make the decision to separate or divorce, explain the situation honestly to your children. Ideally, both you and your partner should talk with the children about the divorce at the same time. Discuss the situation in simple, honest, age-appropriate language they can understand. For example, if you have a child in the younger years of middle childhood, explain the situation simply and directly:

"Mom and I have decided that we are going to stop living together. We don't know yet whether it's going to be forever or for a little while. We're getting what's called 'separated.' That means that Dad will live in one place and Mom will live in another. You are going to live most of the time with Mom and some of the time with Dad. But we both still love you just as much as we always have."

Talking with Your Child About Divorce

When you and your partner tell your child about your divorce, she will have many questions. More than anything she will want to know, "Am I going to be okay? Do Mom and Dad still love me? Will they be able to take care of me?" Keep your discussions honest, simple, and age-appropriate.

Here are some of the specific questions you might expect from your child or that you can bring up yourself.

- ■ "Why are you getting divorced?"

- ■ "Will we ever be a whole family again like before?"

- ■ "Do you still love me?"

- ■ "Was it my fault?"

- ■ "Where am I going to live?"

- ■ "Will I have to change schools?"

- ■ "Will I still spend time with both of you?"

- ■ "Will I be able to see my friends as before?"

- ■ "Will I still be able to see both sets of grandparents?"

- ■ "Will the family still have the same amount of money?"

- ■ "Why can't things be just the same?"

As you talk to your child, explain that despite the changes that lie ahead, everyone hopes that life will be better under the new family arrangement. For instance, if your child has been exposed to constant arguments in the home, this transition should help resolve the arguments. And as you and your partner get a new start on life, the two of you will become better, happier parents in many ways.

Allow your child to respond with whatever she is feeling. She may be upset. She may cry. While some parents try to convince their children that they should not feel sad, this is unwise and is often an attempt to ease their own guilt about the impending family disruptions.

Here are statements to children that some parents have found useful:

- "Hearing about the divorce probably makes you angry."

- "Our divorce seems to make you sad."

- "You probably have a lot of strong feelings about Mom and Dad right now."

These "active listening" statements from parents may give a child who is experiencing divorce an opportunity to express her thoughts and emotions. When such statements are followed by a brief period of silence, the school-age child is more likely to respond.

You might find that your child is not at all surprised by the impending separation or divorce. By the middle years of childhood, most kids are sensitive enough to family dynamics to realize that problems exist in the marriage, and they are probably familiar with divorces in the families of relatives or friends. Your own child may have heard you or your partner make threats about divorce in the past. She may even have already verbalized her fears about divorce ("You and Dad are going to get divorced, aren't you?").

When choosing the best time to have this discussion—whether at the time of the separation or several days or weeks beforehand—take into account your child's maturity level. A 5-, 6-, or 7-year-old has a frame of reference that typically doesn't extend further than a week or two into the future, and she may become confused if you are talking about a separation that won't take place for a month or longer. Keep information honest and simple. Be wary of hiding information for prolonged periods. It may cause further harm by contributing to a child's feeling that she is not being told all the information she needs.

You can give an older child a little more advance notice, allowing her a chance to think about and adjust to the changes ahead and to ask questions. Expect the questions to continue. Most children cannot quite comprehend and adapt to the issues the first or second time they hear them. Additional questions will occur to the child as she grows older and reconsiders what has happened.

Adjusting to the Changes

When a divorce occurs, the family generally moves through a series of stages. In the *pre-divorce* period, as partners argue and the distance between them grows, children may be caught up in the marital conflict, either directly or indirectly, and may exhibit acting-out behavior like fighting, disobeying, talking back, and crying for no reason. Then, during the *separation* phase, as one of the partners leaves the household, children in the middle years may feel quite insecure with the dis-

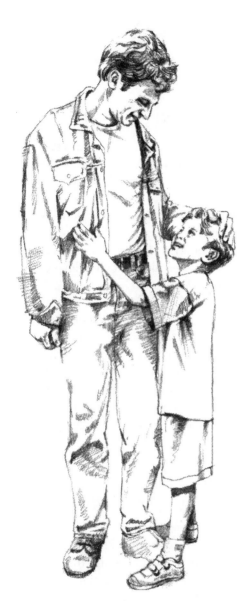

Children cope better with divorce when they have an ongoing relationship with both parents.

ruptions in their daily routines, with one parent no longer around to pick them up from school, help them with their homework, or tuck them in at night.

As the initial turmoil subsides, the *adjustment* period begins, and children start to cope with their new life circumstances, including new routines, visiting schedules, and living arrangements (for example, two homes instead of one). Frequently, the income and financial resources of the custodial parent decrease during this time. This economic hardship can make the child's emotional adjustment to divorce even more difficult, particularly if his parents argue a lot about financial matters. Failure to pay child support is an all-too-common occurrence that can place stress on the entire family and prolong the adjustment process. Sometimes parents are so caught up in grieving over the loss of their marriage and what it represented for them that they are paralyzed into inaction. Professional help may be necessary to get the family's adjustment and recovery back on track.

Next, during the *reorganization* period, both child and parents reach a new equilibrium and the child feels more stable. Consistent routines in both households help a child understand what to expect and boost his feelings of security.

Through these stages, children will experience many emotions, including anger, sadness, loneliness, embarrassment, disappointment, fear, and a sense of betrayal. Each of these emotions needs to be recognized, accepted as real, and discussed between parent and child. Your son or daughter needs to feel free to express these feelings within the family.

Adjustment to Divorce: Different Ages, Different Needs

Children ages 5–7 years: The younger children are, the more naive their view of your family's changes. You may find you need to emphasize the changes and moves happening, as a 5-year-old may believe certain situations to be only temporary. Age-appropriate play therapy is a great idea for this age group even if the situation seems to be progressing smoothly.

Children ages 8–10 years: They will remember what life was like before the family transition and may have particular challenges coping with the changes. Age-appropriate counseling is recommended even if all seems to be taken in stride, as kids this age are able to internalize certain feelings or anxieties, keeping them deeper below the surface.

Children ages 11–12 years: Preteens are experiencing their own hormonal shifts and school adjustments, and the impact of a family divorce can further complicate these transitions. Keep the lines of communication open during this challenging time. Don't expect all conversations to be fruitful with a tangible agreement or result; your goal as a parent during this transition is to be present for your child, allowing her to feel heard as an individual. Counseling is a good idea even if all seems to be progressing smoothly.

All children have fantasies about their parents reconciling. This wish may last for years, representing their desire for the family to be whole again. It is a sign of their loyalty to both parents. Accept this wish without ridiculing it; it is a normal part of the process of coming to terms with the divorce.

An older child in the middle years may ask, "Did you and Mom ever love each other?" You can respond by explaining that people's feelings change over time. "When you were born, things were better between Mommy and me. But things have gotten more difficult, and we couldn't make them better."

A child may pose questions like "Why didn't you work it out?" or "Why did you let him leave?" He may blame one parent or the other for the divorce. If this happens, acknowledge your child's hurt and anger, and tell him: "That may be the way you see things, but there are other ways to look at it. Sometime when you are not so angry, let's talk more about it." You do not need to become defensive or go into the details of why your marriage did not work.

On occasion, children blame themselves for what is happening. The 5- or 6-year-old may feel that he somehow caused his parents' divorce ("They're getting divorced because I was bad"). The child who is a little older may understand that he was not the cause of the divorce but may blame himself for being unable to make things better ("I failed in trying to keep Mom and Dad together").

While you may already have tried to reassure your child that the divorce is not his fault, do not demand that he stop blaming himself. Instead, say something like "I believe you did your best to keep us together" or "I know you are disappointed, but there is nothing you could have done." Let him know that the divorce was beyond his control.

In the weeks and months ahead, keep the lines of communication open. But while you should invite your child to talk, do not force the conversation if he is not ready. In middle childhood kids are doing a lot of analyzing of their own and may not always be ready to share what they're thinking. They need to go through the grieving process as they experience and learn to accept the loss of their original family structure. Sometimes a hug is more important than words. In general, older school-age children are more verbal than younger ones, but if your child has always tended to be withdrawn and quiet, he will probably continue to be that way through the divorce. In times of stress, children's usual ways of interacting may be accentuated. In any case, always make yourself available for discussion ("I know you're upset; would you like to discuss it?").

Some parents feel so guilty about the divorce that they will impose less discipline upon their children during this time. However, if your son or daughter is angry and acting out, you need to set limits and not give in ("I know you're angry, but that doesn't mean you can break your toys or throw things at your sister").

If he is younger, your child may have periods when he seems to be regressing, when sadness and anger that he hasn't exhibited in months resurface, or when he becomes afraid of the dark or asks for help in tasks he has already mastered such as brushing his teeth or doing his homework. Be understanding of this behavior for a while, and reassure your son or daughter that you are still there to care for him.

Sometimes a child's birthday, a special holiday, or a vacation may trigger emotions related to the divorce that he hasn't felt in a while. The need to change schools may do the same. In general, children take about six months to a year to move through the post-divorce adjustment process, although a variety of emotions may resurface from time to time thereafter.

Some factors will help your child cope better with your separation or divorce. A sibling to share the experience with can provide considerable support, because brothers and sisters can understand one another's feelings and reactions on a level that others may not. Research shows that siblings tend to become closer as their parents go through a divorce. However, if siblings fight more during or after the divorce and this problem does not subside on its own, it may be a signal that professional help is warranted.

Relationships with grandparents, aunts, or uncles also can be stabilizing for middle-years children. Give your child access to these relatives, and do not make him feel guilty if he wants to see your former in-laws, for example. If you do not feel comfortable letting him go over to their home, invite them to drop by, but do not deny them access to your child.

Keep in mind that extended-family members often feel awkward talking with you about the divorce and expressing their concern. Give them suggestions on how they can be supportive of your child. For instance, invite them to take your son or daughter to the park or play catch in the yard. Encourage them to call as often as they would like. Even though you and your ex-partner are divorced, your child is still a member of both families and should be able to maintain his status within those family units.

Your child may have friends whose parents are divorced, and he may already be talking with them about his experiences. Children from divorced households often compare notes about their experiences and give one another advice, even at this young age. Some communities have formal support groups for children of divorced families, which can make a child feel he is not the only one in these circumstances. Although this peer support will not remove the pain that may accompany divorce, it can help to normalize the feelings your child is experiencing.

Your child's attitude toward you and your partner may change over time. He might feel a loyalty conflict between the two of you, particularly if you or your partner is trying to pull him to one side of the conflict or the other. Or he might reject the parent he blames for the divorce. In this case, allow your child to have these feelings but still encourage his relationship with that parent. Eventually he will get the message that both of his parents still love him. Your child may ask himself: "How can I belong to two people who don't love each other?" Eventually, however, if both parents continue to care for him appropriately, he will recognize that both his parents love him.

Although some of your child's emotions—anger, for instance—might be directed at you and your ex-partner, he may be hesitant to express them. As much as you'd like to know what's going on inside, you may not be able to help ease every hurt. Respect your child and his feelings, and allow him to select the people (friends, grandparents) he wants to use for support.

Making the Divorce Livable for Your Child

To help your child move through the divorce process as smoothly as possible, keep the following issues in mind:

- Try to make your divorce as amicable as possible. If you and your ex-partner continue to argue over everything from your divorce settlement to child visitation, this ongoing conflict is going to interfere with the healing process. Both of you should be willing to make some compromises for the sake of your child; do not overreact to every issue that remains unresolved between the two of you. Remember that you are modeling healthy behaviors to your child during this process; your child learns her own future behavior patterns in relationships by observing the adults in her world. Whenever possible, avoid a lengthy legal battle, which can frighten and demoralize your child. Many states require divorcing parents to meet with a mediator before custody suits are heard; try to resolve these matters out of court to save everyone time, money, and aggravation.

   Some research suggests that joint custody tends to be a more favorable situation for children than sole custody, but this is true only if both parents can maintain open communication, tolerate their differences, and work cooperatively as a team. Often joint custody arrangements, which force the child to shuttle back and forth and adapt to two households, cause distress and interfere with the child's social life.

- Try your best to understand the feelings of your child and your ex-partner without attempting to change them. Think of your former partner as the co-parent that he or she is, and try to maintain a relationship in which you can talk with each other without a lot of discomfort. This may take some time and patience, but eventually you want to be able to work *with* your ex-partner in raising your child, not to remain adversaries.

   Initially, most divorced parents find it easier to discuss parenting issues by phone, since face-to-face contact may raise the emotional climate to uncomfortable levels. But whether you choose to have these conversations by phone or in person, you and your ex-partner will need to discuss your expectations of each other and establish some ground rules for communicating through the post-divorce period.

   At the outset the most important issues to deal with are visitation and access to your child. Make a schedule of when the noncustodial parent will call and visit. At the same time, you and your ex-partner should set up a regular schedule for speaking by phone about issues pertaining to your child; by routinely keeping in touch with each other, the two of you can deal with your child's problems before they become crises. These discussions should also involve sharing observations about the events in your child's life. As trust builds, you will find it easier to discuss issues related to school, health, morals, religious values, and other important matters. With time you can work out a reasonable co-parenting relationship.

- Respect your child's relationship with her other parent. Allow her to spend time with your ex-partner without making her feel guilty because she enjoys doing so. She needs to have an ongoing relationship with both her parents. No matter what you personally may feel about your ex-partner, unless he or she is abusive to your child, it is better for your child to see both parents *regularly* rather than to have only intermittent contact, or none. The exception to this is if your former partner is physically or emotionally abusive.

  If you are the custodial parent, it is your responsibility to persuade the noncustodial parent to maintain this contact with your child. If your ex-partner breaks off his or her relationship with your child, seek professional help yourself to find ways to reach out and include the noncustodial parent in your child's life. Sometimes former in-laws can help encourage an ex-partner to take the parenting role more seriously. Court-ordered visits tend to be resented by children and do not promote positive relationships.

- Define clearly for your child any changes in her role in the family. If you are going back into the workplace, for example, you might say, "I need you to be more cooperative with Mom, and that means helping me a little more. When we get home after I pick you up from daycare, I need your help in setting the table for dinner." However, do not make your child feel that he or she has to assume a parenting role—that is, avoid statements like "You are now the man in the family" or "Now I have to depend on you."

  Sometimes you or your child can benefit from some emotional first aid during and after the divorce. If you are feeling overwhelmed by the changes in your life, or if your child has long-term difficulties adjusting to the new circumstances, talk to your pediatrician for a referral to a mental health professional. Parents can find books that will help them talk to their children about this. There are also several good age-appropriate books for kids themselves. These books can help minimize feelings of isolation and encourage problem-solving for any issues you may be facing.

  During the grieving process every child may have some difficulties—for example, a B student may get C's in her classes for a while. However, if she is skipping school, getting into fights with classmates, and not completing enough work to get even passing grades, then she may need counseling. Extreme aggression, experimentation with drugs or sex, or signs of depression (irritability, withdrawal, apathy, poor sleep, loss of interest in usual activities) also are signals of a need for help.

The therapist may recommend treating you and your child together on matters that involve both of you. She might also suggest that your ex-partner participate in therapy when problems affecting your child are discussed. The ultimate outcome of divorce for your child depends on how well you can prioritize your child's needs, avoid criticizing the other parent in front of or to your child, maintain consistent and similar routines at both homes, and respect the relationship of your child with his other parent.

~ 31 ~

Single-Parent Families

SINGLE PARENTHOOD BRINGS a distinctive perspective to the parenting experience. Some parents choose single parenthood from the time they first decide to have a child. Other parents have separated from their child's other parent and may not have expected to find themselves in this situation. Some school-age children have experienced the death of a parent. Others may have been adopted by an unmarried individual.

Although single parenthood may be a dramatic change from the life you once had or imagined, it can be a workable, rewarding family situation. Particularly when it occurs in the aftermath of a divorce, it may be a more desirable circumstance than the tumultuous marriage that preceded it. Many single parents describe the contentment they feel in having put the tension and discord of their marriage behind them, and in making a new life for themselves and their children.

Most single parents work. Although looking for work and finding a job to support the family can be stressful, most single parents report that they enjoy the autonomy associated with bringing home a paycheck. In many cases they also enjoy a strong sense of satisfaction from their jobs. Kids with working parents learn life lessons and have a broadened view of what men and women can accomplish in life. As a parent's work schedule may reduce the amount of time she spends with her children, those hours together tend to become much more precious for everyone. Other relationships may become more important too, such as the children's connections with their uncles, aunts, or grandparents.

Supporting Your Family

Unless you are receiving spousal or child support from a former partner, you are likely the sole source of financial support for your child, which can be stressful. Your work obligations may mean that your school-age child sees less of you. Make sure he understands your economic realities and that you need to work more in order to support your family. Reassure him that even when you are away from him, he is a priority for you. A routine after-school phone call, text message, or video chat with him from work, if possible, may ease the distance he feels between you.

Task Overload

A single parent's responsibilities do not stop the moment work ends each day. You may have what seems like a full day's worth of tasks awaiting you at home—from cooking dinner to laundry to helping your child with homework. Although these same obligations are faced by working parents who are married, a single parent faces these responsibilities independently.

If your budget allows, outsource tasks that can be delegated. Kids in any household can and should pitch in with household tasks (for more on this, see page 309). Take a step back and look at the big picture; if there are recurrent problems in the weekly schedule, what creative solutions can help? The same goes for overscheduling kids' extracurricular activities—if scurrying to and from multiple activities is overwhelming, it is time to prioritize the preferred activities and eliminate obligations lower on the list.

Single parents should set aside some downtime to rest and recuperate to prevent burnout. Having emotional support or help around the house from another adult can go a long way toward helping you to manage the big picture.

Personal Pursuits

Single parents often feel they have little personal time, whether to exercise or to have dinner with friends. Even if they can find time for these individual pursuits, they may be so tired that they have no energy for them. Being deprived of sleep will take a toll on anyone, parent or child. Sometimes the best that you can do for yourself and your child is to get more sleep each night.

For some single parents, during or after a divorce or death of a partner, their lack of energy is dramatic and part of a more serious depression. Persistent sadness, irritability, difficulty sleeping, and weight gain or loss are all signs of depression. A depressed parent has much less to offer a child. If you are depressed, speak to your physician or a mental health professional.

Single parents, like all parents, may at times find the responsibilities of child-raising to be overwhelming. Even routine events in their child's life—carpooling, events at school, or normal oppositional behavior—become burdens for parents struggling to squeeze everything into their day. At the extreme, these parents feel they can't deal with their children appropriately and may resort to physical punishment. Or they may give up altogether and agree too easily to their children's demands. When possible, they may need to turn over more of the child-raising responsibilities to the child's other parent and obtain professional counseling to help them cope better.

Child Care

Single parents need to make sure their children are cared for appropriately when they are at work. For middle-years children, many options are available, from commercial child care centers to after-school programs sponsored by community organizations such as YMCAs and Boys and Girls Clubs. Sitters can also give single parents a break to pursue their own interests for a few hours a week. Sometimes employers or various programs will pay part of the cost of child care for working parents. For more information, see Chapter 23, "Child Care."

Decreased Involvement with the Noncustodial Parent

If you are the primary caretaker of your child, you might find that your ex-partner has gradually decreased contact with your kids. After about the first year following a divorce, many fathers in particular stop seeing their children on a regular basis—and sometimes altogether. That increases the pressure on single mothers and interferes with the child's long-term adjustment to the divorce.

Parents drop out of parenting for a number of reasons. Since they are no longer in the house, they may feel they have become less important and influential in their children's lives. They may become so dissatisfied with the noncustodial role that, out of frustration or anger, they may decide to give up parenting altogether. In some cases parents may abandon their responsibilities because they feel they can no longer afford child support. Sometimes they do it in order to avoid paying child support. Or they might have remarried and, in starting a new life, feel they have less time to devote to the children of their former marriage. Some parents feel unwelcome and struggle with how to proceed in developing a separate relationship with their child.

If you are a noncustodial parent, you should remain actively involved in your children's lives. In general, children from divorced families who maintain a relationship with both parents tend to be better adjusted than those who have contact with only one parent. How much time should you spend with your child? As much as possible, given your living arrangements. If you live close to your kids, maintain regular contact, preferably both during the week and on weekends. It is a good idea to have your child spend at least one night a week at your home in order to give him a sense of his place in your life. This avoids you (the noncustodial parent) developing into a parent who only visits him to have fun. It also enables him to receive guidance and regular discipline from you.

If you don't live near your child, you need to maintain regular contact via telephone calls, text messages, and video chats, and you should plan visits for extended periods of time (such as weekends and holidays) so that you both have the chance to maintain emotional closeness. Children can accept and adjust to these schedules if they are given appropriate explanations, and if they perceive that they are still important to the noncustodial parent.

Intensified Involvement with the Custodial Parent

The custodial parent may develop stronger ties to the children, particularly if the noncustodial parent plays a smaller role in the child's life. Sometimes this intensified relationship can be a positive influence upon the child, provided it remains within reasonable bounds and allows the child to pursue friendships and activities outside the home. It can become harmful, however, if the kid assumes too much of an adult role in the family and therefore gives up his own separate life and privacy for the sake of the parent. This may happen if the single parent asks him to take on more responsibilities around the house or to become the parent's confidant. If parent and child become too closely enmeshed, perhaps because both are lonely in the aftermath of the divorce, their relationship can become so intense that other relationships cannot develop for either of them. At the same time, it may become harder for the parent to maintain authority, even over simple matters like what time the child should go to bed.

While a close relationship with your child is encouraged, avoid a situation in which you are spending virtually all your free time together. Your child is not an adult friend; both of you need your own friends and outside interests. In some cases, when parent and child have become closely intertwined, jealousy and resentment can surface when one of them develops other relationships—for instance, the daughter who, as an adolescent, finds a boyfriend and leaves her mother home alone on Saturday nights. Such closeness can be confining.

Changes in Children's Behavior

A child's difficult behavior in the aftermath of his parents' separation tends to be temporary and will probably diminish as the crisis of divorce subsides. However, there are a number of troublesome behavioral patterns that, if persistent, are signs of more serious problems. Boys and girls in middle childhood often respond differently in these situations as they adjust to living in a single-parent household.

For example, boys may become aggressive after a parent moves out, challenging the custodial parent's authority. In this situation the custodial parent needs to work hard to maintain his authority as soon as this behavior becomes apparent, or matters could get out of control as the child's aggressiveness escalates. Both parents should support the ex-partner's position as an authority figure; however, a parent should not be called in to "rescue" a former partner, since this will tend to undermine the other parent's authority position and could even cause additional misbehavior by the child as a way of forcing more contact with the noncustodial parent. Occasionally, boys will develop some of the departed partner's behavior and assume an adult-like relationship with the mother. He may become jealous if she starts to date, or may otherwise attempt to assume an adult role in the family.

Girls, by contrast, tend to become more reserved and withdrawn as their response to the changing family structure. They may assume a maternal role in relation to their mother and siblings. An 11- or 12-year-old girl may actually run the household while her mother is working, which may create an unhealthy relationship between her and her siblings. If the girl is living with her father, she might also develop some of the departed mother's behavior and function as a "wife" to her father. These are not healthy patterns. To reduce the stress on an older daughter, involve the grandparents and extended family for help; alternatively, when financially feasible, hire a part-time housekeeper to assume some of the household responsibilities. The younger children in the family can also begin taking responsibility for more chores.

When You Start to Date

Most middle-years children need some time to adjust to their parents' separation before their parents begin to have new romantic interests. In general, a good guideline is about a six-month wait from the time you separate from your child's other parent to the time you start to date, although dating will often occur sooner. You should talk with your child about your new adult friends. Allow your son or daughter to express her feelings and opinions.

Here are some other suggestions to keep in mind:

- You don't need to introduce your child to all your dates—only to those with whom you are developing a serious relationship. Although your older child may be curious about a man you are going out with, she might form an attachment to him before it is appropriate to do so. She may want you to marry this person immediately in hopes of creating a new family unit. Be sure to explain to your child the differences between dating, developing a relationship, becoming engaged, and getting married; she should understand that not all dating and friendships end in marriage.

  Discuss with your partner the best time for him to meet your son or daughter. Do not put pressure on your new partner to meet your child before he feels ready to do so.

- Prepare both your new partner and your child for their first meeting with each other. Tell your child about this person, and explain why you like him—for example, he is smart, or he is funny. Then say something like "I was thinking that you might like to meet John. Would you like him to come over for dinner, or would you like the three of us to go out to dinner together?" Show her that you would like her to participate in arranging this first meeting. In telling your new partner about your child, share what your child likes to do, what sports she enjoys, her hobbies, what she likes in school, and other information you think might help your new partner in conversation with her.

- Don't expect miracles during the first encounter. There may be some anxiety during the first meeting between your new partner and your child. The goal of the initial get-together should be only to say hello—not for the two of them necessarily to like each other. Don't rush things; they will need to develop their own relationship over time. Discourage your new partner from trying to impress your child, or from attempting to get too close too quickly.

- Help your child deal with any negative feelings she has. Sometimes children may see their mother's new love interest as a threat to their fantasy that their parents will someday reunite. When this person becomes a serious enough part of your life that you are introducing him to your child, you also need to deal with any unrealistic ideas your child has ("Dad and I are divorced, and it is important that you understand that we are not going to get back together again").

Your child may still prefer her other parent to your new partner. But with time, she might come to see this new man as a nice person with whom she can be friends. Any jealousy she feels over your dates with another man should resolve after an initial period of adjustment.

Also, let your child's other parent know that you will be introducing your child to your new partner. Your child should not feel that this is a secret she has to keep, or that she will have to be the one to disclose this information to her other parent, which she might find painful to do. Children should not be keepers of secrets.

- Show some discretion about intimate relationships with your new romantic interest. Children learn about the adult world through example—particularly from parents. As you develop a relationship with a new person, keep in mind that your child is learning about intimacy at the same time. Open, age-appropriate communication during the development of a romantic relationship will allow your child to experience a new level of awareness about grown-up behavior; however, direct exposure to frankly sexual conduct is not a good idea.

When school-age children are exposed to these new relationships, they need a clear statement from you about your feelings toward your new friend and your wish to be close to him, and also about the differences between adult relationships and those between children or adolescents. When you have a discussion with your child about a new intimate relationship, encourage her to express her feelings, good and bad, and help her feel comfortable with asking you questions about your new friend and the ways in which you relate.

Parent-Child Disagreements

If you and your child are increasingly at odds with each other, creating more stress in the household, you may not have anyone else to turn to for support now that your ex-partner is out of the house. If you are beginning to feel overwhelmed by this situation, here is a strategy for regaining control.

Stop arguing. Step back from the problem at hand and try to understand what is really at issue between you and your child. Then, without operating in the heat of the disagreement, try to clarify with your child what is preventing the two of you from getting along with each other. Perhaps changes in the family circumstances will force both of you to make adjustments. Calmly explain the new situation now that your child's other parent is no longer living with you. For example:

"We cannot afford a housekeeper any longer, so I need your help in keeping your room clean."

Avoid arguing about situations in which there are no options. Your child may complain that he can't go to the summer camp he would like to, but your budget simply may not make that camp possible. He needs to understand that everyone in the family will adapt to the new demands brought on by the one-parent family. Help him take part in the problem-solving; use the situation as a learning experience. This can be an important lesson in resilience and creative problem-solving. Single parents, just like all parents, should adjust any expectations about what children need in terms of material possessions; be realistic in order to minimize unnecessary stress. Studies show that material possessions do not contribute to long-term happiness; rather, emotional connections and experiences do.

Children are resilient and adaptable, and will rise to the occasion if you give them the opportunity. The more often you and your child can sit down and talk, the better. Have discussions of what each of you envisions for the future, taking into account your changing circumstances. It is better to talk *regularly* when issues arise, rather than yell at each other when you reach an impasse. Tell your child, "When you and I don't agree on something, let's sit down and try to understand what our disagreement is all about. Then let's both try hard to come up with a solution." (For a discussion of family meetings, see page 268.)

Support

It is hard to raise a child on your own; don't be hesitant to ask for support. Investigate if your parents, siblings, other relatives and friends, or sitters are able or willing to care for your child for a few hours a week, or help with specific tasks such as a carpool on a certain day. Others may not realize what it is that you need help with—if you receive offers of "How may I help?" be specific in terms of what tasks they can assist with. Parent groups through your house of worship or community may prove helpful as well.

~ 32 ~

Stepfamilies

THROUGH DIVORCE AND remarriage, a child may share a household with a new stepparent and his or her children. Most stepfamilies function quite well. In blended stepfamilies, parents can turn to each other for support and share parenting responsibilities. It takes time and honest effort, but stepparents and their stepchildren can develop a genuinely positive regard for one another, and the new family can provide an enriching experience for everyone. Along with a new stepparent may come new stepbrothers and stepsisters, and a new extended family. These relationships require some negotiation, but they broaden each child's experience with people and may introduce him to new social and cultural influences.

Becoming a Stepfamily

When you and your new partner are ready for a more committed relationship, discuss these plans with your children to prepare them for the changes that are about to take place. If you are planning to get married, your son or daughter will want to be part of any celebration. The wedding ceremony itself is generally a positive experience for children, one in which they should be given a special role. The more that children feel a part of the process of becoming a stepfamily, the more smoothly things will progress for all concerned.

Next, a new household will be established, and the blended family will learn to live together. This is a period of establishing who you are, what you are willing to share, and what each individual's role in the new household will be. This process takes time, conscious effort on the part of all family members (especially the parents), and occasionally outside help. From the child's perspective, the new stepparent is a guest in the house. The stepparent needs to develop his relationship with the child gradually and independently from his relationship with the child's parent.

Once the transition period is over, people settle into routines as any family does. Later, there may be changes and transitions that can force adaptations in family life—for example, if the remarried couple has a new baby of their own, or an older child leaves for college.

The success of stepfamilies depends on a number of factors, but especially on the quality of the new marriage. If the new partners begin having difficulties with their own relationship, that will affect nearly every aspect of family life, including how the children fare.

As the children themselves adapt to the new family arrangement, some will do better than others. Sometimes, the fit between stepchild and stepparent is a good one. However, there are situations in which problems may arise. Perhaps the child is jealous of the new partner in his mother's life, or he may resent the intrusion of stepsiblings into his home. Sometimes members of the blended family have minimal tolerance for their differences, creating dissatisfaction and tension that can undermine the family's equilibrium.

What Your Child Is Experiencing

For a child, remarriage can have positive aspects, although she may be looking forward to different things than her parent is. However, there are also some difficulties that can arise as members of two families begin living under the same roof. Here are some of the most common concerns for school-age children:

Dealing with Loss

As their parents date, develop serious relationships, and eventually decide to remarry, children may be reminded of their original family and of the life they once had with their parents. Now, with the prospect of a new marriage, they must confront the reality that their parents really are not going to reconcile and that they will not have their original family back. This can be a source of sadness. There are other losses to deal with as well. Children who have built a particularly close relationship with their own parents during a period of single parenthood must now learn to share that parent not only with a new partner but perhaps with stepsiblings whom the child barely knows.

As the middle-years child experiences this kind of loss and pain, she may show signs of increased attachment to the parent who is getting married. For instance, she might not want to leave the parent's side in certain social situations, or she might express jealousy when her parent shows attention to the new partner and his or her children. She might even verbalize some of her hurt and anger ("I don't think he's the right guy for you, Mom"). Some children wonder to themselves: "Where do I belong?" As they see their parent starting a new family, for example, they may feel more like an outsider than part of the new family structure. With time, however, most children adjust to their new family circumstances. As they get to know their stepparent and stepsiblings better, their level of acceptance will grow too.

Divided Loyalties

Many children feel that if they like and show affection toward their new stepparent, they will be demonstrating disloyalty or a lack of devotion to the original parent whom this new stepparent, to some extent, is replacing in their home. They may worry that if their parent remarries, bringing a new parenting figure into the household, they will lose the love and attention of their other parent.

Your child may still feel awkward for a while, having to get used to two fathers or two mothers. Particularly in the beginning, allow her to view your new partner in the most comfortable way for her—perhaps as a second father but sometimes just as Mommy's husband. You need to reassure her about these concerns, saying something like "Your stepfather is different from your dad, and no one will ever replace your own dad."

Along the way, you can expect your child to make some comparisons between her real parent and stepparent, in both positive and negative ways. She might blurt out statements like "You're not as nice as my dad." Comparisons are normal during this adjustment period. Eventually your child should stop making them.

If possible, the child's parents and stepparents should make contact with each other to begin working toward talking comfortably about your children. This can begin with a phone call just to say hello and to share observations of the child. Both parties might decide to have lunch or some other informal meeting. Although these two adults may run into each other at special events, such as birthdays and graduations, these occasions may not be opportune times to do much talking.

The more comfortable these two individuals become with each other, the more reassured she will feel that she does not have to choose between the love of her parent and the developing relationship with her stepparent. It will show the child that the adults are pulling together on her behalf, and that they all care and have her interests at heart.

Do not expect your child to solve her loyalty conflicts if you have not resolved your own differences with your ex-partner. For example, when remarriages occur, the issue of child custody often resurfaces; if a noncustodial father marries a woman with children, he may return to court, requesting that his own child now live with him. In the midst of an ongoing custody battle, the child will find it much harder to deal with her own loyalty conflicts.

Difficulty with New Rules

As children move from a household with a single parent into one that is occupied by a stepparent and perhaps stepsiblings, they will probably be confronted with changes in the way their family operates. Routines will be altered and new chores may be imposed. With more people in the home, privacy issues may become more important. It may be harder for children to carve out a personal space they can call their own.

In a sense, the entire household is in transition, and everyone—including the children—needs to participate in the reorganization and adapt to the way it runs. The majority of family members adapt, but it may take some time.

Unreasonable Expectations

All couples want their new marriages to be as harmonious as possible. Hopefully, having learned from past experiences, they can achieve their expectations. However, within stepfamilies it is unrealistic to hope that the children will immediately respect and love their new stepparents. In the real world, relationships develop more slowly. Children need time to really get to know and feel comfortable with a stepmother or stepfather.

In general, good relationships develop most quickly with younger children. Older children, who are more set in their ways, may rightly feel that their established lifestyles are being disrupted by this new person entering their life.

Stepsiblings

One of the most challenging aspects of a blended family is for the children of each parent to become comfortable living together as brothers and sisters. Children who are brought into the same household with minimal preparation and are expected to function as a congenial, loving family are unlikely to succeed. Storybook relationships may appear to be developing in those first few weeks of getting to know one another, but this is generally only a honeymoon period until the children feel comfortable enough to express their disagreements and conflicts with one another.

As with any siblings, there will probably be some competition between the children in stepfamilies, much of it for their parents' attention. Stepsiblings should not be expected to spend all of their time together, and in fact each child will need some time spent just with his or her own parent. This is particularly important for the child who may live with her mother and whose father remarries. The child may recognize that her dad is now spending less time with her than with the stepchildren who live with him. She may think, "Why do they get to live with Dad and I don't? Does he like them better? I don't get to do as much with my dad anymore because of them."

Children in this situation should have some special time with their fathers on a regular basis. Parents must acknowledge and respect this need, finding afternoons or entire weekends that they can devote solely to their own children, who may live across town or in another part of the state.

Other problems can occur with stepsiblings who live together. Sometimes a child is asked to share a room with a stepbrother or stepsister when, in the past, that same room was hers alone. Or when her stepfather's children come to visit him on the weekend, they may move into her room for a couple of days, sometimes creating anger and jealousy.

Privacy and personal space become important issues in blended families. Whenever possible, children should have their own rooms. Even if they share a room, however, each child should have her own toys and other possessions; she should not be forced to turn them all into community property.

In some cases, the remarried couple will have one or more babies of their own, who will become the existing children's half siblings. While most school-age children generally like having a baby around, they may also complain about the drawbacks. A newborn is often the center of attention of family and friends, and that means a loss of focus on the older children. More important, the older children may feel jealous that their parent is starting a new family, and that the baby gets to live with both of her parents, while their own parents are divorced. Even so, most new additions to the family are treated with love by the other children. (See Chapter 22, "Sibling Rivalry.") With time, stepsiblings tend to become good friends and companions, and their relationships are enriching and rewarding.

Who Will Handle the Discipline?

All children need discipline. But in stepfamilies, parents often are unsure of who should administer it. Should a stepparent, for example, discipline his partner's children, or should she be the only one to handle it?

Stepparents may attempt to assert authority and directly discipline their stepchildren, rather than letting their partners take the lead with their own children. Particularly in the initial few months, stepparents should play a supportive role in discipline but allow their new partner to continue being the primary disciplinarian. They should avoid sweeping statements like "From now on, we're going to do things this way." The new couple should gradually make a transition to shared authority. This transition can be accomplished by a delegation of authority from the child's parent to the stepparent, with the parent saying something such as "While you're with him, you need to mind what he says—or answer to me."

If a new stepparent becomes too assertive in parenting his partner's children, the children may resent him and complain to their parent. She may find herself caught in the middle between her partner and her children as conflicts escalate. And if she takes her partner's side, her children may feel betrayed. It is a position that can and should be avoided.

If the new partners disagree on disciplinary issues, the child may begin undermining and challenging the stepparent's authority, which is not good either for the child or for the new relationship. When parents disagree this way, they need to negotiate their differences, or problems will escalate.

Advice for Stepparents

In most blended families, children challenge their stepparents from time to time. Some children may become openly aggressive; others may keep an emotional distance from their stepmother or stepfather. If this happens in your family, don't take it personally; it is the child's way of testing you and perhaps dealing with his own feelings over having a new adult in his life.

If your stepchild criticizes you, don't overreact; this will become less common as the months pass. In general, the older the child, the more critical and judgmental he is likely to be of you as a stepparent. While letting him express his feelings, you can be comforted by the fact that, if you are fair and making a sincere effort to get along, the negative feelings will eventually be outweighed by more positive ones. It is a sign of progress and a developing relationship that he feels comfortable enough with you to voice his feelings.

To build bridges, find some interests that you and your stepchildren share, and invite them to join you in these activities. You might hold regular family meetings to pull together on some issues and to iron out differences (see page 268 for more on family meetings). Above all, treat your stepchildren with respect, and you will ultimately win their trust.

Sometimes the difficulty children have within stepfamilies is really a continuation of their unresolved feelings over their parents' separation. Children's responses to the divorce of their parents can take many forms—and those feelings are not easily or quickly resolved. They may linger and then disappear, only to resurface in times of stress, especially when new relationships such as stepfamilies are formed. Most communities have support groups to help remarried couples and their children deal with the various issues that can arise in stepfamilies. If you are in need of resources or further direction, discuss this with your family's pediatrician.

~ 33 ~

Adoption

TODAY ABOUT 2 PERCENT of the children in the United States are adopted. Children may be adopted by extended family members, by single parents, by same-sex parents, or by more traditional families. In all types of families, adopted children can and do thrive. If you have adopted a child, you prepared for your child in a unique way—not with a nine-month pregnancy, but rather through the lengthy legal process involved in adoption. Your family's adoption experience was possibly preceded by years of trying to become pregnant yourself, or alternatively, you desired to expand your family with an additional member in a different way. Your child has biological relatives outside of your family somewhere in the world. You and your child may be similar in some ways, and different in others—her race may not be the same as yours, and her temperament might be different. These differences occur in all families, but they may have a specific impact on families who have adopted a child.

Even if you adopted your child as an infant, prenatal experiences of malnutrition, drug or alcohol exposure, or inadequate healthcare may have lasting impacts on her. If you adopted your child not in infancy but rather during the preschool, elementary school, or teen years, her life experiences before you became part of her life could present challenges. Some children may have been denied affection, or even basic nutrition or medical care, in their prior living environment. Others may have been physically, sexually, or emotionally abused and may have physical or emotional scars from those experiences. While the adoptive family's loving care is hugely important in helping children to heal, many children and families benefit from working with a mental health professional who is experienced in early childhood adversity and adoption. The long-term consequences of these early experiences are often difficult to predict, and can occur at any time in a child's life, as new circumstances bring up old memories.

No matter what the reasons for and circumstances of the adoption, most adopted children are well-adjusted and happy. Nevertheless, adoptive families often feel different and at times socially isolated. Indeed, these differences are real, and there are issues unique to the family who adopts a child. These issues need to be acknowledged and addressed.

There is no better camaraderie and advice than from others who have had similar experiences. Connect with other families who have adopted children in your immediate community as well as greater geographic area. Many family networks are found on social networking sites: these can be an excellent source of emotional support and a great format in which to exchange notes and share stories. There are many books and magazines dedicated to families who adopt a child and the unique situations faced, whether it's a domestic or international adoption.

Explaining Adoption to Your Child

All children need and deserve to know about their own histories, and like everything else children learn, it is important that they come to understand their own stories over time. Parents should start talking about adoption with their child right from the beginning of their time together, whether the child is a newborn or an older infant or child.

Your explanations should be simple, direct, and honest. Explain that he was not born to you. Tell him that he was born to other parents who could not take care of him or any baby at that time. Then describe why you chose to adopt a child. Talk about how much you wanted him, and talk about the process you went through to get him. If your child was relinquished by his birth parents involuntarily, talk about the fact that they were having hardships that prevented them from being able to take care of a child, but that there were adults who made sure that he found a family who could take care of him.

Allow your child to ask questions. For example, he might want to know, "What happened to my first mommy and daddy? Where are they?" You can share as much as you think your child will understand right now, and add more details over time as he comes to understand his story. Your comments should answer his questions in ways appropriate for his maturity level, and follow his lead with what details he is or is not interested in at the moment. At the time of the adoption you may have been given some basic information about your child's biological parents—from medical issues (a family history of heart disease, for example) to personal characteristics. You may also have ongoing contact with your child's birth family, and so may learn more over time. This is all information that is valuable to your child and which you will want to share and protect for him. One useful way to address all kinds of adoption questions is with a "life book," a scrapbook of all of the information you have about your child, from his past through his transition to your family and his ongoing story with your family. This can be especially helpful to a child with a complicated history of multiple moves. This book can be updated creatively with your child over time as he matures and as his interests and questions evolve.

If you are reading this and realize that you have not yet been talking about adoption with your child, there is no time like the present to start. Adoption should never be a secret. Every child needs to have an honest understanding of his origin. The longer you wait to talk about adoption, the harder it will be to discuss it with your child. Also, he is liable to find out from someone else—perhaps by overhearing the conversations of relatives, or from teasing by neighborhood children who have learned from their own parents that he is adopted. Children who learn about adoption "by accident" or later in life often feel betrayed and lied to, and may have real struggles trusting their parents in other areas of life as a result. Working with a family therapist who is experienced in adoption-related matters can be very helpful if you find yourself in this situation.

Sometimes parents who struggle to talk about adoption with their children have difficulties of their own in accepting that their son or daughter is not their biological child. Sometimes they might feel inadequate, and they avoid explaining the adoption to their kids so that they will not have to revisit that issue. Sometimes parents are hesitant to talk about the adoption because they are trying to be protective of their child's feelings, sensing that he might be hurt at finding out he was adopted. They might also be afraid of being rejected by their adopted children. They might think, "What if my son says, 'I don't want to live with you anymore; I want to go live with my real mommy'?" These are all normal feelings for adoptive parents, but it is important to work through them and be ready to talk with your child about adoption regardless. Here too, working with a therapist experienced in adoption can be very valuable.

Keep in mind that it is important for the child to know about his adoption from his earliest memories. Your honest communication about this important issue early on can strengthen the relationship you have with him, building a strong bond of trust. Your child will have questions over time about his birth family, and about why he was not born to you. His questions are normal and do not reflect a lack of affection toward you. The more your child talks about it with you, the more comfortable he will feel with the idea, and the stronger his relationship with you will become.

Your answers to these questions should be direct but still sensitive to the emotional maturity level of your child and to what he has already learned and understands about the adoption. Do not dismiss these questions and concerns, but do not overreact to them either. Acknowledge the fact that his family situation is different from that of many of his friends. At the same time, do not magnify the significance of his special circumstances or dwell upon them. You can follow your child's lead on what is important to him at the moment. Your child's basic needs are the same, regardless of whether he is living with his biological or adoptive parents. Most aspects of his life will be the same as those of his peers, but frequently are also colored by his knowledge of his own and his family's unique history.

Children think about adoption in different ways, and with different frequencies and intensities, at different times in their lives. Some children think and talk about adoption on an hourly basis, while others may have times where they are really not very concerned with the issues at all. Some children will think a lot about adoption but not talk with their parents about it for fear of hurting their parents. You should not leave it to your child to continue the conversation. Raise issues naturally and as opportunities present themselves. For example, at his birthday you might say, "I'm sure your birth mom is thinking about you today. I'm sure she is very proud of you." Another time you might comment on a physical characteristic, as in, "I bet those broad shoulders came from your birth dad. I remember when I met him. . . ."

There are some normal stages through which your adopted child is likely to pass. These may happen at certain ages, but more often they are related to his developmental maturity and his particular interests. In early childhood, for example, he may understand that he has "two mothers" and "two fathers," but the social customs and the full meaning of adoption are probably still a bit unclear. He is likely to ask questions about why his birth mother did not keep him. And he may have anxiety-generating thoughts like "Since my first mother left me, maybe my second one might too."

When your adopted child is a little older, typically in the early school years, he will continue to develop a better understanding of being adopted. You can expect to be asked specific questions about his biological parents, if he does not have an ongoing open relationship with them. In a sense, he will be trying to construct a more accurate "memory" of his original family, which is a normal part of coming to understand himself.

Later in the middle years, all children, including those who are adopted, become increasingly concerned with their appearance and fitting in. Your adopted son or daughter may become more curious about and sensitive to differences in his own skin or hair or eye color if they are not the same as your own. He will also become even more interested in his biological parents, and what his original cultural origins may have been. Expect many more questions about both his biological and adoptive relatives and his family tree.

"Sharing" Your Child

As you raise your adopted child, she is yours in every sense of the word. At the same time, however, there is an aspect to her life—the fact that she has biological parents elsewhere—that may make it critical to think more broadly about "family." Many adoptive families today have ongoing contact with their children's biological families—sometimes just with a birth parent, but often even with extended families. While it can be tricky to grow these relationships, establish boundaries, and work out problems when they arise, these relationships have been shown to have tremendous benefits for adopted children, who can have many of their questions answered.

During middle childhood your son or daughter will probably have questions, fantasies, and feelings about her biological parents. Most adoptive families can deal with these matters well. Children at this time may feel more psychological and emotional conflict about being adopted. At various times they may test and challenge their adoptive parents with statements like "My real parents wouldn't . . ." Adoptive parents often become anxious if their child says things like this, but don't panic. These challenges are a normal part of your child adapting to and accepting her unique family circumstances. Children who are not adopted test their parents with similar kinds of statements too.

In middle childhood, adolescence, and young adulthood, your child may become interested in learning more about her biological mother and father and even may consider searching for them. This may be a function of curiosity, or she may want to get a sense of completion about her own identity. There are avenues available for pursuing this search, usually through support groups, state-mandated confidential intermediaries, or the adoption agency or lawyer. Although you might feel threatened by her desire to learn more about her birth parents or even to meet them, remember that her interest is normal and appropriate for her developmental stage. We all want to know where we came from and what our roots are, even when we know that our adoptive family is truly our real family. Children and young adults who feel supported in this search process often report even stronger ties to their adoptive parents.

Discipline and Your Adopted Child

Some parents find it difficult to discipline a child they have adopted. They may set fewer limits than they would for a birth child. They might react less strongly to misbehavior.

What are the reasons for these patterns of parental inaction? Some adoptive parents are afraid their child might stop loving them if they discipline her. Or they may doubt their own right or ability to parent the child fully. Some children who have experienced adversity before their adoption may react differently to standard disciplinary strategies, and this can complicate things as well.

Despite these concerns, you should feel empowered to fulfill this part of parenting as well as all of the others you perform. One of your tasks as a parent is to help your child grow and mature by providing structure and boundaries and by helping her adjust to the limits you set. It can be helpful to look at the obstacles that may be preventing you from assuming this parental role, such as being fearful of losing her affection to a birth parent who is in close proximity, or feeling uncertain of how to proceed due to your child's history or previous adversity. For children who have experienced significant hardships in the past, you may need to use different parenting and discipline strategies than you would use with a child who has not had those experiences, but you still need to provide the structure and rules that will help your child to grow.

Keep in mind that even though you did not give birth to this boy or girl, he or she is your child. That means you have the right and the obligation to say "It's time to go to bed now" or "No, you can't have your brother's toy right now." Your child's well-being depends on your willingness and ability to function as a full parent.

When your child says to you, "I don't have to listen to you; you're not my real parents," respond calmly, and don't take it personally. All children wish they didn't have to obey their parents—adopted children just have an easy out! Let them know that you understand they wish they didn't have to do whatever it is you are asking them to do, but they do. A parent is someone who parents and who loves his or her child, and that is what you have been doing for years, in both happy times and times of struggle.

International and Interracial Adoption

A significant number of families adopt children from other countries, cultures, or ethnic groups. If you have made this conscious decision to become a multiracial or multicultural family, there are things you can do to assist your adopted child's adaptation and development. You have the responsibility as a parent to instill in your child pride and knowledge about his ethnic origins. This will also help give him tools to combat discrimination and stereotyping.

Here are ways you can incorporate his heritage and customs into the family:

- Have multiethnic toys, clothes, objects, artwork, food, and music in your home as a part of daily life.

- Learn to cook signature dishes from your child's country or culture of origin together.

- Follow news and events from his country or culture of origin.

- Visit ethnic restaurants, stores, cultural programs, and exhibits as an ongoing part of family life—not as special events.

- Make diversity among your adult and family friends a priority, as an example of how you value your child's origins and people of many different origins.

- Select books for your child that feature diverse people and families, from your child's country and culture of origin as well as others. Encourage your child's school and local library to build a similarly diverse collection.

Others' Responses

When you adopt a child, it is important for your relatives to accept him as a part of the family. Most do, but unfortunately there are exceptions to the rule. For a child to feel loved and welcomed, he needs to be treated like a full member of the family. If your parent, brother, sister, or other relative has difficulty relating to your child as part of the family, you need to talk with this relative about it. Explain how important it is for your child to feel accepted. Do not settle for anything less.

If your adoptive child happens to be of a different race or ethnicity than you, be prepared for insensitive comments when you are out as a family—for example, at the grocery store. Some adoptive families share uncomfortable stories in which strangers have asked them, "Where are her real parents from?" Remain calm and have a pleasant yet direct and simple response ready for these individuals who may be genuinely curious without realizing how rude they sound. Look at these interactions from the perspective of your child—your response is more important to your child than it is to the person asking the intrusive questions. Respond simply and matter-of-factly, and if you feel uncomfortable, leave the situation. Your child learns how to navigate these tricky circumstances by modeling your behavior.

Sibling Rivalry

Some families have both children who were adopted and children who were born into the family. This can sometimes create conflict, anger, and hurt feelings. Remember, all children will find reasons to argue. Each child in your family should understand her own origins and those of her brothers and sisters. But no matter what her background, every child should be treated the same by you, your spouse, and the other siblings. Diversity within your family can create wonderful opportunities for all of your children to celebrate differences as well as similarities, and to learn to accept others for who they are, not what they look like or what abilities or challenges they have.

Sometimes academic or athletic differences between your children can seem exaggerated because of their different origins. For instance, if your adoptive child does not do as well in school as your biological child, their differing backgrounds can heighten any tensions that might emerge because of their respective school performances. Having a chronically ill or physically impaired child in the home can add to the usual stress within families. Sometimes the adopted child may feel "different" to begin with, and if her sibling excels in areas where she doesn't, she could feel that she is less than a full member of the family.

With all of your children—whether they are born to you or adopted—look for their strengths, and focus on those as much as possible. As one mother told her child: "Yes, you are having a hard time with math right now. But I know you are working hard and will be able to learn it. And there are many things you can do that make you very special."

As you raise your adopted child, keep in mind that adopted children are, first and foremost, children. In the same way, adoptive parents are parents. There is a lot of joy and satisfaction in raising children, and your relationship with your adoptive child will be as deep, loving, and long-lasting as any parent-child relationship.

~ 34 ~

A Death in the Family

BY SCHOOL AGE, children understand that death is an irreversible event. Even though they recognize that death is something more than going to sleep for a long time, they still may have many unanswered questions they may not verbalize: "Where did Grandma go when she died? What is she feeling? Is she in pain? Why did she die? Can we ever see her again? Are you going to die too? Who will take care of me if you die?" Offer opportunities for your child to ask these questions. The more open, honest, and straightforward your answers are, the better he will fare through the grieving process.

The reactions of children to death are highly personal. One child might quietly and sadly express his grief. Another might become rambunctious and oppositional. Still another might become extremely anxious. Children often take their cues from watching the reactions of other family members, particularly their parents. In some families, death is a taboo subject, and children sense that they should not talk about it; in other families, death is discussed openly, and children feel comfortable expressing their sadness.

Some adults believe that children should be shielded from death. They keep children away from funerals. They try not to cry in front of their children. They may make up stories in an attempt to protect children from sadness and grief. They may avoid all discussions of the deceased. Despite good intentions, though, these "shielding" actions are counterproductive. As with most topics, communicating with children about death should be honest and direct. Children need to grieve as much as adults do. They need to be able to share their feelings with others (particularly with their parents and other trusted adults), tell stories from the person's life, and talk about how they are going to miss the person who has died. By school age, children have already been exposed to death, even if only indirectly, through media or hearing about it from friends. Hiding death only makes it more mysterious and scary for children, and can inadvertently leave the children feeling alone in their sadness and grief.

A Child's Reaction to Death

What can you expect your child's response to be to the death of someone in her life?

Death of a pet. If a child is attached to her pet, she may find its death quite difficult. Even so, this event will prepare her for later encounters with death by giving her experience and understanding.

Death of a grandparent. When a grandparent dies, children may not find it as devastating as the loss of a parent or a sibling. To them, their grandparent is an older person, and when people get old, they die. However, if the grandparent has provided day-to-day companionship for the child, perhaps even living with the family or residing nearby, the death will be much harder.

With the passing away of a grandparent, children often think, "Now that my dad's dad is dead, does that mean that my dad is going to die next?" If you sense this kind of reaction, reassure your child that you and your spouse are healthy and will live for a long time.

Death of a parent. Whenever a child loses a parent, the event is traumatic and alters the course of her development. You cannot protect the child from what has happened, but you can help her face the reality of it.

If you are a surviving parent, in addition to dealing with your own feelings of loss, you need to help your child through this experience. Expect reactions ranging from regression and anxiety to anger and depression.

Be honest and open about what has taken place. Provide your child with comfort, both verbal and nonverbal. Reassure her that you are not going to leave her too, and that life will get back into a routine as soon as possible.

If the parent who is the primary caretaker has died and the other parent must return to work, find someone to assume a caretaking, nurturing role—perhaps a relative or a nanny. While these substitutes can assist with day-to-day functions, the surviving parent will still need to spend more time with and give more attention to the child to help her adjust to their new life. Talk with your pediatrician, as all family members would benefit from professional counseling at this time.

Death of a sibling. When a brother or a sister dies, children can find it just as difficult as losing a parent, sometimes even more so. In some ways a sibling is the person to whom a child is closest. They have been constant companions, sharing many life experiences. Perhaps they even shared a bedroom.

When a sibling dies, children may feel guilty, as all siblings have had arguments at some point. Or they may have survivor's guilt ("Why did he die and I didn't?"). They may even feel guilty because of the jealousy they experienced if their sibling was ill and got extra parental attention.

If one of your children dies, make sure the other children are not sidelined during the grieving process. You may be overwhelmed with your own sadness, yet your other children will also need a lot of attention, comforting, and understanding. Mobilize extended-family members and friends to help give your children support. Try to avoid putting the deceased child on a pedestal, or your other children may feel they can never be as perfect or as good in your eyes. Talk to your pediatrician to ensure everyone in your family is receiving appropriate professional counseling during this difficult time.

To help your child, you need to feel comfortable with your own grief reaction over the death of a loved one. It is appropriate for your child to see you cry when you feel sad; he will take comfort knowing that you are expressing your feelings so openly. This will make it easier for him to do the same.

How Is Your Child Reacting?

Unlike adults, children usually learn about the death of a loved one from others. They probably were not at the hospital when the person died, and they must rely on adults to tell them what happened.

Give your child prompt and accurate information, and answer her questions in language she can understand. If possible, as in the case of a terminal illness of someone she loves, give her a chance to prepare for the death in advance. You might say something like "Grandma is very sick and may not get better; the doctors think she might die soon." By contrast, if the death is sudden and violent—for example, in an automobile accident—your child's grieving process likely will be more difficult.

Children grieve in a manner similar to adults. They may experience a variety of feelings—sadness, anxiety, anger, guilt, shock, and helplessness. They may be confused and disbelieving. They may be restless and have trouble sleeping. They might cry, lose their appetite, and withdraw from friends. Especially during the first months of acute grieving, many children are fearful and anxious about both their own safety and that of their surviving family members.

Some younger school-age children may view death as something reversible or temporary. They might even deny that the person has died at all. In their play and fantasy they may continue to speak about the deceased individual as though he or she were still alive.

In the later years of middle childhood, however, as children are better able to understand the death and what caused it, they will be able to deal with it more directly. They may express their feelings about the death openly (through crying, for example), or in their play or daydreams. At times their reactions may be quite severe.

The intensity of your child's grieving also will depend on his relationship with the individual who has died. If the deceased is an aunt or uncle whom your child was not particularly close to, your child may not have much of a reaction. However, if the child has lost someone whom he was dependent upon—for example, a parent or, in some cases, a grandparent who frequently cared for the child—then he will be more devastated by the death, and it will take him longer to adjust to the passing away of this person. Children who lose a parent or a sibling often end up dealing with that death for the rest of their lives.

Once a death occurs, accept your child's response, whatever it is. If the child is upset, be respectful of that reaction. If the child is quiet, that should be respected as well. These individual responses will reflect the child's own development and maturity, the circumstances of the death, and the child's own personality.

Some factors seem to make it more difficult for the child to cope with the death of a parent. The death of the primary caretaker is harder on children. When the surviving parent's functioning becomes chronically impaired, children lose a critical source of support. Unanticipated deaths are more difficult to cope with than when the family has time to plan and the child can say goodbye.

Grieving is a process. It takes time. Don't expect it to come all at once and be over with quickly. However, since grieving is a healthy process, you can help it along by talking to your child about what she is feeling, answering her questions, and not hiding your own grief in order to protect her from pain.

The Funeral

Many parents are hesitant to take their children to funerals. However, by the time a child reaches school age, he should be given a choice as to whether he wants to attend the funeral. Explain to him what a funeral is—that it is the time when the person who has died is put to rest according to your culture's funeral rites, and when those who knew her get together to remember her. Step by step, describe what will happen logistically with the events of the funeral. Tell him that people will be sad and crying.

If the child decides to go, an adult should stay with him during the entire funeral. If he becomes too upset to remain (especially a younger school-age child), the adult accompanying him should go with him out of the ceremony. At the funeral he will see other people grieving, which will make it easier for him to express his own feelings. And despite parental fears, he won't be traumatized by attending the funeral.

Adjustment Afterward

After the death of someone close, like a parent or a sibling, your middle-years child may want to stay home from school for a few days. She may need to be close to you and other people who can provide her with comfort and support.

Before long, however, you need to get the family back into a routine. While allowing the grieving process to continue, also try to redirect your child's attention to the normal life events that can give her a sense of continuity. Returning to school can make her feel that her life is getting back to routine. Some children, in fact, work extra hard at school as a way of dealing with their grief.

Make sure you sit down with your child each day to talk about what she is feeling. Some symptoms related to the loss can continue or resurface after many weeks and even months. Perhaps holidays or the anniversary of the death will remind children of their loss. Sometimes they may be afraid to go to sleep. They may have fears of separation from their surviving parent. They might refuse to go to school, or become chronically depressed.

When these conditions linger, your child may need professional counseling to put the healing process back on track. Family therapy may be useful if family members feel so overwhelmed by grief that they cannot get their lives into a regular routine. Also, ask your doctor for a referral to a support group for children whose sibling or parent has died.

PART VI

· · · · · · · · · · · ·

Children in School

~ 35 ~

Making School Choices

A CHILD'S EDUCATION should be a top priority for families. The years from 5 to 12 are a critical period in a child's development. Quality educational programs lay the foundation for learning more than just facts—in addition to expanding their knowledge, children learn social skills, cultures, physical health, and other intangibles that benefit the child as a whole person. Girls and boys who have the strong support of their families as well as access to quality educational programs can achieve their unique potential for the future. Decades of research have shown a strong link between level of education and positive outcomes.

Education does not simply take place between the student and the teacher. Parents have an enormous role to play in encouraging and supporting the child, providing the resources needed to attend school regularly and stay organized, as well as the appropriate nutrition to maximize the school day. A partnership among the student, teacher, parents, principal, school, and society as a whole will best benefit the child.

Before the age of 5 years, your child may have already attended preschool for one or more years. There he socialized with other children and perhaps got a start on learning the alphabet and other fundamental academic and social skills. Even so, as you contemplate signing up your child for kindergarten, you may have questions about his readiness for what lies ahead. Does your child demonstrate the appropriate skills and maturity to begin school?

Evaluating Your Child's Readiness

By law, children must be enrolled in school or an approved alternative program by a particular age. In most parts of the country, these age requirements are 5 years old for kindergarten and 6 years old for first grade. Cutoff dates for birthdays for age and grade assignments can vary from state to state.

The idea that because of their birth date some children are "ready for school" and others are not merits discussion. Just as children begin to walk or talk at different ages, they also develop the psychological and social aptitudes necessary for school at varying ages. In addition, many parents and educators feel that schools need to be ready for children. This newer approach emphasizes how school programs can be designed so that all children of a chronological age to enter school can benefit from the program.

When determining when your child should start school, consider your child's unique abilities. Gather accurate information about your child's development, especially communication skills, including language development and the ability to listen; social skills and the ability to get along with other children and adults; and physical skills, from running and playing to using a crayon or pencil. Talking with your child's pediatrician, preschool teachers, and child care providers can provide useful, objective observations and information.

Some schools may conduct their own tests to evaluate your child's abilities.

WHERE WE STAND

School readiness includes not only the early academic skills of children but also their physical health, language skills, social and emotional development, motivation to learn, creativity, and general knowledge. Families and communities play a critical role in ensuring children's growth in all of these areas and thus their readiness for school. Schools must be prepared to teach all children when they reach the age of school entry, regardless of their degree of readiness. Research on early brain development emphasizes the effects of early experiences, relationships, and emotions on creating and reinforcing the neural connections that are the basis for learning.

So-called readiness tests tend to concentrate on academic skills, but most usually do evaluate other aspects of development. These tests are far from infallible; some children who do poorly on them still fare well in school. Even so, you can use them as one of the yardsticks in determining how your child's development has progressed relative to other children of the same age. Often, your own parental intuition about your child's capabilities is an accurate measure of how well she is prepared to enter school, particularly if you have an older child with whom you have had experience.

If you or the school identify some areas of your child's development that are of concern, use this information to help you and the school plan for the special attention that your child may need. By sharing information with your child's teacher and other school staff, you can help the school be ready for your child. At the same time, you are establishing a partnership for your child's education that can and should continue throughout her childhood. Talk with your pediatrician regarding special concerns, as she may suggest you contact the school district ahead of time to determine if testing is needed for an Individualized Education Program (IEP).

Parents can encourage their children's cognitive, physical, and emotional development before they enter school. Kindergarten teachers are prepared to teach children who are enthusiastic and curious in approaching new activities, can follow directions, are sensitive to other children's feelings, and can take turns and share. Some specific skills that will make your child's first year at school go smoothly include her ability to:

- Play well with other children with minimal fighting or crying

- Remain attentive and quiet when being read a story; participate in circle time

- Use the toilet on her own

- Successfully use zippers and buttons

- Say her name, address, and telephone number

There are great benefits to reading to your child beginning in infancy. Help your child acquire some basic skills, like recognizing and remembering letters, numbers, and colors. Expose her to enriching and learning experiences such as trips to the local museums or zoo, or enroll her in community art or science programs. To promote social skills development, encourage her to play with other children of both sexes in the neighborhood and to participate in organized community-sponsored activities and park district programs.

Some parents consider intentionally delaying their child's entrance into kindergarten. They believe that their child may gain an advantage and be more likely to succeed in academics, athletics, or social settings if she is older than average for her grade. Delaying school entry in order to obtain an advantage is not necessarily a winning strategy. Although there is some evidence that being among the youngest in a class may cause some academic challenges, most of these differences seem to disappear by the third or fourth grade. On the other hand, there is evidence that children who are old for their grade are at greater risk of behavior problems when they reach adolescence.

Registering Your Child for School

To enroll your child in school, you will need to demonstrate that he meets the school district's age requirements for kindergarten. Some schools require that a child be 5 by September of his entry year; others use different cutoff dates. If proof of age is requested, bring a birth certificate or a physician's record. If you feel convinced that your child is ready for kindergarten and you want him to attend but he has not reached the designated chronological age, explore the exemption process that may be offered in your school district.

Visiting the Pediatrician

Before your child enters school, make an appointment with your pediatrician. This can be accomplished during the routine annual examination in the year leading up to school entry. The doctor will make certain your child is properly immunized and can discuss with you the various issues related to this important transition.

Since many schools register new kindergarten students in the spring, schedule this doctor's visit by late winter or early spring so the important readiness issues discussed earlier can be addressed well in advance, and also so that you avoid the late-summer busy season in the physician's office. Ask for a copy of your child's immunizations to bring with you to school during registration.

Immunizations

When you register your child, you will be asked for his immunization records. Specifically, the school staff will want to see either a copy of the record from your child's pediatrician or the clinic where the immunizations were given, including the doctor's signature, or a summary copy from the physician's office. Many states have a specific form that will need to be completed, including immunization dates and information as well as the physical exam; many school districts keep these forms available for families on their website.

If you do not have a record but are sure your child has had all the necessary shots, it is important to take steps to obtain the records well before the first day of school. Most schools will not be able simply to take your word for it; the immunization requirement is a state law, and the state dictates which types of records are acceptable.

A fully immunized 4- or 5-year-old will have had two MMR (measles, mumps, rubella) vaccines, five DTaP (diphtheria, pertussis, tetanus) vaccines, three hepatitis B vaccines, two varicella (chicken pox) vaccines, four polio vaccines, four pneumococcal vaccines, two hepatitis A vaccines, and three to four *Haemophilus influenzae B* conjugate vaccines. All these immunizations are important not only to keep your individual child healthy, but also to keep the school community protected in case of an infectious outbreak such as measles. (See page 633 for more information on childhood immunization.)

If your child is not yet fully immunized for her age, your pediatrician will recognize this and can address the issue during the prekindergarten appointment. The needed immunizations can often be given at that visit. If additional immunizations are needed to catch up, your child will probably be admitted to school with a note from your pediatrician that the immunizations are "in progress." School personnel are aware that time intervals (such as six weeks) are often needed between some of these immunizations, but may allow only that amount of time, so it is important to stay prompt with any catch-up schedules.

Vaccines are safe and save lives. The safety and efficacy of immunizations, the greatest public health advancement of the twentieth century, has been studied in great detail; ongoing studies continue to ensure their safety and efficacy. Herd immunity, meaning a community with strong vaccination rates, helps to protect those who are either too young for vaccines or unable to receive them because of particular medical problems or because they are receiving immune suppression medications. Discuss vaccines with your pediatrician if you have questions or concerns. For more information, see Chapter 61, "Immunizations."

Choosing a School

You may have a choice of which school your child will attend within your community. In addition to public schools, there may also be private or parochial schools to which you might decide to send your child; for these there will be tuition payments. It is important for you to familiarize yourself with the schools from which you are choosing. Once you understand the differences among the schools, you will be better able to make an informed decision. Knowledge about your child's school is important both to prepare her for the year ahead and to equip you to work with the school as an advocate for your child to ensure that she receives the best education possible.

Elementary schools have traditionally included kindergarten through the sixth grade (K–6) or kindergarten through the eighth grade (K–8). In some districts, children have been grouped in different ways to accommodate their developmental needs, as well as to make better use of the school district's resources. In some districts students may be attending schools with structures such as stand-alone kindergarten, primary school (first through third grades), intermediate school (fourth through sixth grades), and a separate middle school or junior high (seventh and eighth grades).

Educators are aware that pre- and early adolescents (ages 10 to 13) have particular educational needs. These children can benefit from more autonomy and an increased ability to experiment than is available in most elementary schools, yet they need a safer, more structured, and more overtly supportive environment than that of the usual high school. Middle school, also called junior high, addresses these needs.

What to Look For

When selecting your child's school, there are issues to consider.

Expectations. What are the school's academic and social expectations for students in the grade your child is entering?

Individuality. Is learning individualized? That is, are each child's individual skills and needs considered by the teachers, or is the entire class taught the same material at the same pace at the same time? Some children fare well in a highly organized atmosphere, while others thrive in a more individualized environment. You need to assess what type of environment is best for your child, given her particular temperament and learning style.

Special needs. Is the school able to meet the special needs of your child in compliance with the federal statutes protecting individuals with disabilities? Are special education services available? Most important, do you feel your school is welcoming to those with different physical, educational, and emotional needs?

Grouping. Within a grade level, are children grouped by ability, or do all classes have children at different levels?

Climate. What is the climate at the school? If you visit the school during the academic year, you will learn a lot. Do students and teachers treat one another with respect? Do teachers communicate a love for and an excitement about teaching and learning? Is the school an orderly but not repressive environment? Are the children well behaved but still allowed to be playful individuals? Is the work of students displayed on the classroom walls and bulletin boards, showing that their

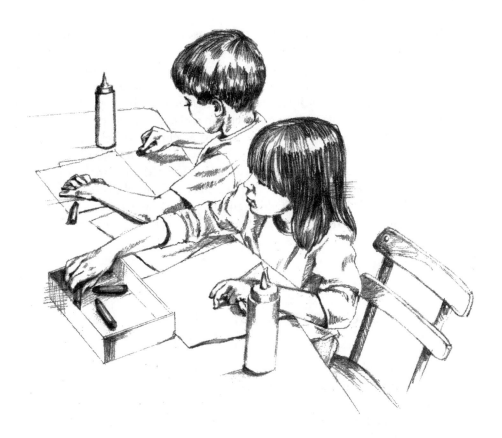

efforts are valued? Is praise from teachers commonplace? Do you sense a positive relationship between the school and the surrounding community?

Cultural variety. What is the school's racial, ethnic, and socioeconomic composition? There are many lessons that a child can learn from developing friendships with children of different backgrounds and cultures. Does the school consider differences in race, religion, and culture to be assets of which everyone is proud? Does the school handle holidays with religious significance sensitively?

Do programs exist for meaningful study of different cultures (curriculum units, appropriate educational trips)? Are students provided with opportunities to interact with students from different backgrounds through visits, school-to-school pen pals, and the like? Are parents from the school interested in working together to provide their children with these experiences?

Are children treated equally regardless of their family's income? For example, do all children go on field trips regardless of their ability to pay? Are children who receive free or reduced-cost lunch made to stand in separate lines?

The principal. Is the principal a visible presence at the school? Do you see her welcoming children in the morning, visiting classrooms, or walking through the halls? The principal's leadership is one of the most important factors in contributing to a school's effectiveness and sets the tone and standards for the school.

Student-teacher ratio. What is the student-teacher ratio? Most educators believe that, from kindergarten through the fifth grade, a ratio of 25:1 or less is adequate. When the ratio exceeds 30:1, the ability to teach can be impaired. Even so, there is more to the story than these numbers. In a classroom with many children who need a significant amount of individualized attention to help them control their behavior, a ratio as low as 15:1 may still be too high and might be improved by, for example, the presence of a teacher's aide. Conversely, if the majority of children are capable of independent work, then a higher ratio might be acceptable.

Teachers. How do teachers and children interact? Do teachers spend most of the classroom time lecturing? Or does the teacher coach the students' learning,

School Experiences and Opportunities Through the Years

Your child's school years from kindergarten through middle school are an exciting time of opportunities and new experiences.

Children ages 5–7 years: At this age, children are adjusting to full-day school with increasing academic expectations. A large part of these years is early socialization. Expectations should be kept age-appropriate and there should be opportunities for recess breaks with open-ended play to help kids stay focused during class time. (For the AAP's position on recess, see page 408.)

Children ages 8–10 years: They have typically moved on to a more rigorous curriculum that includes chapter books and longer-term school projects. Parents should continue to serve as a guide while providing increasing opportunities for the child to gain experience with taking responsibility for her own work.

Children ages 11–12 years: Now children have expanded opportunities for extracurricular activities, such as student council positions and school sports teams. Kids in middle school should be showing more self-responsibility in terms of staying organized and taking ownership over schoolwork and longer-term projects.

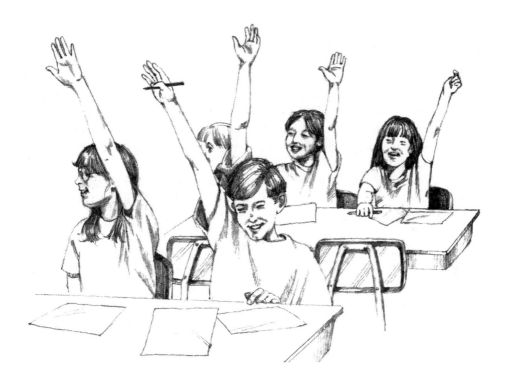

and does the school day consist of a mixture of talking to and with the students, and include student input? Are small-group activities encouraged, with or without direct teacher participation? Students can learn a great deal by helping one another within a structured setting.

Resources. In addition to academics, what is the quality of other aspects of the school, such as the library or resource center, art and music classes, guidance counseling, and physical education programs? What is the access to computers, tablets, and the internet, and how are these incorporated into the curriculum? Are there periods in the daily schedule reserved for recess, and are these more frequent for the younger children? It is important for children to have opportunities throughout the day for free play, exercise, and the ability to regroup for the remainder of the school day. The STEM fields (science, technology, engineering, and mathematics) should be well represented, and even young kids are ready to learn the basic concepts of computer sciences such as coding.

Physical education classes should be more than a time to blow off steam. There should be a balance between fitness activities and skill development. In some schools, classroom teachers are responsible for PE classes, while in others, where formal PE instruction is provided, classroom teachers may supplement it with coordinated activities that have been designed by the PE teacher.

With reductions in school budgets, physical education programs are often one of the first areas to be cut back or even eliminated. In schools where this is occurring, classroom teachers frequently have taken on more responsibility for these programs, particularly those teachers who have some training in this area.

Nutrition. How seriously does the school take good nutrition? Is the food served in the cafeteria consistent with the principles of good eating that are taught in the classroom? Many schools have implemented innovative, cost-effective programs to boost the nutritional value of cafeteria meals. Nutritious snacking is important as well; schools should encourage students to bring healthy snacks to school such as fresh fruit, and to drink water.

Some schools take part in a government-funded breakfast program in order to help low-income families supplement the nutrition of their children. The presence of this kind of program can indicate the school's commitment to students' nutritional needs.

Safety. Are the children physically safe at school? Safety should be a high priority in the classrooms, the playgrounds, the parking lots, and on campus. Many schools keep a daily log of injuries and accidents on playground equipment and elsewhere on the school grounds and review these records to implement programs for greater safety.

How are health services delivered in the school? Who provides emergency first aid? How do children or parents gain access to the nurse or health aide? (See "Dealing with Health Problems at School," page 482.) Does the school have a clinic? A dental screening program?

WHERE WE STAND

Recess is at the heart of a debate over the role of schools in promoting the optimal development of the whole child. A growing trend toward reallocating time in school to accentuate academic subjects has put this important component of a child's school day at risk. Recess serves as a necessary break from the rigors of concentrated academic challenges in the classroom. Equally important is the fact that safe and well-supervised recess offers cognitive, social, emotional, and physical benefits that may not be fully appreciated when a decision is made to cut back. Recess is unique from, and a complement to, physical education, and is not a substitute for it. The American Academy of Pediatrics believes that recess is a crucial and necessary component of a child's development and, as such, it should not be withheld for punitive or academic reasons.

For children with life-threatening food allergies, autoinjectable epinephrine should be stored properly and in close proximity to where the students spend time. Are faculty and staff trained in recognizing the signs of anaphylaxis? Is there a school nurse on the premises some or all of the time? What are the school's policies about food brought from home in terms of snacks, lunches, and classroom treats on special days?

School Safety During Emergencies

School safety is a big concern for families today. It is important for parents to know that their children are safe while they travel to and attend school. Some important questions parents have may include: What plans are in place to help kids stay safe? What kind of training does the school do to prepare for an armed intruder? What happens if there is a fire or a blizzard at school? How do I talk to my child about school safety without making him worry?

Peanut-Free Lunch Tables, Peanut-Free Schools?

Food allergies are an epidemic. The rate of food allergies has tripled in the past two decades. How can we help keep children with food allergies safe? Kindergarteners and first-graders are at a developmental stage where they share generously, including food at lunch; for these grades, a designated peanut-free table, while not a 100 percent perfect barrier, can help keep 5- and 6-year-olds safe.

For older kids with food allergies, the concept of a "peanut-free school" may lend a false sense of security. As kids grow, they need to learn to be proactive—to protect themselves by reading labels and asking about ingredients. Kids 7 and older, especially by 10 and 11 years of age, can and should learn to only eat food that they brought from home or that has been determined to be safe. One of the challenges for families of children with severe food allergies is to help their child navigate a world in which the food allergen exists. Kids can keep safe by learning and remembering to eat only food that was prepared at home or has a thorough ingredient list that has been closely examined. If the safety of the item cannot be guaranteed, the child *should not eat it.* For more on food allergies, see page 542.

All schools should have an organized emergency operations plan in place to reduce risks or prevent, prepare for, respond to, and recover from a crisis situation. Many school districts have a safety coordinator or director assigned to them. School staff are trained to assess the seriousness of incidents and respond according to the plan's established procedures and guidelines.

During a crisis situation, misinformation can often be spread quickly. Parents should always know how to get updated information from their child's school in

Talking with Children About School Safety

For some children, even participation in a drill may cause some emotional distress, especially if it reminds them of a prior crisis event or if they otherwise are feeling vulnerable or anxious. As a parent, you are in the best position to help your child cope. Any conversation with a child must be developmentally appropriate.

Children ages 5–7 years: Young children need brief, simple information that should be balanced with reassurance. This includes informing children that their school and home are safe (once these are secure) and that adults are available to protect them. Young children often gauge how threatening or serious an event is by adult reactions. Young children respond well to basic reassurance by adults and simple examples of school safety, like reminding them the exterior doors are locked.

Children ages 8–10: They may be more vocal in asking questions about whether they are truly safe and what is being done at their school. They may need assistance separating reality from fantasy. Parents can share the information they have about the school's safety plan and any other relevant communication to ease their child's mind.

Children ages 11–12: Many 11- and 12-year-olds have strong and varying opinions about causes of violence in school and society. Parents should stress the role that students have in maintaining safe schools by following the school's safety guidelines (e.g., not providing building access to strangers, reporting strangers on campus, reporting threats to school safety made by students or community members).

case of an emergency. Usually schools have a system in place. For example, some schools will send updated information via text, email, or phone. Always make sure your school has your updated contact information so that you can be notified directly of an emergency.

Before- and after-school programs. Are early morning activities or an after-school program available at the school? If not, are there any school-based resources to help parents find this needed child care? If programs are scarce in your community, consider joining with other parents and approaching YMCAs or other agencies to encourage them to start an after-school program.

If your efforts to find out more about a school—public or private—are not met with open arms or do not answer most of your questions, do not allow yourself to be put off or intimidated. If you show some flexibility, such as making an appointment for a day that is less busy than others, the school staff should be willing to accommodate your visit. Most principals, in fact, will be proud to show you their school, and will welcome your interest and involvement in your child's education.

New Learning Structures

While you research school options, you may be surprised at the variety you will find. Some schools have an open structure, in which classes are all under one roof without walls between them. Teachers might have their own distinctive style of teaching. While some prefer having their students in assigned seats, others work best with an approach that seems less structured, with students free to roam through the room during particular assignments. Some teachers utilize learning centers for independent learning or solitary study. To some degree, your child's success will hinge on the match between his need for structure and choice, and the teacher's own approach to teaching. Even if your child is growing up in a fairly structured home setting, you might be surprised to find that he does quite well in a relatively unstructured classroom environment. In any event, a high-quality teacher will adapt his or her own teaching style so that students are more likely to learn. In addition to teaching style, evaluate how well your child's teacher communicates and resolves conflicts in the class. Also, what are the teacher's areas of special skill or interest?

If magnet schools are available in your community, consider them as another option. As their name implies, these schools attract students from surrounding areas. They tend to emphasize a particular area of the curriculum—for instance, science, the arts, or foreign languages—and students may choose them because of a special interest or talent. In some school districts students are assigned to these magnet schools. Free transportation may be provided.

School Lunch Preparation

Early involvement of your child with school lunch preparation is a wise idea. Meals brought from home are usually healthier, more affordable, and able to accommodate different dietary guidelines or restrictions (e.g., food allergies). Don't expect a perfect system right away; your child's lunch preparation will occur in stages and will be a process that evolves over time, helping your child develop a lifelong relationship with food. In a rut, bored with the same options? With your child, search the internet for "school lunch ideas"; you'll find plenty of inspiration!

Bento boxes and other similarly divided, reusable, dishwasher-safe containers are a fun way to present food and are a nice choice for kids who prefer that their foods not touch. Often these require an initial investment, but they are reusable and will last for quite some time.

A key step to help your kids pack their own lunches: ensure the fridge and pantry are kept stocked with essentials and supplies. Keep a pad of paper in a central location of the kitchen so all members of the family can add necessities when supplies are running low. Post a list of lunch ideas to serve as inspiration.

Guidelines for a complete lunch and ideas to inject some fun:

- **Fruit or vegetable.** Sliced apples are an easy start, but you can branch out from there.

- **Main course.** A sandwich is a typical and easily packed entrée, but don't be afraid to try other options for the main course, such as a thermos of leftover soup, pasta, or a mixed salad.

- **Beverage.** Water is best! A reusable water bottle is ecofriendly and saves on costs.

- **Assemble homemade finger foods.** Some ideas are rolled deli ham or turkey, cheese sticks, hummus for dipping, and whole-grain crackers.

- **Something sweet.** A sweet treat is okay if it is small. Don't underestimate the sweetness of natural fruits.

Children ages 5–7 years: Younger children will likely require a bit more adult assistance, especially if new to the idea of preparing their own school lunches. Consider designating different drawers in the refrigerator for different, pre-prepared elements of the school lunch, for easy grab-and-go on weekday mornings. You and your child can work together on weekends to wash and prep fruits or veggies to store in bags for this purpose.

Children ages 8–10 years: Increased kitchen skills help kids this age get a bit more creative with school lunches. Consider making extra batches of pasta on the weekends; the pasta can be mixed with veggies for easy weekday pasta lunches.

Children ages 11–12 years: Kids this age should have increased independence in the kitchen (on age-appropriate kitchen skills, see page 28) and correspondingly can get creative with their school lunch ideas. Remember to promote creativity. There's nothing wrong with breakfast for lunch—for example, hard-boiled eggs with whole-grain waffles and fresh fruit. Dinner leftovers make for the base of many excellent lunch options. Layered salads can be made ahead of time, with heavy and wet ingredients (cannellini beans, vinaigrette dressing) on the bottom and lighter veggies and lettuce on top, to be shaken when ready to eat.

Private or Religious School

Private and religious schools come in different sizes, philosophies, and affiliations. Parents consider a private or religious school for their child for many reasons: a particular educational philosophy and method of teaching, a reputation for high student achievement and academic success, a religious affiliation and an education with a religious orientation, a military orientation, or a family tradition.

If you are deciding whether this type of school is right for your child, there are other issues to consider besides the factors mentioned above. For instance:

■ What are the expectations of the school's staff and students?

■ What are the educational styles and characteristics of the principal and teachers?

■ What is the student-teacher ratio?

- What additional educational and student service resources—such as special education, nursing, physical and speech therapy, and audiology—are provided?

- What safety and nutritional services are available?

- Is financial assistance available to help meet tuition and fees?

While comparing private/religious and public schools, other criteria may help you make your decision. Ask about licensing requirements for teachers, administrators, and healthcare personnel, since they are sometimes less stringent in private and religious schools. Check to see whether the private or religious school has fewer resources, and whether teachers are trained specifically in art, music, physical education, guidance counseling, and special education. Determine whether high tuition costs keep the private or religious school from attracting a mix of students from different backgrounds. Finally, find out if parents are required to make a substantial time commitment to volunteer at and fund-raise for the school.

Homeschooling

Homeschooling has been in existence since the pioneer days due to necessity, and it has had a renaissance in modern times. Families may decide, for a variety of reasons, that instead of public or private education, they can themselves direct their child's curricula and education. Families may decide that homeschooling is a good fit for their special-needs child, wish to foster a positive social environment, or want to pursue a more particular curriculum. One family may decide to incorporate more of their faith into their child's education. Another family may have a dedicated ice hockey player with an erratic practice and game schedule and would like to modify the education to accommodate their competitive athlete's schedule.

Some may think of homeschooling as a solitary pursuit; however, in this day and age homeschooling families are more connected than ever, joining together for cooperative efforts to expand on their children's opportunities. Homeschooling laws and regulations are based in each state; therefore, it is extremely important to check existing laws in your state. Homeschool co-ops work well for combining science experiences, as an example, with an added bonus of socialization with other children.

If you are interested in learning more about homeschooling, there are a number of resources to help you. The Home School Legal Defense Association (www.hslda.org) is an online resource to learn about all aspects of the homeschool experience. You do not need to become a member to utilize the website. You can learn about each state's individual homeschooling laws, curriculum choices, conferences, and homeschool support groups. Also keep in mind that your school decisions are not absolute and binding; you may decide that homeschooling in the younger grades suits your child's needs better, with a plan to mainstream into public schools by the middle school or high school years.

~ 36 ~

Preparing for a New School Year

THE START OF a new school year brings excitement: new classes, different teachers, fresh faces, and new friends. If your child is starting kindergarten or middle school, or if your family has moved into a new community, a new school year is a transition for the whole family.

In the days and weeks immediately preceding the first day of school, find out some basic school information to prepare for the adjustment.

- What will her daily schedule be like? What time does school begin and when does it end each day?

- Should your child bring a bag lunch and a snack to school, or are meals provided, or does she have the option to purchase them? If lunch is scheduled relatively late, your child may need a more substantial morning snack.

- Are certain clothes required for physical education classes and recesses? Children will go outdoors for recess, and in the winter that may mean hats, gloves, boots, and snow pants, even if the children do not need to wear them in the car or on the bus. Inquire as to whether your child should bring shoes to change into.

Starting a New School Year: Age-Specific Ideas

Children ages 5–7 years: Since they are new to school, they may benefit from "meet the teacher" opportunities and school walk-through days. It can be helpful for younger kids to visualize what their day, and the classroom, will look like. Make connections with classmates in your neighborhood to ease the transition.

Children ages 8–10 years: Some children may be returning to the same school, while others may be transitioning to a new school if their family has moved or if the district groups the elementary grades into primary (kindergarten or first grade through third grade), intermediate (fourth grade through sixth grade), and middle schools (seventh and eighth grades). Take advantage of opportunities before the first day to visit the classroom ahead of time. Participate in your public library's summer reading programs to boost literacy, promote a love of reading for pleasure, and prevent the "summer slide," a slight backtracking of skills seen for children who have three-month-long summer vacations.

Children ages 11–12 years: With the transition to middle school may come your child's first experience with a school locker or PE uniforms. Kids are resilient and will learn the new routine quickly. Reassure your child that the routine is new for *all* the students; there may be hiccups the first day or so, but just a week or so in, the new schedule should feel like a regular routine.

If it is possible in your school district, visit the school with your child to see her new classroom and meet her new teacher before school officially starts. Many districts offer a "walk-through" day to help families get oriented and see the classrooms before the first day of school. Many kindergartens also have school buses present on this day so the children can practice boarding a bus and finding their assigned seat.

Safety

If your child will be walking to school, walk the route with him for his own comfort level as well as to assess its safety. Find out about traffic patterns and crossing guards. Instruct your child to stay on sidewalks and main roads rather than cutting through alleys and wooded areas that may be somewhat deserted.

Although safety rules will likely be discussed in class, do not wait for that instruction; make your own rules specific to your child's situation. In a low-key but firm manner, tell your child: "These rules are one way we take care of ourselves." Reassure him that he can keep himself safe. Review these safety issues several times throughout the year.

If an older sibling goes to the same school, have the children walk together. Otherwise, talk with a family with a responsible older child from your neighborhood who would be willing to walk with your child to school. As your children grow older, remember to look around your neighborhood for young children you can help in this way.

What is the school's policy on reporting school absences? Call your school early in the morning whenever your child is absent. This will provide an additional measure of safety for your child, since if he does not show up for school, school staff will be more likely to check with you.

Does the school have rules regarding bikes or skateboards? Some schools require helmets and locks for cyclists, which is a great idea. Before the first day of school, review the basic safety rules with your son or daughter. By insisting your child wear a helmet and abide by all bicycle safety guidelines, for example, you will be encouraging a behavior that is potentially lifesaving and hopefully will become a lifetime habit. Ask the school staff if your community has a program offering low-cost or even free helmets for children; if there is no such program in your area, talk with other parents about starting one to increase the number of children wearing helmets. Wear your own helmet whenever you bike or skateboard to model appropriate safety behavior.

The School Bus

Is bus transportation available for your child? Many parents have questions or concerns about bus rides, especially for the first day of school. What happens if a child misses the afternoon bus?

On your child's first day of elementary school, you might be tempted to drive her to school, particularly if she seems apprehensive about the bus ride or about starting school in general. However, except under unusual circumstances, strongly encourage your child to ride the bus that first day. Your son or daughter should be there if seats on the bus are assigned, and the driver needs to get used to the stop where your child will be picked up. Remind your child that it is *everyone's* first day, and that *everyone* is adjusting to the new routine; she is not alone! You can take your child to the bus stop and meet her there when she returns. If your work schedule doesn't allow you to be there, arrange for another adult or an older sibling to take on this responsibility.

Review the basic bus safety rules with your child: Wait for the bus to come to a full stop before approaching it from the curb. Do not move around on the bus; this will help avoid injuries if the driver needs to stop quickly. When getting off the bus, cross at least ten feet in front of the bus and only when it is fully stopped, the red lights are flashing, and the driver has signaled that it is safe. Of course, the child should also check to make sure that no other traffic is coming.

You won't be allowed to ride on the bus with your child, even on the first day of school. Take advantage of a district walk-through day, as often buses are available for children to experience before the first official day. School staff are prepared to help children navigate through the school grounds on the first day.

If your child reports any issues occurring on the bus during the school year, whether the issue is a rowdy classmate or something else, find out what the particular problem is and take appropriate action. Keep in mind that time at the bus stop or on the bus itself is considered school time. If your child is being teased or harassed, work with her to brainstorm potential solutions in hopes that she can resolve the difficulty herself. If she is being hurt or is afraid for her safety, call the principal for assistance. To minimize problems, discourage your child from bringing expensive or popular toys or electronic devices to play with on the bus, since they can easily become damaged when other children want to try them. Bear in mind that drivers need to concentrate on driving the bus; they have neither the time nor the training to serve as disciplinarians.

WHERE WE STAND

The American Academy of Pediatrics would like to see changes in laws to reduce the number and seriousness of school bus injuries. We believe that seat belts should be required on all newly manufactured school buses, regardless of their size and the number of students they transport. We also urge that seat backs be elevated to 28 inches—4 inches above the federally mandated height—so as to support and cushion a child's head and neck. In addition, padding designed to adequately absorb impacts during crashes or fast stops should completely cover the rears of seats and the top rails.

Each school district will have its own guidelines and regulations regarding the use of electronic devices, tablets, and other screens on school buses. As a family, you should examine your own values and feelings on the subject; even if it may seem the norm in your community for kids to use an electronic device on the bus ride to school, your family may decide this is not the right choice for you. Keep in mind that many kids develop motion sickness on a swaying school bus if their eyes are focused on a screen rather than their surroundings. Kids, especially kindergarten through the younger grades, often use bus time as a social, interactive time with friends, which is lost if screens are being used. If your child is going to be using screens on the bus, you should review your family's rules and guidelines on appropriate photography—that is, not taking pictures of others without their consent (for more on media and technology, see page 315). Also, parents and child alike should be aware of consequences should the electronic device be damaged or lost.

Expectations

As a general rule, children *rise* to expectations. Your child's goals, and your family's goals, for the school year should be optimistic as well as realistic. Expectations can be a powerful influence on the kind of school experience your child will have. Even when they are communicated in casual conversations, they can have a significant effect on your child's outlook. Past experiences can also influence a child's outlook and expectations. While he may have had some problems in the previous year, you and he should try to approach each new school year with a clean slate and a positive attitude. Kids and adults alike will benefit from a *growth mindset*, as opposed to a *fixed mindset*; this means that they are eager to learn from experience and continue to develop as the years pass.

Making the First Day Easier

Most children are excited and perhaps a bit anxious on the first day of school each year. You can help make the day easier for your child by keeping the following guidelines in mind:

- Point out the positive aspects of starting school: It will be fun. She will see old friends. She will meet new friends. Refresh her memory about previous years, when she returned home after the first day in high spirits because she had a good time.

- Remind your child that the first day is *everyone's* first day; she is not the only student who is a bit uneasy about the first day of school. Teachers know that students are anxious and will be making an extra effort to make sure everyone can appropriately adjust. You can share stories from when you had a case of the jitters in your own life, such as making a presentation at work; it helps your child to know that everyone feels nervous from time to time.

■ Review all your child's accomplishments from last year, and talk about the kinds of interesting things she will learn in the months ahead. You can even show your child pictures and video from last year's first day so he can see how far he has come.

■ Put a note in her lunch box that will remind her you are thinking of her while she is at school.

■ Find another child in the neighborhood with whom your son or daughter can walk to school or ride with on the bus. If your child is older, have her offer to walk to school or wait at the bus stop with a new or younger child. Over the summer invite these children to your home so everyone can get better acclimated with each other, which will in turn increase everyone's comfort level on the first day of school.

A Checklist for the First Day of School

As you and your child prepare for the first day of the new school year, use this checklist to help make sure you have taken care of the necessary tasks and learned the information you need.

■ Is your child registered? Many school districts hold registration for returning students the spring of the prior school year, often online.

■ When is the first day of school?

■ What time does school start?

■ How is your child going to get to school? If your child is biking, does he know the school rules for bicycles? If he is walking for the first time, with whom will he walk? Have you reviewed with him safety precautions regarding traffic and strangers?

- Does your child know his teacher's name?

- What will his daily schedule be like?

- Will he need to bring a snack? What kinds of snacks are allowed and encouraged? Are refillable water bottles allowed? Water is the perfect beverage, an inexpensive and healthy choice.

- What time is lunch? Can your child buy it at school, and how much will it cost?

- What clothes will your child need to wear? Are there any restrictions on what can be worn? Will he need a different set of clothes for physical education or art classes?

- Does your child need to bring pencils, paper, notebooks, and other supplies? Often school districts will publish grade-specific school supply lists online ahead of time, and supplies can be brought in during the school walk-through day. Many parent-teacher organizations hold online fund-raiser supply kit sales as well. Does your child have something in which to carry his books and supplies back and forth to school? Will he have a place (besides his desk) to keep his things at school?

- Have you filled out all health forms and emergency contact forms that have been sent home or are found online on the district website?

- Have any new health problems developed in your child over the summer that will affect his school day? Does the school nurse know about this condition, or is an appointment set up to discuss it?

- If your child will need to take medication at school on the first day, have arrangements and necessary paperwork, usually requiring signatures from your pediatrician, been made for this?

- Does your child know where he is going after school (e.g., home, sitter)? Does he know how he will get there? If you will not be there when he arrives, does he know who will be responsible for him, what the rules are, and how to get help in an emergency?

- Does your child have your cell and work telephone numbers memorized and accessible?

- Encourage her to look for new students in her classroom or on the playground, invite them to join the group for a game, and ask them about their interests.

- When you and your child reconnect after the first day of school, give her a hug and ask about her day. Did she have fun? Did she meet new people? Does she need any additional school supplies (notebooks, rulers, erasers) that you can shop for together?

In addition to the suggestions listed above, your child may need some extra support if she is starting at a new school. Here are some suggestions to make the transition easier.

- Talk with your child about her feelings regarding the new school—both her excitement and her concerns.

- Visit the school with your child in advance of the first day. Teachers and staff are usually at school a few days before the children start. Peek into your child's classroom and, if possible, meet the teacher and principal. You might be able to address some of your child's concerns at that time. She may not have questions until she actually sees the building and can visualize what it will be like. When you formally register your child in the new school, bring her immunization record and birth certificate; or school records usually can be sent directly from school to school once you sign a "release of information" form.

- Try to have your child meet a classmate *before* the first day so they can get acquainted and play together, and so your child will have a friendly face to look for when school begins.

- Do not build up unrealistic expectations about how wonderful the new school will be, but convey a general sense of optimism about how things will go for your child at the new school.

- If your child sees another student or a group engaged in an activity she is interested in, encourage her to ask if she can participate.

- As soon as you can, find out what activities are available for your child in addition to those that occur during school itself. Is there a back-to-school picnic or party planned? For community sports programs, sign-ups often begin weeks or even months before the start of the season, but if your family is new to the area coaches may make accommodations.

During the first few weeks at a new school, your child's teacher will probably conduct some informal assessments. You should be able to get some idea of how your child's academic and social adjustments are going at that time. If you have any concerns, reach out to your child's teacher via email or phone to set up an appointment.

See also "Family Moves," page 274, and Chapter 35, "Making School Choices."

~ 37 ~

Getting Involved in Your Child's Schooling

ONE OF A child's greatest assets is a family who is involved in his education and his school. When parents care and become active participants and partners in the educational process, both their own child and other children at the school benefit enormously.

School success begins in the home. A consistent bedtime to ensure adequate sleep, healthy meals, exercise, and limited screen time will all contribute to a child's school success. Studies show that students who live in homes with healthy habits, regular routines, and good communication have a higher degree of school performance.

Designate a specific area of the home to keep all school supplies organized, including backpacks, school projects, and lunches. This will help your child know where to find things when getting ready in the morning for school. A specific zone to do homework will help kids complete their homework efficiently, whether it is a desk or the kitchen counter with a basket of supplies.

Read together for pleasure, and have your child read aloud to you as well. Above all, have fun. Look for teachable moments together. For example, cooking combines math and science elements. Make dinner together and read recipe instructions aloud, discuss fractions as you measure ingredients, make hypotheses ("What will happen when I beat the egg whites?"), and examine results.

Children learn by example. Read for pleasure yourself, whether it is books, the daily newspaper, or other print media. Show your children that you put away your own screens (phones, laptops) for designated periods, especially for family meals. Take time to learn a new skill and discuss the experience with them. Sit down and pay bills or do other "homework" while your kids do their schoolwork. Participate in the public library's summer reading program to boost a lifelong love of reading simply for the joy of it. If you seek out learning opportunities for yourself, using a growth mindset, your kids will model that behavior in their own lives.

Really *listen* when your child talks about her classroom, her teacher, and her classmates. Put down your phone and other distractions and give her a chance to express her anxieties, excitements, or disappointments about each day, and continue to support and encourage her by praising her efforts and resilience.

Meet your child's teachers and stay in regular contact by phone or email so that you can discuss any concerns as they arise. Not only will it pave the way for you to ask questions, but it will also help the teachers feel more comfortable with calling you if they have concerns about your child.

If a family's home environment promotes learning and education is a priority, then your child will have a greater chance of achieving his academic potential.

Communicating Effectively with School Personnel

Parents should be knowledgeable about the educational program their child is receiving and should be actively involved with the school. The first step toward productive involvement is to know the members of the school staff. These are the people with whom your child spends a large percentage of her days and on whom you and she depend for her getting a good education. Many parents meet their child's teacher, principal, and the school administrative staff during an open house at school or at the first parent-teacher conference. However, you might find it helpful to meet these individuals earlier in the school year. Demonstrate your interest and involvement early.

Keep in mind that the first few days and weeks of the school year are quite busy; if you would like more than just five minutes to introduce yourself and exchange brief greetings, respect the demands on the teacher's time by calling or emailing and setting up an appointment beforehand. Teachers cannot stop their classroom activities when a parent arrives.

During the first week of school many teachers explain their expectations for the child's work and classroom behavior, as well as the consequences of not complying with these rules. For this purpose, many school districts hold a formal "expectation night" or "back-to-school night" for parents during the first week or two of school. If you make sure your child understands the guidelines early, you can help her get off to a good start in the class. If she does not know what the teacher's expectations are after a week or two, contact the teacher. Some teachers have the class participate in setting expectations for classroom behavior and consequences, so there may be a natural delay.

Teachers vary in the way they communicate their plans for the year to parents. Some will send out a memo in the first two weeks. Others do not present that information until parents' night. Many teachers maintain a website on the district's home page to post classroom updates. Ask when you will be receiving information about the curriculum and plans for homework and various projects. If you feel you need the information sooner, email the teacher to set up a meeting or perhaps a phone call for a quick overview.

While most schools will encourage you to stay in touch with your child's teacher, be aware of some of the difficulties involved in doing so. Emailing or sending a note to the teacher is an excellent way to establish contact about many issues. Let the teacher know specifically what you need. (This is preferable to "Please give me a call.") Teachers may have limited access to telephones. They must remain with their students most of the day. Many times, teachers can reply via email or send home a note with the information you need. If you would like to be called instead, let the teacher know your phone number and convenient times to reach you. During your first contact, ask how the teacher would prefer to be reached in the future.

Becoming an Involved Parent

Fortunately, the relationship between parents and the school staff is usually quite good. In most instances teachers and principals welcome your input and your hands-on involvement in the school. Active involvement in the parent-teacher association (PTA) or parent-teacher organization (PTO) is an excellent way to provide the school with your help and input in an organized way. With school budgetary restraints and two-career families, a parent who is able to volunteer even an hour or two a week is much appreciated.

Many parents enjoy volunteering in the classroom, working with students at a regular time each week, perhaps helping a small group with reading, arts and crafts, or computers. If you can volunteer in your child's classroom on a weekly basis, let the teacher know early in the year, and work out a convenient time for both of you—a time when the children you will be working with are readily available and will not be out of class for a special education program or band practice.

Schools often need help preparing and serving meals or refreshments for special events. Make sure your volunteer efforts coincide with the curriculum or the philosophy of the school or the teacher. If you have agreed to bring refreshments for a class party, the teacher might want them to be healthy snacks to reinforce the nutrition education at school. Rather than cupcakes, the teacher might prefer a fruit platter.

Field trips and educational trips are important means of giving children diverse experiences in the community, which they can then use as springboards for writing and discussions. However, without parent chaperones, these excursions may not be possible. If you are able to volunteer, you will probably be responsible for a particular group of children. If you need lead time to plan your participation in these trips or block out your work schedule, ask the teacher for as much advance notice as possible.

Even if you cannot help out at your child's school very often, try to do so at least once in a while. Even participating in one activity a year—accompanying a class on a field trip or helping out backstage on the day of a talent show—can mean a lot to your child. It will make him feel that his activities at school matter to you.

Many parents try to attend school events of which their children are a part. However, if there is an important event in your child's school life that you simply cannot attend because of work or other commitments, try to have someone else there—a grandparent, an uncle, or a friend—who can give your child moral support and maybe even take pictures for you.

Some parents are getting involved in the schools in another way—namely, on the policy-making level. Many schools have site councils, parent advisory councils, or Healthy School Teams, which help determine the direction of each school. Also, school boards need candidates for their seats, as well as volunteers to serve on special committees that evaluate everything from curriculum to school safety.

Occasionally the relationship among teachers, administrators, and enthusiastic mothers or fathers becomes strained and frustrating for all parties. Whether parents are lobbying for a new program for their child's school or are trying to serve as an advocate for their own child, who might be having difficulty with a particular subject area or teacher, their input can sometimes be perceived as more disruptive than helpful, no matter how well-intentioned it may be. To make your relationship with the school productive, show the staff respect, listen to their point of view, exhibit some flexibility, and find compromises whenever possible. Both you and the school have the same goal in mind—to educate your child—so try to work *with* the teacher and staff rather than assuming an adversarial stance.

The Parent-Teacher Conference

During the school year you will have the opportunity to have a scheduled conference with your child's teacher—an opportunity to discuss your child's capabilities and progress, and your mutual goals for her for the school year. Together, you and the teacher can develop plans to make the school experience as positive as possible.

Before these conferences, parents sometimes worry that they themselves are being evaluated and judged as parents, or that they might ask a silly question or embarrass themselves in some way. They may even experience the same type of general anxiety that they feel when visiting the doctor's office, anticipating that something is wrong.

If those feelings sound familiar, remind yourself of the positive nature and intent of these conferences. You are in a partnership with the teacher and other school personnel. You are an expert on your child and family, and certainly have information to share with the teacher that can be helpful in enhancing your child's classroom experience. At the same time, the teacher can tell you what is going on in the classroom, as well as suggest appropriate plans and goals for the remaining school year and possibly for the next year.

Before each conference, think about the questions you have and the issues you want to raise. For instance:

- Are there areas in which my child is not working up to her capabilities?

- What can I do at home to help her improve in the subjects in which she is weak?

- Does my child get along well with her classmates? Does she tend to be overly shy or aggressive?

- Have you noticed any learning problems or behavioral difficulties?

- Is there a need to formally assess my child's capabilities or further explore the course of her difficulties?

- Has my child had any unexplained absences or tardiness?

- Are her homework assignments being turned in, and are they well done? Am I supposed to help my child do homework or correct it?

- What are my child's strengths and interests, and are they being nurtured?

Since the time allotted for the conference may be short, you may want to make a list of your questions in order of importance. If both parents cannot attend, talk about the conference with the other parent in advance, and go over the issues he or she thinks should be raised.

Ask your child too if there is anything she would like you to discuss. Are there particular reasons she is continuing to have difficulty with math, for example, or science? Is she having any problems with classmates? Reassure your child that the conference is designed to help her do better at school and for you to better understand her school experience, not to find things about her to criticize. In some schools the students attend all of these parent-teacher conferences; find out your school's philosophy about this in advance, and if you would like a conference without your child, it can usually be arranged.

Arrive on time for the conference. Meetings with parents usually are scheduled at precise intervals. If you feel you need more time with the teacher, make

Parent-Teacher Conferences: As the Years Pass

Children ages 5–7 years: Make sure you check with the school ahead of time to determine what days and times conferences are held so you have plenty of notice to block work schedules or arrange child care for other siblings. Teachers will often have samples of your child's work in various subjects to show you her progress. Bring a list of questions or concerns with you; if the list has more than two or three items, you may consider contacting the teacher by email in case more time is needed for the conference.

Children ages 8–10 years: Even if there are no specific questions or concerns, parents should make every effort to arrange their work and child care schedule to attend these important meetings. Ask your child's teachers, based on their individual reading level, what books are recommended for reading for pleasure or for other ideas for home projects to reinforce what is being learned in the classroom.

Children ages 11–12 years: Many junior highs will let parents know that conferences are needed only if there are concerns. Parents should still strongly consider attending these important meetings, knowing that usually at the middle school level, conferences may only be five or ten minutes long. It is helpful to attach a name to the face and have that initial contact in case issues arise during the school year. Teachers at this level usually welcome emailed questions or concerns if you are unable to attend conferences.

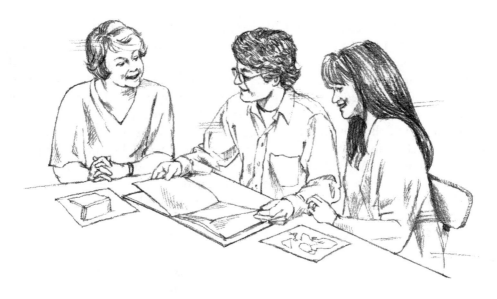

contact with the teacher ahead of time; indicate that you believe you'll need more time, and state the reason or issues. You may need to ask for a special time of sufficient length so all of your questions can be discussed. Also, if your time is up and you still feel there is more to discuss, schedule a second meeting or a phone call to continue the dialogue. Between meetings, if there is a problem with your child that you are trying to resolve, collect as much information as possible and come to the next meeting with some ideas and solutions in mind. Be respectful of the fact that your child's teacher has dozens of student families to communicate with.

After the conference, discuss it with your child. Tell her what you learned and what you and the teacher decided about future plans and strategies. Consider sending the teacher an email or note of thanks, particularly if the conference proved helpful or you sensed a special thoughtfulness or commitment to your child's educational progress and well-being.

Questions Commonly Asked by Parents

"MY CHILD IS HAVING CONTINUED DIFFICULTY WITH HIS SCHOOLWORK. WE'VE TRIED THINGS THE TEACHER HAS SUGGESTED. SHOULD I CONSIDER HAVING HIM TESTED FOR SPECIAL EDUCATION SERVICES?"

Schedule another meeting with the teacher with this specific question in mind. Review with the teacher any extra help your child is now receiving and other strategies that have been tried. Talk about the problems that still exist and what other approaches might be considered. If the conference does not produce any significant new directions to pursue, be prepared to request that your child receive further evaluation, including consultation with the reading specialist, special education teacher, school nurse, guidance counselor, and your child's pediatrician. You might also request that the principal or special education teacher join you at this meeting to answer your questions and provide input.

At the end of the conference, make sure that a plan has been established and that you are clear about the next step. If a testing or other evaluation or consultation meeting has been scheduled, tell your child about it and why it is being done. He should understand that the testing is designed to determine additional approaches to help make learning and schoolwork easier for him.

"WHY DOES MY CHILD'S SCHOOL GIVE STANDARDIZED TESTS?"

In many school districts, children routinely undergo a battery of standardized tests, designed by university, state, or private educational services and scored by computer. They are intended to provide a measure of a child's achievement or skill level in certain subjects. In other districts the results may be used to place children in particular classes or programs, and to measure their need for extra services. Some schools report that the collective test scores are used only to examine the school's overall direction and needs and to evaluate teacher performance.

Opponents of these tests argue that they measure only certain components of a child's achievement and intelligence and neglect other important ingredients of success, such as creativity, motivation, and a practical approach to life.

You need to know what your child's scores are and how they are being used in his school. If he does not do well on these types of tests and your school makes extensive use of their results, you should consider several options. If your child learns well despite his test scores, you might have him tutored in taking tests. Also, ask that appropriate information be added to your child's file about his strengths and successes.

"SHOULD MY CHILD BE ALLOWED TO USE A CALCULATOR?"

Most children need to be able to perform the mechanics of math without a calculator. Once they have mastered these skills and can set up problems, then the use of a calculator may be appropriate—but only if the teacher approves. Talk with the teacher about it, and ask the reasons for his or her decision.

Bear in mind that whether or not children use calculators for school and homework, they need to learn how to use one. Also, it is always appropriate to play number games with the calculator. For example, you can compute a problem in your head while your child checks your answer on the calculator; switch roles for the next problem.

"SHOULD I BUY MY CHILD A COMPUTER OR TABLET?"

It is important that your child learn basic keyboard and computer skills. Many schools train elementary school students in computer skills. There are many computerized learning programs that students use at school to practice and review math and language art skills.

Most schools consider a family home computer essential, but not that the child herself needs to have her own device. Here are some factors to consider:

- Does your child have a special learning problem that could be helped by working with a computer? For example, does he have a muscle or neurological problem that makes it difficult for him to write with a pencil and paper, and thus could a computer make it easier for him to do his homework and term papers? A child with dyslexia benefits from hearing written passages read aloud, an option with a computer.

- Do you have the time and money to find, buy, and teach your child educational programs?

- Will the computer be used almost exclusively for videogames?

- Will it interfere with family time?

Parental time and interest, not a computer, are the critical ingredients for learning at home. Parents must carefully monitor computer and internet use—supervision is a must. Keep the computer or laptop in a central location in the home. Computers can consume time otherwise available for homework, play, and physical activity. For more on computers and media usage, see Chapter 25.

~ 38 ~

Problems at School

AT SOME POINT during the school years your child's teacher may call, email, or ask you to come to school to discuss a specific concern or issue regarding your child. If this happens, schedule the meeting as soon as possible, since most problems are best dealt with early.

During this parent-teacher meeting, some parents feel they are on the defensive and are unsure how to react. Here are some guidelines to bear in mind:

- Do not feel threatened. The development of most children is uneven, and there is often one area of a child's performance that could use improvement. Withhold judgment and listen carefully to what the teacher has to say.

- Ask for specifics. For instance: "Could you give me an example of what is taking place? How often is this happening? How do the teacher and the other students respond to this particular behavior? Is this an isolated episode or a pattern of behavior?"

- Be open to the idea that situations within your family might be contributing to your child's difficulties, and share them as you deem appropriate (such as a recent parental job loss or death in the family).

- As you discuss the problem and possible solutions, approach the situation as a partnership, and look for ways to work together for improvement.

- If the problem is relatively uncomplicated, you and the teacher may decide during your conversation what action needs to be taken.

- Before the meeting ends, determine how and when you will follow up with each other to evaluate the success of the interventions and the progress of your child. What are the things you will be looking for to judge her progress (for instance, misbehaving less in class)? And how will this progress be communicated to you?

- If you feel that the opinion of another professional would be helpful in evaluating the problem or suggesting possible solutions, speak with the principal or another member of the support staff (counselor, nurse, psychologist), either with or without the teacher present. You also might decide to seek out an independent opinion from someone outside the school system. Ask your pediatrician for her opinion or for a referral.

Special Concerns About Peers

Difficulties may arise at school that will require your intervention. A common concern is when a child feels rejected by classmates. If your child comes home upset that "everyone is being mean to me at recess and in the cafeteria," keep in mind that most children have conflicts with their friends at some point and end up feeling pushed away. Parental reassurance can comfort these children until things return to normal at school.

However, if a pattern of rejection exists, let your child know that you are sensitive to how difficult this situation is for him, and that you are going to help him figure out ways to make things better. Give him a clear message that you are on his side and are going to help. Rejection by a child's peers may be a group reaction to someone they see as different. It may also result from inappropriate behavior on the part of one or both parties, and the behavior needs to be modified.

For older students who have internet access or smartphones, social networking can contribute to bullying even when school is not in session. Schools have become very aware of and proactive regarding students' online interactions. Delay purchasing your child an electronic device; it is easier to begin with limits and restrictions on any device before loosening the reins, so to speak. Minimize your child's usage of electronic devices; be aware of your child's apps and social networking accounts, including apps that aim to keep information away from parents. For more on internet usage and online bullying, see page 322.

If there seems to be a pattern of rejection, schedule an appointment with your child's teacher. Consider requesting that the principal or guidance counselor attend the meeting. Have them obtain information from the recess and lunch aides about what is happening. Follow the steps described in "The Parent-Teacher Conference," page 430. After this initial meeting, or whenever you feel you have enough information, you may want to consult with your pediatrician, who is familiar with your child's developmental pattern. (See also "Friends," page 157, and "Children Without Friends," page 161.)

Academic/Teacher Issues

At one time or another, nearly every child does poorly on a particular test or has difficulty with a subject or two in school. These situations can often be dealt with successfully by working one-on-one with your child, or through a three-way interaction involving you, your child, and her teacher, with a focus on helping your child develop good preparation strategies.

If there is a concern with certain aspects of the learning environment in your child's classroom, or if you feel she is not receiving proper guidance with a particular subject, approach the teacher first with your concern. Explain the problem without being accusatory. Give the teacher a chance to explain what is taking place, to share another perspective, and to suggest a solution. If you are dissatisfied with that encounter, or if you feel that sufficient progress is not being made after trying the teacher's plan, then bring your problem to the attention of the principal. The principal may suggest a meeting with you and the teacher. In many instances the difficulty can be resolved with input from the principal.

The principal can become your ally in other situations too. Approach her for problems unrelated to the classroom—for example, difficulties with a bus driver or a playground aide. At times, other school personnel such as guidance counselors or psychologists may be helpful too.

If the principal and teacher, or others, have initiated a specific plan to improve the situation, give things a reasonable chance to improve. It will not change in a couple of days. However, if after a reasonable amount of time the problem still remains unresolved, then continue up the educational hierarchy, which may lead you to the superintendent's office. For an issue involving school district policy, the superintendent and his or her associates will be the decision-makers. If you still remain dissatisfied, approach the school board members. They may be able to get action on your problem or put you in touch with the person who can.

As you move up the administrative ladder, gather, organize, and stay focused on the facts; save your emotional reactions for someone else who can acknowl-edge them. Be persistent and remain as pleasant and objective as possible. You will not make progress by losing your temper and by alienating the people who might help solve the difficulty. At some point along this path of seeking help, con-sult your child's pediatrician for advice or for a referral to another professional outside the school system.

Does Repeating a Grade Help?

Teachers and parents are sometimes faced with the question of whether to have a child repeat a grade because he seems unprepared to learn the material in the next grade. When making this decision, keep in mind that research shows that low-achieving students tend to progress at the same rate, whether they are retained or promoted. Retained students do not necessarily score better on achievement tests at the end of the repeated grade, compared with similar students who are pro-moted. Even if retained students improve on standardized test scores, their overall learning does not appear to increase.

You must also consider the negative effects of grade retention on social and emotional development. Quite often these students have fewer friends and a poorer self-concept. If a child already has emotional or social difficulties and has an academic deficit only in a particular area, he might benefit more from special services rather than retention. Experts believe that grade retention increases the risk of behavioral issues.

Teachers may mention a child's immaturity when they recommend retention. Ask for specific examples of this problem. Is it in the physical, emotional, or so-cial realm? Ask if retention is the only or the best solution. If your child's school-work is on track but he has difficulty controlling his impulsive behavior with his friends on the playground, then a consistent approach at both home and school to help him change his behavior may be appropriate.

Other issues also must be considered. Rigid, test-based policies regarding pro-motion and retention often do not take into account issues beyond the student's control, such as a poor teaching environment, learning disabilities, emotional problems, or family difficulties that may cause students to miss school. In general, retention does not help children learn and may contribute to a poor self-concept, diminished self-esteem, and emotional or social difficulties.

Other practical solutions may be alternatives when retention is being consid-ered for your child, whatever the reason.

- Some schools have instituted a policy that prevents students from entering the first grade before they are ready to read and write. By creating a "read-iness first grade" for 6-year-olds who are not quite ready for the usual first grade, they have eliminated the need for students to repeat the same first-grade curriculum. For example, the content of the reading materials varies between the readiness class and the regular class, so students do not repeat the same work. Teachers report fewer behavior problems in the more positive learning environment of this approach.

■ Multiage grouping, or mixing children from two or more grade levels in the same classroom, can be beneficial. In this way, a child stays in the same classroom with his friends—continuing to develop socially and emotionally—but receives the appropriate academic work that he needs. It also allows the child to do grade-appropriate work in those areas in which he is capable.

■ Some schools make adjustments during the school year itself, moving the child to a different class or involving a tutor if it is obvious he will need extra help.

■ Sometimes children are permitted to repeat a failed semester instead of a full year, which requires the teacher and student to be flexible.

School staffs tend to be very knowledgeable and experienced in decisions about retention, and do not lightly make the recommendation to hold a student back. Some students do benefit from retention, particularly those who already have strong self-esteem and are emotionally healthy but are still having difficulty keeping up academically with their classmates. That said, if retention is recommended and you are not comfortable with it, seek an additional opinion. Talk it over with your child's pediatrician, another teacher, or a psychologist. Consider whether an outside evaluation would be helpful.

If you and the teacher ultimately decide that it is necessary to retain your child, ask for the teacher's suggestions on the best way to explain that to your child. Also, inquire about the program that will be in place next year to address your child's problems. In preparation for the next school year, help your child figure out positive ways to discuss his grade retention. Role-play how he can answer the inevitable questions from his friends and classmates. For the middle-years child, the optimal times to retain him are at the end of kindergarten or first grade, or upon moving to a new school or a new city.

School Discipline

When students know what expectations are in place for appropriate behavior and classroom routines, education can proceed smoothly. Schools will monitor students who consistently talk out of turn, peek at another student's paper during a test, or interact with classmates inappropriately online, as examples. All of these situations warrant some disciplinary action. Most schools have a policy about discipline, and in many cases it is available in writing, often published in the school handbook. Although both students and parents tend to think of discipline as a form of punishment, it actually means to teach in a correct way and has a highly desirable purpose: providing an orderly, safe environment to promote learning.

Disciplinary efforts work best when clear explanations are given to both children and parents about:

- The behavior that is expected

- The behavior that is unacceptable

- The consequences of unacceptable behavior

The American Academy of Pediatrics feels strongly that while departures from expected behavior should be dealt with appropriately and firmly, teachers and school staff should also take into account each child's individual temperament, attention span, and cognitive abilities. For example, a child with attention deficit hyperactivity disorder (ADHD) may have more difficulty sitting still in class than most of the other children. In all cases, disciplinary actions should show respect for the child and take into account the student's capabilities, effort, and ability to improve and respond positively. While discipline may include an extra homework assignment or a loss of privileges, physical punishment should *never* be used, nor should a child ever be humiliated in front of others. If your own child has disciplinary problems at school, you need to take a more active role in determining the reasons and ensuring that she behaves appropriately. Make certain she understands the type of behavior you and the school expect from her in the classroom and on the playground.

On occasion you may not agree with the school's approach to discipline. In that event, address your concerns directly to the teacher, principal, or other school personnel. Do not make negative comments about the school directly to your child. Your own attitudes and behavior are a powerful role model for your child, and if you do not appear to have much respect for the school, your child will not either. As an example, if your child is being kept inside at recess as a form of punishment, and you feel he needs to get outside and burn off excess energy, be careful how you express your dissatisfaction to your child. Talk directly with the teacher and suggest another form of punishment that might be more appropriate. You and the teacher should try to find a common ground so your child receives a consistent set of expectations and positive reinforcement both at home and at school.

In general, a child should not be kept from play at recess to complete classroom assignments at her desk. She will dislike her work even more if she misses out on outdoor activities that she enjoys. And since her attention will probably be on the playground, she may not learn much from what she is doing. It is very important for children to be outside playing with others at times during the day. For more on recess, see page 408.

In all cases, ask the teacher or principal to keep you aware of disciplinary problems with your son or daughter. Some principals call home immediately upon the child's first visit to their office; others believe that by the upper grades of elementary school, the child should take more responsibility for her own behavior, and thus these principals may try to help the child work out the problem without parental intervention.

If there is a serious problem, you will likely be notified at once, but for more routine behavioral difficulties, you cannot necessarily count on being called. If your child tells you she has been to the principal's office and you want to know exactly what happened, feel free to call the principal. On the other hand, many issues can be resolved effectively without your involvement and without your also punishing your child at home for something that she is already being disciplined for at school. Keep in mind that behavior problems are often a signal of stress or a call for help or attention. Consider the underlying causes of the behavior difficulties as well as the problems themselves.

~ 39 ~

Homework

DURING THE ELEMENTARY school years, most children begin to have homework. Precisely when it starts will depend on the school and the teacher. In addition to homework, all grade levels will encourage students to read independently at home, either with a parent or on their own. When homework is assigned, it will average about fifteen to twenty minutes per night in the early elementary school years, but depending on your child's capabilities, he may need more or less time to complete it, sometimes up to about an hour.

As a general guideline, some educators believe that the number of minutes a child should spend on homework is equivalent to his grade level times ten. Thus, a third-grader should complete his nightly homework assignments in about thirty minutes; a fifth-grader in about fifty minutes. Keep in mind that in addition to homework assignments, children of all ages are encouraged to spend time daily engaging in either independent reading or, for younger children, reading with a parent. Find out early in the school year what the teacher's philosophy is regarding homework, and plan accordingly. Ask the teacher questions about how much homework is assigned, how often, and how involved the teacher prefers parents to be.

Developing Good Homework Habits

Help your child develop good homework habits, including designating a regular location and time to work on daily assignments. She does not necessarily need a desk in her room; the kitchen island or table can work just as well. No matter what place you choose, it needs to be well lit and quiet, without the distractions of the television or other screens, other children playing, or people talking on the telephone. Keep your child's materials (paper, pencil, dictionary) nearby so she can get started quickly and on her own each afternoon or evening.

Some children get right down to work without needing much encouragement. Others need help making the transition from playing to a homework frame of mind. Sometimes providing a ten-minute warning is all it takes to help a child get ready mentally as well as to move to the place she intends to work. Some teachers give a week's worth of homework as a packet on Mondays, which allows the child to plan ahead and divide the work among the weekdays. This is particularly helpful if extracurricular activities occur on certain evenings, as it allows for a greater portion of the homework to be completed on the other weeknights. Some younger children may feel the need to complete the entire week's packet on Monday nights; for these kids, you may need to reinforce the fact that the work is meant to be spread out over a few days and is too much for a single evening.

There is no universally right time to do homework. In some families, children do best if they tackle their homework in midafternoon, shortly after returning home from school; other kids may do best if they devote the after-school hours to unwinding and playing, leaving their homework until the evening, when they may feel a renewed sense of energy. Let your child have some say in the decision. Homework can become a source of conflict between parent and child—but if you agree on a regular time and place, you can eliminate two of the most frequent causes of homework-related dissension.

Some parents have found that their children do not respond well to having a regular study time, such as four o'clock every afternoon. Instead, these kids are given guidelines ("No videogames until your homework is done"). Find out what works best both for your child and for the family as a whole, and once this is determined, stick with it. A fair amount of homework may need to be completed online; if this is the case, monitor the situation to ensure that your child is staying on task as opposed to being distracted by unrelated online activities.

Some children prefer that a parent sit with them as they do their homework. You may find this an acceptable request, particularly if you have your own reading or paperwork to complete. However, do *not* actually do the homework for your child. She may need some assistance getting focused and organizing her approach to the assignment. Occasionally, you may need to explain a math problem; in those cases, let your child try a couple of problems first before offering to help. But if she *routinely* requires your active participation to get her everyday homework done, then talk to her teacher. Your child may need stronger direction in the classroom so that she is able to complete the assignments on her own or with less parental involvement. One area where children may need parental help is in organizing how much work will have to be done daily to finish a long assignment, such as a term paper or a science project.

If your child or her teacher asks you to review her homework, you may want to look it over before she takes it to school the next morning. Usually it is best if homework remains the exclusive domain of the child and the teacher. However, your input may vary depending on the teacher's philosophy and the purpose of homework. If the teacher is using homework to check your child's understanding of the material—thus giving the teacher an idea of what needs to be emphasized in subsequent classroom teaching sessions—your suggestions for changes and improvements on your child's paper could prove misleading. On the other hand, if the teacher assigns homework to give your child practice in a particular subject area and to reinforce what has already been taught in class, then your participation can be valuable. Some teachers use homework to help children develop self-discipline and organizational and study skills. Be sure to praise your son or daughter for her efforts and success in doing her homework well.

In general, support your child in her homework, but do not act as a taskmaster. Provide her with a quiet place, supplies, encouragement, and occasional help—but it is her job to do the work. Homework is your child's responsibility, not yours.

As the weeks pass, keep in touch with your child's teacher regarding homework assignments. If you determine that your child is having ongoing difficulty understanding what the assignments are and how to complete them, or if she breezes through them as though they were no challenge at all, let the teacher know. The teacher may adjust the assignments so they are more in sync with your child's capabilities.

Whether or not your child has homework on a particular night, make time to read aloud with a younger child after school or at night, and encourage independent reading for an older kid. This type of shared experience can help interest your child in reading, as well as give you some personal time with her. Also, on days when your child does not have any assigned homework, this shared reading time will reinforce the habit of a work time each evening.

To further nurture your child's love of reading, set a good example by spending time reading on your own, and by taking your child to the library or bookstore to select books she would like to read. Many families turn off the TV each night for at least thirty minutes, and everyone spends the time reading. As children get older, one to two hours may be a more desirable length of time each day to set aside for reading and other constructive activities.

Many families obtain news and information online, but consider a daily print newspaper subscription that gets delivered to your home. When screens are turned off, kids naturally gravitate to the comic pages, followed by other parts of the newspaper, learning valuable reading skills as well as gaining information about current events. A particular advantage of a print newspaper over online news is that you are exposed to articles and commentaries that you otherwise may not have encountered, which is a great way for children to learn about the world around them.

As important as it is for your child to develop good study habits, play is also important for healthy social, emotional, and physical growth and development. While encouraging your child to complete her assignments or do some additional reading, keep in mind that she has already had a lengthy and perhaps tiring day of learning at school and needs free time. Help her find the play activities that best fit her temperament and personality—whether it is organized school sports or music lessons, free-play situations (time at the playground, riding her bike, playing with friends), or a combination of these.

Homework for Children Ages 9 to 12: Developing Responsibility

As children enter the fourth grade, the purpose of homework changes to some extent. In grades one to three, students are learning to read; thereafter, they are reading to learn. In fourth grade both schoolwork and homework become more challenging. Learning tasks require more organization and more sustained attention and effort. Because of this change, homework becomes a more integral part of children's learning and is reflected more in their academic record. This shift comes at a good time, since at about the fourth grade, children are ready for and want more autonomy and responsibility and less parental hovering and involvement.

Homework for older children has a number of purposes. It provides an opportunity for review and reinforcement of skills that have been mastered and encourages practicing skills that are not yet mastered. Homework also is an opportunity for children to learn self-discipline and organizational skills and to take responsibility for their own learning.

Many of the same suggestions for approaching homework that are recommended for younger children apply to older children as well. Homework is best done when the child has had a chance to unwind from school or after-school activities, is rested, and is not hungry. You and your child should agree upon a regular schedule for when homework will be done, and the length of time that should be devoted to it. This schedule should provide predictability and structure but should be sufficiently flexible to respond to special situations. Just like adults, some children do best if their work time is divided into several short sessions instead of a single long session.

Usually parents can be helpful by assisting their child in getting settled and started. You can look together at each day's homework assignment and decide what parts might require help from you, a sibling, or a classmate. The most difficult parts should be done first. Often homework needs to be completed online; ensure children are staying on task and not engaging in distracting unrelated online tasks. Reviewing for tests and rote memorization tasks also should be done early and then repeated at the end of the homework session or first thing the next morning. As is the case for younger children, homework should be done in a location with few distractions (no screens, telephone, videogames, loud conversation) and where all the necessary supplies and reference materials are available.

Here are some specific suggestions on how to approach homework of different types.

Reading Assignments

1. Divide chapters into small units or use the author's headings as a guide.

2. Find the topic sentence or the main idea for each paragraph and underline it or write it down.

3. Write a section-by-section outline of the reading assignment, copying or paraphrasing the main points; leave some room to write in notes from class discussions.

Writing (Composition)

1. Begin by recognizing that the first draft will not be the last, and that rewriting will produce better work.

2. Make a list of as many ideas as possible without worrying about whether they are good or correct.

3. Organize these "brainstorm" ideas into clusters that seem reasonable, and then arrange the clusters into a logical sequence.

4. Write down thoughts as to why these clusters were made and why the order makes sense.

Talking About Your Child's School Day

"What did you do in school today?"

"Nothing."

This is a familiar exchange between parent and child. And it can be a frustrating one for an interested parent who genuinely wants to keep abreast of a child's activities at school. Children will usually be more responsive about their day at school if they are asked fairly direct questions at a time that is appropriate. For instance, when a child first arrives home from school, he might be tired and want a snack, or want to relax or play with a friend rather than rehash the day. It might be better to talk with him about school later in the day or evening. Often the best conversations are when you are performing a task such as driving in the car or preparing dinner together.

Make your questions as focused and nonjudgmental as possible. For instance:

- "What new thing did you learn in school today?"

- "What questions did you ask in class?"

- "How is that book you've been reading in class? What's happening in the story?"

- "Tell me three things about your day that I don't know yet."

- "Do you have any papers or artwork in your backpack that we could look over?"

- "Tell me about the spelling test. Was there a word or two you had trouble with?"

- Also see "Get the Conversation Started" on page 188.

Knowing that students may have trouble remembering everything that happened in school, teachers often communicate about class and school issues by maintaining a classroom website with updates and posted weekly assignments, as well as through written notes. Looking at the class website together with your child may prompt more conversation.

At times your child might want to talk about school when you're right in the middle of something else. As much as possible, try to catch these opportunities, saying something like "I want to hear about school—help me make this salad for dinner while we talk."

5. Use this work as an outline and write a first draft; at this stage, do not worry about spelling or punctuation.

6. Revise the first draft, paying attention to detail.

Check the following:

Meaning. Does it make sense and meet the purpose of the assignment?

Paragraph formation. Does each paragraph have a topic sentence, and are the other sentences logically related?

Sentence formation. Does each sentence express a complete thought? Are capitalization and punctuation correct?

Word. Was the best word chosen? Is it spelled correctly?

Neatness. Is the paper easy to read? Does it follow the format and style the teacher expects?

STEM (Science, Technology, Engineering, and Math)

1. Work toward mastering the basic facts and operations (addition, subtraction, multiplication, and division) until they become automatic. Do this work in small doses, and limit the number of facts to three to five each session. Use writing, flash cards, and oral quizzes.

2. Be sure the basic concepts of computation are well understood. Do computation homework slowly and check the results, since if the facts are understood, most errors come from being careless.

3. Use money examples when learning decimals.

4. For fractions, use visual or concrete aids rather than oral explanations.

Studying for Tests

1. Gather together homework assignments, class notes, outlines, quizzes, and handouts, and arrange them chronologically (by date).

2. Four days before the test, read the information through in a general way.

3. Three days before the test, look at major titles of sections in notes and books.

4. Two days before the test, review the titles of sections and read the information and organize it into related clusters.

5. The night before the test, repeat the process of the night before and recite as much as you can from memory.

Other Ways to Reinforce Learning

In addition to doing homework, your child should spend time reading not only with you but on his own as well. When a child finds pleasure in reading, it will become a lifelong habit. His teacher or school librarian can help you and your child select some books for leisure reading. Make sure he has a card at the public library. Peruse the nonfiction shelves pertaining to topics your child finds interesting—for example, robots or dinosaurs. Consider joining a children's book club or subscribe to a magazine for children in the appropriate age group (such as *National Geographic Kids* or *Stone Soup*). If your child sees you reading regularly, there is a good chance that he will follow your lead and sit down with a book himself. Set aside some time to talk with him about what each of you is reading. If you have been regularly reading aloud to your son or daughter, by school age they'll probably want to read aloud to you too, perhaps alternating chapters in a book you both enjoy. Do not worry if your child occasionally picks up a book intended for younger readers; there is joy in having mastered a book. Similarly, you don't need to shy away from more advanced reading; a daily print newspaper, combined with a household using a minimal amount of screen time, results in awareness of world events and advancing reading skills.

Find time to converse with your child about your respective days, including what he did at school. Even on a night when you are particularly busy, you should still be able to find a time and place to talk. (See Chapter 14, "Communicating with Your Child.")

You should encourage your child to write or draw without any educational purpose in mind other than to express himself. Perhaps he can compose original stories, or write cards, letters, and invitations to friends and relatives. Keep paper, pencils, crayons, markers, and tape in a convenient, accessible location so he can sit down and use them without advance planning or special permission. Many researchers believe that writing improves a child's reading skills and vice versa.

Plan some activities—an art project, for example—that you can do with your child. Put away screens and keep phone call interruptions to a minimum during this period; make it time you spend with each other. Some children say they wish they could call their parents on the phone, because screens or a phone call often get first priority.

Put a map on the wall in your child's bedroom and refer to it frequently. You might ask, "Where does Aunt Jennifer live? . . . Can you find the city where the president lives?" You can also use the map to talk about history, especially around a historical holiday.

Many children enjoy going to the library. Because they use the school library frequently, children almost instinctively feel at home when they go to the community library. In schools, libraries are now often called "learning centers," because they have video and audio materials as well.

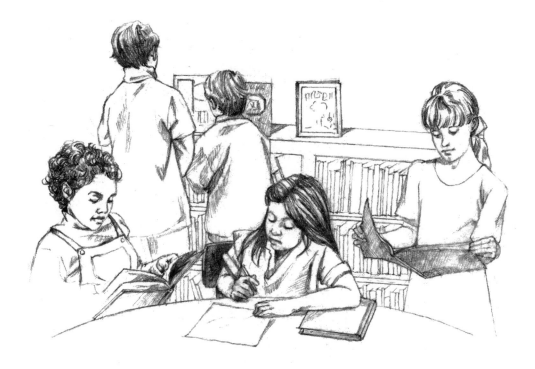

Make it a routine to visit area museums, zoos, and aquariums to enrich what is being learned in the classroom. Find some community activities that are pure fun. Despite their recreational nature, they can still be viewed as providing support for what is being taught in school, since they will broaden your child's base of experience and give him something new to write about.

Try to reinforce your child's health education at school in a number of ways—for instance, by making healthful food choices when you shop. No matter what is taught in the classroom and served in the school cafeteria, these influences are much less likely to have an impact upon your child if you do not follow the same health-promoting guidelines in your own food selections. Actively involving your child in the process by having him read recipes and measure ingredients can reinforce nutrition education. (See Chapter 2, "Nutrition.")

Capitalize on your child's physical education program at school too, by scheduling some weekend or after-school activities that are appropriate for the entire family. Swimming, tennis, bicycle riding, and skiing are some of the sports that children can participate in for their entire lives and that can keep your child fit long after he has left school. Do not overlook walking as a perfect way for the family to enjoy physical activity together. (See Chapter 4, "Physical Fitness and Sports," for a thorough discussion of fitness and exercise.)

~ 40 ~

Learning Disabilities

IN THE MIDDLE years of childhood, there comes a time when kids leave the protective confines of the family and enter the world of school and peers. If a child learns slowly—or if she needs to work harder than her peers to learn—both children and parents can feel disappointed, frustrated, and confused. There is a wide spectrum of typical development within any particular grade of students. If your child seems to be struggling academically or is underachieving, it is possible she has a learning disability, which can also be called a learning disorder, learning difference, or learning difficulty. When present, learning differences may cause emotional, social, behavioral, or family problems, especially if the disability is not diagnosed or is misdiagnosed, or if the interventions or treatments used are not appropriate or do not achieve results.

The earlier you become aware of a possible learning issue, and the sooner your child is evaluated, identified, and assisted, the better the chances for a positive outcome.

What Are Learning Disabilities?

Learning disabilities are a diverse group of disorders in which children who typically have at least average intelligence have problems process-

If your child has a learning disability, there are a variety of interventions and supportive services available to assist him.

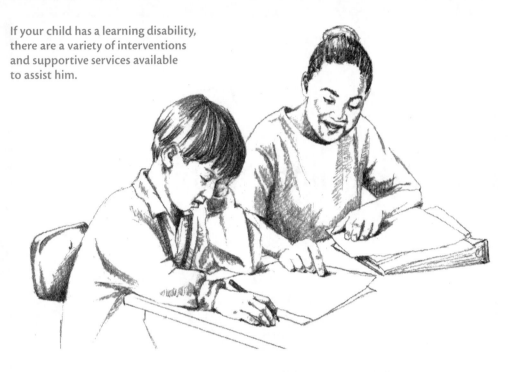

ing information or generating output. Learning disabilities can result from a variation in your child's central nervous system functioning. Children are built in different ways and there is a wide range of typical. Some learning issues run in families. In some cases, a previous head injury or brain infection might cause learning difficulties. In most instances, children are born with the tendency for learning problems; the cause is unclear, and the affected children look and act like other children and are in other ways no different from them.

Learning disabilities tend to run in families. About 50 percent of these children have a parent, sibling, or extended family member with a similar difficulty, although this may not be known to the family, as in the past certain learning difficulties were frequently misdiagnosed or mislabeled.

Learning disabilities can range in severity from mild to severe. They may affect a single learning task, like spelling, or they can influence many of them, like reading, writing, and listening comprehension. In some children, their presence may be obvious even before school age; in others, they may become apparent later and then only in subtle ways. Parents may not even be aware that their child has a learning issue until his learning capabilities are challenged and he is unable to keep up with classroom demands and expectations. Learning disabilities can last a lifetime, becoming more or less obvious depending on the academic and other learning demands that kids can face. With identification and intervention, they often do improve.

When a child does not perform to expectations at school or seems to lose his motivation to learn, he might be responding to other issues in his life. He might be experiencing problems with peers, or there may be family transitions that he finds distracting. As with learning disabilities themselves, social and emotional problems that mimic learning disabilities require immediate and appropriate help.

The Impact of Common Learning Disabilities

When learning disabilities occur, they generally affect three general skill areas:

- Academic skills, such as reading, writing, spelling, and arithmetic

- Language and speech skills, encompassing areas such as listening, talking, and understanding

- So-called motor-sensory integration skills, such as coordination, balance, and writing

When problems exist in any of these areas, there is a breakdown in one or more stages of learning. For instance, the child may have difficulty taking in information through hearing or sight. Or he could have problems remembering the information he has heard or read. Finally, he may be unable to utilize this knowledge in a productive way. There may be overlap between these skill areas, as a child with reading challenges may struggle in math story problems.

Diagnosing a Learning Disability

Learning disabilities are diagnosed by a variety of means. A traditional method is to conduct two tests and note a discrepancy between their scores. These tests are an intelligence (or IQ) test and a standardized achievement (reading, writing, arithmetic) test. Most children found to have a learning disability have typical or above typical intelligence but do not fully demonstrate that potential on achievement tests. For example, a child might score 112 on the full-scale IQ test but her math score might be 90; this discrepancy of 22 points between her potential ability (IQ) and actual achievement (in math) might qualify her for special services at her school. State-mandated definitions sometimes exclude a range of learning difficulties that do not produce wide discrepancies in these test scores.

When a learning disability is not detected early, diagnosed correctly, or treated effectively, it can cause a number of other problems. These additional difficulties may be emotional, and a child may show signs of low self-esteem, frustration, or disappointment. Behavior problems such as acting out might occur. Or the learning problems may show up within the family, causing, for example, misunderstandings, increased stress, or the blaming of others.

Does Your Child Have Attention or Learning Problems?

Attention deficit hyperactivity disorder (ADHD) is a problem closely associated with learning disabilities. About 25 percent or more of children with learning disabilities also have attention difficulties, which can affect their academic, language, speech, and writing skills, as well as all other areas of learning.

If your own child has been diagnosed with a learning disability, you need to consider whether attention problems are present as well. If he has been diagnosed as having ADHD, he might also have a learning disorder.

For more information on attention problems, see page 558.

Common Learning Disabilities
Language and Speech Disabilities

These are among the most common learning problems and can be quite significant, as so much of learning is dependent on language. If your child has such a disability, it can affect his reading, spelling, writing, speech, and ability to understand what he hears or reads. Even a mild language disorder can lead to later reading troubles. A language issue may also affect his memory or comprehension—that is, the ability to recall or understand information previously heard or read. Your child may have difficulty following instructions, understanding explanations, or expressing himself. These problems not only can affect his learning but also may impede his social interactions, which require good listening and speaking skills. As a result, he may become embarrassed, confused, or quiet and withdrawn. He might even resort to acting out his feelings, thoughts, or frustrations with inappropriate behavior.

Writing Difficulties

Like children with other types of learning disabilities, children with writing problems may be bright and creative but may have difficulty expressing themselves on paper in a coherent manner. This may cause frustration or even a writing phobia. Since any written document is a semipublic, permanent display of one's work, these children sometimes feel extremely embarrassed or self-conscious, and they often try to avoid writing assignments or don't make much of an effort when doing them. Writing is a complex task that requires the simultaneous use of many skills, including letter formation, grammar, vocabulary, spelling, the mechanics of writing (punctuation, capitalization), and organizing ideas into sentences and paragraphs. While some children may master each of these skills separately, carrying all of them out at the same time may prove to be too difficult. Writing problems are complex and may have several causes, including visual, fine motor, language, or memory difficulties.

Visual Learning Difficulties and Dyslexia

When children have a weakness or disability in understanding visually presented information, it may affect their ability to read, spell, interpret, or remember the printed word, graphs, tables, illustrations, and maps. These are learning problems; the children's vision is normal and unrelated to the specific problem.

Sometimes visual learning difficulties occur along with another weakness—for example, in conjunction with fine motor difficulties—which can affect handwriting. When that happens, the child's writing may be illegible. He may have difficulty forming letters or numbers, or keeping numbers properly aligned in columns. He may write letters or numbers backward. This can affect not only his writing ability (including legibility and speed) but also his proficiency in mathematics, causing him to make miscalculations.

Dyslexia is the most common learning disability; it has been reported to affect as much as 20 percent of the population, with a range of severity. Difficulty reading can be a presenting symptom; however, it is more than simply letter reversals, as is commonly thought. Dyslexia is characterized by difficulties with accurate or fluent word recognition and by poor spelling and decoding abilities. Younger children may present with difficulties learning "sight words" in kindergarten or first grade, as rapid word recognition and recall can be impacted.

Dyslexia can impact more than just reading skills; affected children can have spelling and writing challenges and troubles with multistep math problems or story problems as well. If your child has problems learning the alphabet, difficulty identifying letters or letter sounds, or challenges reading at an age-appropriate level, discuss your concerns with your child's teacher. Many school districts have a reading specialist who may be able to assist in evaluating your child for dyslexia. It is often helpful for parents to specifically mention dyslexia as a concern for which you wish the child to be tested.

Dyslexia: Signs at Different Ages

Children ages 5–7 years: Affected kids may have trouble learning the alphabet, numbers, days of the week, and how to spell and write their own name.

Children ages 8–10 years: Affected kids may have difficulty connecting letters and sounds, or decoding single words; they may make reading or spelling errors frequently; they may have difficulty learning to tell time.

Children ages 11–12 years: Affected kids may struggle with word math problems in addition to reading and language subjects. Listening to audible forms of written assignments may be helpful for these kids.

Any child suspected to have dyslexia should be tested by a qualified testing examiner. Speak with your school and your pediatrician for more information.

Memory and Other Thinking Difficulties

As children move through elementary school, they are increasingly asked to remember, retrieve, and use more and more information rapidly. They need to recall specific information in a very detailed manner, as well as to recall and assemble information in a creative and open-ended way. The first, more specific type of memory (called convergent) is useful in short answers or multiple-choice tests and in analytical, fact-oriented reasoning. The second, more general memory (divergent) is useful in essay writing, retelling a story, interpreting a poem, or describing a character in one's own way.

Memory involves taking in information, classifying it, associating it with previously learned information, and consolidating it. Many children understand what they read or are taught but can't remember it later, perhaps for a test, or they can't recall it in a different context. While a memory problem can be subtle and difficult to assess, you should suspect this type of difficulty if your child is underachieving.

Some children have particular trouble remembering several pieces of sequential information, such as multiple instructions or a series of words or numbers like a telephone number. As a result, a school-age child may have difficulty doing a three-step math problem, organizing events, learning the alphabet, remembering multiplication tables, or recounting a story in the proper sequence. Even learning the days of the week, months of the year, and class schedules can be hard.

A number of factors can make memory problems even worse. These include too much or overly complex information being presented at one time, or an excessively rapid rate of incoming information. Attention problems, emotional disorders (depression, anxiety), boredom, loss of motivation, and fatigue (poor nutrition, inadequate sleep, mental exertion) can also contribute to memory difficulties.

Difficulties can occur with other higher-level thinking as well. Some children have problems with a skill called abstract reasoning, meaning that they are unable to determine the general meaning of a particular word or symbol—perhaps the symbol for an unknown quantity in a math problem. They also cannot make inferences by going from a specific, concrete fact to a more general type of thinking.

Children may also have difficulty with organization and thus be unable to assemble information into a usable form. Good organizational skills can also help children associate newly learned information with their existing knowledge, making it fit in with something familiar so it can be more easily retrieved and utilized.

Summarizing skills are another possible problem area. Children may have trouble taking a large amount of information and condensing it to a more manageable size so it is easier to remember and use. Children with this skill are not able to separate major facts and concepts from lesser ones, ascertaining which ones are most worthwhile.

Inadequate Social Skills

These often occur in conjunction with learning disabilities and usually result in difficulties interacting with other children or adults. Children with this problem may have trouble interpreting the messages or intentions of others and responding appropriately to others, even to parents and teachers who are trying to be helpful. Recognizing and alleviating these difficulties is critical, because peer acceptance and a successful social life are important to kids in middle childhood and greatly affect their self-image and self-esteem. (See Chapter 11, "Developing Social Skills.")

What Parents Can Do

If your child is performing below grade level, is failing or struggling to maintain barely passing grades, or is not achieving to the degree to which you think she is capable, here are some suggestions for beginning to get her the help she needs.

- Trust your instincts. You know your child best, and you are your child's strongest advocate. If you suspect something is wrong, it should be investigated. Don't assume that learning disorders don't matter or that your child will "grow out of it." Early recognition and treatment are important.

- Ask the teacher for his or her opinion about the possibility of learning disabilities in your child, specifically mentioning the term "dyslexia," for example, if that is a concern. Listen to any concerns the teacher may have. Rely on his or her experience and training.

- If your child appears frustrated, unmotivated, or bored, or is acting up in school, these could be signs of an underlying, undiagnosed learning problem that needs diagnosis and treatment. Also, if your child is failing, underachieving, or working extremely hard just to keep up, this could also be a symptom of a learning difficulty.

- Is your son or daughter devoting adequate time and energy to her schoolwork? Is she interested and involved in the learning process? Could your family's everyday functioning and expectations be affecting her adversely? Is she preoccupied with peer relationships or with problems at home? Are academic and emotional stresses causing frustration and a loss of confidence and motivation, almost to the point of helplessness ("No matter how hard I try, I still can't learn")?

- Think back to your own childhood. Many parents experienced similar learning difficulties when they were younger, and these problems tend to run in families. Your own empathy, understanding, and acceptance will influence the course of your child's learning problem, as will your attitude toward schools and learning.

- Speak with other adults and professionals. Seek out information and guidance from your child's principal, guidance counselor, school psychologist, or coach, or from the parents of your child's friends.

- Your pediatrician's advice will also be helpful, because he or she understands typical child development, knows your child, and has experience in these common childhood problems. He or she may also be able to send questions to school to try to clarify an apparent problem with learning, or advocate on your family's behalf to obtain necessary testing.

Your pediatrician can also determine whether any physical problems (including a vision or hearing deficiency) could be playing a role in your child's learning difficulties. He or she can refer you and your child to the appropriate professionals, perhaps suggesting that your child have a formal learning disability evaluation, either by the school or by independent psychologists and educators not affiliated with the school system. In most states, if a child is failing or otherwise performing below grade level, the public schools are obligated to conduct such evaluations and may be required to provide special services. (For children with ADHD, see Chapter 49, and for children on the autism spectrum, see Chapter 41.)

Your Right to Special Services

Once a learning problem is suspected, ask your child's school staff about special educational services, such as evaluation and, if appropriate, treatment. Sometimes teachers or principals are reluctant to request a consultation or make a referral. If you feel strongly that your child's needs are not being met, you need to be your child's advocate. It's the law: public school systems must make special services available under the Individuals with Disabilities Education Act, a federal statute enacted in 1975. In order to receive federal funds, every state and school district must have a procedure for identifying, assessing, and planning an educational program for these children, from age 3 to 22. This law covers not only children with learning disabilities but also those with perceptual problems (hearing or visual impairments), cerebral palsy or other brain injuries, mental retardation, orthopedic problems affecting mobility, and serious behavioral and emotional difficulties that can interfere with the process of education.

This law provides five basic rights:

1. The right to a free, appropriate public education

2. The right to an Individualized Educational Program (IEP) based on a complete developmental assessment and approved by parents (for more on IEPs, see page 473)

3. The right to access records or the right of parents to review the child's educational records

4. The right to due process, or giving parents the right to participate in the evaluation and decision-making process

5. The right to the least restrictive educational environment (placing the child in a learning situation that is as normal and convenient as conditions allow)

The Evaluation

A minimal evaluation includes a psychological assessment of cognitive function (an IQ test) and an educational assessment of academic achievement (a standardized test). Other testing might evaluate neurodevelopmental functions (such as language, memory, attention, and motor skills), the emotional status of your child, and a social assessment (family and environment).

This evaluation process can be complicated, time-consuming, and difficult for parents and child to understand. Sometimes it is quite expensive if you obtain the evaluations outside the school system. In most cases, you should start with the full evaluation provided by your child's school. If it cannot be done within a reasonable time or if specialized testing is needed, request payment from the school system before you get a private evaluation. However, regardless of where they are done, these evaluations can be both informative and productive.

Because the entire evaluation process may be complex and involve many people, a case manager or services coordinator (such as a pediatrician, neuropsychologist, or learning disability educator) may be helpful. The coordinator can also assist you in planning appropriate interventions or treatments, making referrals, monitoring the effect of treatment upon your child, and arranging for follow-up evaluations. Frequently this takes a team effort.

Once an evaluation is completed, schools usually arrange a meeting to fully discuss the findings and your child's educational plan. This meeting might be attended by your child's teacher(s), a guidance counselor, the special education teacher, the principal, the school psychologist, and the school nurse. Sometimes children attend the meeting. Occasionally you may want to ask your pediatrician to attend to provide support for you and your perspective. If you wish, bring someone with you who might serve as the child's advocate and who is familiar with these evaluations and meetings and understands the implications of the findings and interventions. Make sure the results are explained to you in terms you can understand.

In explaining the learning problem to your child, avoid simplistic, negative labels such as "learning disabled," "handicapped," and "hyperactive"; instead, help him look at himself in a comprehensive and positive manner that acknowledges weaknesses but also emphasizes strengths and special attributes.

Children with learning disabilities generally respond well to a sensitive and appropriate evaluation and treatment plan. This is particularly true if this plan is supportive, removes blame from both child and parent, focuses on the present problems, attends to other associated concerns, allows the child to achieve at a higher level than before, and results in his feeling more confident, self-reliant, and motivated. It can be helpful to point out successful adults who also have learning disabilities.

What Interventions Are Available?

After you and your child understand the results of the evaluation, ask the school for a description of the various interventions or supportive services it can offer. This will begin to provide you with a clear, comprehensive view of what may lie ahead for your child.

Your decision about interventions will depend on the evaluation results and the school district's resources, including the specific resources of your child's school.

Resource room. Your child may qualify for part-time or full-time special services in a resource room for certain specific academic subjects, while being mainstreamed for other subjects and activities. Make sure goals and expectations are set appropriately, with a timetable for achieving them. If needed, your child may also receive help for language problems (speech or language therapy) or motor problems (physical or occupational therapy).

Inclusion mainstreaming or partial inclusion. This is a system in which a child is educated alongside her peers to the greatest extent possible. For students who do not meet the discrepancy criteria for special services under federal law but still need some help, their regular classroom teachers should make changes in the classroom to meet the child's needs, such as modifications in the child's curriculum, the manner in which subjects are taught, homework assignments, and overall expectations. Throughout this process it is essential that the child's strengths, including in extracurricular activities, be nurtured and maintained.

Accommodation interventions. Besides direct intervention, accommodation strategies also are quite effective for some children. This is a method in which weaknesses are circumvented or bypassed. For instance, a child with writing problems might use a word processor to write reports. If she has good oral expressive skills, she could be allowed to give oral reports rather than written ones, and take tests orally.

Children with dyslexia benefit from audiobooks, voice-to-text technology, and keyboarding accommodations. Parents of children with dyslexia should reach out to local and national dyslexia advocacy groups for further support and information. There are multiple excellent resources for adults and kids alike to learn more about this most common learning disability.

Home-based support. At home you can modify the environment or the emotional climate, keep expectations realistic, and generally be supportive of your child. Develop homework routines, be available for help, maintain quiet in the house during homework hours, and, if necessary, monitor your child's commitment to extracurricular activities to allow more time and energy for studies. Nurture and maintain other avenues of success and gratification.

Hiring a tutor experienced in your child's particular disability, if financially feasible, may be helpful and often can reduce or eliminate homework-related tensions between parent and child. However, be realistic and do not overload a child's capacity to perform, or deprive her of time to pursue interests and activities unrelated to school.

Other interventions. If your child is feeling depressed, anxious, or discour-

Children and Learning Disabilities

Here are some points to keep in mind about learning disabilities.

- Children with learning disabilities are a very heterogeneous group. Their disabilities vary in degree, nature, and complexity.

- Learning disabilities may affect more than just learning. Some of these children may also have issues with social skills. Behavior problems, emotional difficulties, low self-esteem, and family stresses may occur as well.

- Learning disabilities change with time. They may diminish or resolve themselves with intervention and maturation; they may appear when certain demands are placed upon the child in a vulnerable area; or they may last a lifetime.

- Children with learning disabilities are often misunderstood. They are sometimes accused of being lazy or not trying. They may be subjected to humiliation and inadequate teaching methods. They, their parents, or their teachers may not really understand their learning problems; in these situations, the difficulties need to be clarified and explained by a professional in a nonjudgmental manner. Emphasize that these problems are not the fault of the child, parent, or teacher.

- Learning disabilities affect families, and families affect learning disabilities. Children who are failing or struggling feel confusion, disappointment, anger, and guilt, as do their parents. Parental attitudes and parenting style affect the children and their attitude toward learning.

- Determine whether emotional, social, or family problems are causing or contributing to your child's academic problems, or conversely, if his academic and learning problems are really the root cause of emotional, social, or family problems. Professional help for family or emotional difficulties must be sought, but it should not divert attention away from the learning disability.

- Children with learning disabilities are entitled to the full support of the school system and require a good advocate and long-term follow-up.

- Be sure your child has other activities and interests that serve as avenues for success and gratification.

- To ensure the best results for your child, recognize learning disabilities early, arrange for the appropriate intervention, and make sure that he is followed over the long term. Also, instill a sense of optimism and hope in your child that together you will work toward a solution to these difficulties.

aged, psychological counseling may be appropriate. Sometimes family counseling is very helpful so family members can better understand each other's feelings and needs, reassign roles and responsibilities, and diminish sibling rivalry.

If your child has attention problems, or hyperactive-impulsive tendencies, she might be helped by medication that reduces distractibility and increases attention span. This medication should be part of a therapeutic package that might include educational and behavioral intervention and psychotherapy. (See Chapter 17, "Seeking Professional Help.") Also, any medical conditions that may be contributing to the learning difficulties or that cause school absenteeism must be treated. These might include central nervous system illnesses or injuries (such as seizure disorders) or a hearing or vision impairment.

Controversial treatments. Often learning disabilities are difficult for the public to understand and for educators to treat. As a result, a wide variety of scientifically unsupported, vision-based diagnostic and treatment procedures have emerged over the years. Other unproven treatments for learning problems include megavitamins, patterning exercises, eye exercises, special glasses, and diets that eliminate certain types of foods or additives. These treatments can be misused by unsuspecting parents once the child is diagnosed. The American Academy of Pediatrics does not recognize any of these treatments as being effective and therefore does not recommend them. Seek the advice of your pediatrician and other professionals about any treatment you are considering.

Vision problems can interfere with the process of reading, but children with dyslexia or related learning disabilities have the same visual function as children without such conditions. Learning disabilities, including dyslexia, are not caused by physical eye problems, but rather are complex language processing difficulties. Review the benefits of any purported "vision-based therapy" with your pediatrician, especially before you make a financial investment.

Monitoring Your Child's Progress

Your child's status should be reevaluated periodically, since a child's development is an ongoing process, changing over time and in the face of new demands. In some cases, a learning disability may be obvious only in specific situations when the child is called upon to perform a particular function. Also, as some children mature, they outgrow or learn to compensate for their difficulties. These children may develop excellent coping skills and develop an unusual degree of insight about themselves. On the other hand, some learning disabilities may become more significant and disabling as the child matures or faces greater challenges.

Regular meetings with teachers are an effective way to monitor your child's status and discuss his progress. They also are a way to let the school and the teacher know that you remain an advocate for your child and that you appreciate what the school is doing. Furthermore, your involvement sends a strong message to your son or daughter that you are willing to stand up for him and seek appropriate services and support. Children with IEPs should receive quarterly progress reports in addition to annual reviews of the IEP and goals. In some cases, change and improvement may not fully raise your child's abilities to age- or grade-appropriate levels, even though the situation may improve. Many children eventually experience success once they complete high school, because they can then select the higher education, vocational training, or job that best suits them and provides them with gratification.

~ 41 ~

Other Educational Concerns

Intellectual Disability

About 1 to 2 percent of children have an intellectual disability. The term "intellectual disability" refers to general intelligence quotients significantly below average. Affected children may also have delays in adaptive functioning in the community.

Intelligence quotient, or IQ, is measured by standardized tests; the typical range is from 90 to 110. The degree of intellectual disability depends upon how far below this normal range a child's IQ falls. The majority of children with below-average IQ scores, those between 70 and 89, are not considered to be intellectually disabled, but instead are termed "below average." For IQ scores less than 70, experts describe intellectual disability as mild, moderate, or severe. The combination of tested IQ score and a measure of adaptive abilities are considered together in evaluating a child's functional levels.

The diagnosis of intellectual disability is usually made by a certified psychologist capable of administering, scoring, and interpreting a standardized intelligence or cognitive test. Adaptive behavior is usually measured as well. Adaptive behavior enables children to interact with, adjust to, and meet the demands of other people and day-to-day living.

A child's cognitive, motor, and communication skills contribute to her ability to learn self-help and independent living skills and other everyday skills.

Intellectual disability can have a variety of causes, including hereditary disorders of metabolism (such as phenylketonuria or PKU), genetic disorders that impact brain development (Down syndrome and others), exposures to toxic substances that alter brain development (such as alcohol or lead), and infections that affect the fetus before it is born (such as Zika virus). Severe stress during labor or delivery may injure the baby's brain, resulting in impairment in specific areas such as motor function or language. In most cases the cause of disability is not known, having no specific identifiable source.

Screening for developmental delays and impairment is a central part of pediatric care from birth onward; however, some children with mild impairment and developmental disabilities are not identified until the early school years. Most children with intellectual disability (ID) are identified as preschoolers because of language delays. Some children with milder symptoms are not identified until they have trouble learning in early elementary school. Early identification is critical to a better outcome, as children at a young age can respond better to appropriate treatments. Children with ID are entitled to a free and appropriate public education under federal law. Federal law mandates evaluations to identify children with suspected handicaps and to provide appropriate services for them.

As children with intellectual disability progress through the school system and through their own developmental stages, they require an evolving training or educational program that is appropriate for their abilities and responsive to their needs and the needs of their families. Initially, these children may need help in promoting basic developmental skills (fine and gross motor skills, speech, and language skills). As children acquire competence in these areas, they are better able to learn academic and other school-related skills.

Children with ID will need an Individualized Educational Program (IEP; see page 473) that will tailor their education to their own learning needs. This may require a smaller, more supported class setting with more individual attention. This is especially true of children who also have challenging behaviors. However, it is important to include children with special healthcare needs, including ID, in school and community activities with typically developing peers—for example, in sports, physical education, art, and singing—as much as possible. School districts are encouraged to educate children with ID in the "least restrictive environment"; this may include regular classrooms with supports for some students.

Preparing children with ID for as much independence as possible in employment, leisure, and self-care requires a partnership of schools and families. Even in the elementary school years, a child with a particular interest or talent might benefit from special training in or exposure to relevant vocations. Specialized vocational training is a major goal in the high school years.

Children with severe degrees of intellectual disability constitute a small percentage of intellectually disabled children. These children may have more limited self-care skills. They have more challenges with communication and may have behavioral challenges. Adults with ID are not likely to be able to live and work independently: those with more severe disability are more likely to require more support. This may include residential care.

Families of children with ID need to plan for transition to adulthood starting in early adolescence. They need to consider issues such as where their child will live, where he will work, and if their child can make his own medical decisions. Talk to your pediatrician and see if she can provide resources. The school must discuss transition needs as well and include a plan in the IEP. Family support organizations and the service coordinator through state agencies for individuals with developmental disabilities also may be helpful in planning for the future.

Autism Spectrum Disorder

Autism spectrum disorder (ASD) is a neurobiologically based disability that affects a child's social skills, communication, and behavior. Children with ASD exhibit a variety of behaviors, including communication deficits and difficulty interacting with others; there can be great variability in developmental skills. Language, social, and self-help abilities are usually impaired; motor impairments are noted on some. Sometimes these children do not acquire speech; other times their language may be delayed or unusual. They may use words without attaching the usual meanings to them or may echo what they have heard. They often are not able to understand other people's facial expressions, perspective, or inferred meanings.

As children with ASD get older and with appropriate intervention, their symptoms may evolve. Frequently children with ASD have other developmental, learning, language, or behavioral issues or diagnoses. ASD is identified in about one in sixty-eight children. Boys are diagnosed with ASD about five times more often than girls. The number of children reported to have ASD has increased since the early 1990s. The increase could be caused by many factors. Families are more aware of ASD and express concerns they have to their doctors. Pediatricians screen for ASD routinely now, as recommended by the AAP, and children are identified earlier—which is a good thing. Also, there have been changes in how ASD is defined and diagnosed. In the past, only children with the most severe autism symptoms were diagnosed. Now children with even milder symptoms are being identified and referred for intervention.

Children with ASD often interact with other children and adults in unconventional ways, and they may not use toys and other objects as intended. Their play may be rote and repetitive; pretend and imaginative play is likely to be rote or very limited. Some children exhibit self-injurious, repetitive, self-stimulating, and oc-

casionally aggressive behavior. Tantrums may occur because they do not understand what is expected of them or cannot communicate effectively. Children with
ASD may be socially withdrawn or inattentive to their surroundings. They may
appear not to hear well, but hearing tests are usually normal.

Each child with autism has different needs. The sooner autism is identified,
the sooner an early intervention program directed at the child's symptoms can
begin.

The American Academy of Pediatrics recommends that all children be
screened for ASD at their 18- and 24-month well-child checkups. Research shows
that starting an intervention program as soon as possible can improve outcomes
for many children with autism.

The diagnosis of autism needs to be made by a qualified professional—usually
a developmental-behavioral pediatrician, psychologist, psychiatrist, or neurologist—
who has experience in the assessment of children with ASD. It is important that
all children being evaluated for ASD have a formal evaluation of their intelligence,
communication, adaptive skills, and hearing. These evaluations may be done by a
single team or through consultation across community and health system resources.
The evaluation should include an observation of play and of interactions between
child and caregiver (for younger children, a detailed history and physical examination including neurologic exam and evaluation for any features of genetic disorders), and evaluation of intelligence, expressive/receptive/social language, self-help,
and motor skills. There are areas of the country in which school teams consult
with medical centers, and other areas where the school team and school psychologist will work in conjunction with the primary care pediatrician.

Children with autism require specialized services within the community and
within the school system. Contrary to previous beliefs, early and ongoing intervention can significantly improve the functioning of many children with autism.
Their families need and should seek out information and support. Families benefit from local support organizations as well as national groups. Their pediatricians, school teams, and state service coordinators from agencies serving children
and adults with developmental disabilities can direct families to local resources.
Parents can visit HealthyChildren.org, which is the official AAP website for reliable, pediatrician-approved children's health and safety information.

It can be difficult to learn that your child has a lifelong developmental disability. Naturally, you, other caregivers, and extended family need to grieve about this.
You will undoubtedly worry about what the future holds. Keep in mind during
these difficult times that most children with ASD will make significant progress in
overall function. Some children with ASD can do exceptionally well and may even
remain in a regular education classroom. Many will have meaningful relationships with family and peers and achieve a good level of independence as adults.

Individualized Education Program (IEP)

To determine exactly which services your child needs in the school environment, you will work with a team of educational professionals through the school to complete a written document known as the Individualized Education Program (IEP). Every child who receives special education services must have an IEP. The IEP is an educational road map for children with disabilities. It spells out your child's goals and outlines the exact education, services, and supplementary aids that the school district will provide for your child.

Parents who feel their child might benefit from special education services should request an IEP evaluation in writing to the school. Your pediatrician can also help draft a letter of request. An IEP is written after an evaluation. During the evaluation, current performance levels are established and documented. To be eligible for special education services, your child must be identified with a recognized disability (there are fourteen different disability categories under the Individuals with Disabilities Education Act) and the disability must adversely affect her educational performance.

In addition, should your child qualify for extended-school-year services, the IEP should lay out the kinds of interventions that your child should receive when school is not in session. The IEP establishes dates and locations of when services will begin, where they will be held, and how long they will last. The IEP should also discuss what will be done when your child's needs change. In addition, the IEP may outline whether your child gets related services such as special transportation, speech therapy, occupational therapy, and counseling.

The IEP is written collaboratively by a group—often called an IEP team—typically made up of:

- The child's parents

- Regular education teacher

- Special education teacher

- Psychologists

- Therapists involved in assessment or ongoing intervention

- School administrator

- Possibly a parent advocate (parents can request the presence of a parent advocate)

- Possibly other school personnel

- Any outside specialists who are treating your child (developmental pediatrician, neurologist, etc.)

A meeting to discuss the IEP must be held within thirty days after a school determines that a child needs special education services via testing. Parents may invite anyone to this meeting, including personnel such as an advocate. The IEP is evaluated at least every year to determine whether goals are being met, and it may be adjusted if your child's needs change.

An IEP should be specific in stating the student's goals and how success is to be measured. How the goals will help the student should be clearly stated. It is helpful to document, in language that new members of the team can understand, how the instructional team should promote the student's engagement in the program and how to address behavioral challenges. The IEP should include the parents' concerns and how the team will communicate with the parents.

When formulating your child's IEP with your school district, it is important to know exactly what your rights are and what to do if you are not happy with the resulting IEP. Before going to your first IEP meeting, do your research. Become familiar with your state's education laws, and know the types of interventions available to your child based on her needs. Talk with your pediatrician for further information.

~ 42 ~

If Your Child Is Gifted

GIFTED AND TALENTED children have abilities beyond those expected for their age and developmental stage, and are potentially capable of high performance. Their giftedness can occur in a variety of areas, including general intellectual aptitude, specific academic capability and achievement, creativity such as in art, music, or the performing arts, leadership, and athletics. Gifted children have special needs in their own way and deserve special educational programs and services beyond those normally provided by the regular school curriculum in order for them to realize their potential talents and avoid boredom.

In middle childhood, gifted children are often noted to have advanced abilities in reading, language, math reasoning, science, literature, or the arts. They often have a variety of interests and tend to read more, read more challenging books, and be involved with collections, activities, and hobbies. These traits tend to be of long standing and may become more apparent with age.

Identifying a Gifted Child

Parents are usually aware that their gifted child has unique abilities or talents. Occasionally, however, teachers are the first to point out that a child is exceptional in some way. Unique aptitudes may not be apparent until the child is in a setting that allows the demonstration of these talents. Academic talent can be documented via achievement testing. Alternatively, a child who is gifted in a nonacademic domain such as music often requires the support and advocacy of the teacher. Parental support is critical for a gifted child to receive appropriate services and opportunities.

Providing Services for the Academically Gifted Child

To meet the needs of gifted or highly intelligent students, schools should include programs to help them master the important concepts in various content fields; develop skills and strategies that allow them to become more independent, creative, and self-sufficient learners; and develop a joy and enthusiasm for learning. Some may also benefit from being with similarly talented peers so they have a social group with which they are comfortable. Programs and classes for gifted children should provide them with stimulation and challenge in their areas of strength and should encourage more creativity and originality. These are the same opportunities that should be provided to all children, but what distinguishes educational programs for gifted children is their accelerated pace of learning and the increased breadth and depth of topics covered.

However, both schools and parents often find it a challenge to provide the appropriate services and stimulation for gifted children. Teachers are faced with a diverse group of students and must meet the needs of all of them; teachers may not have enough time to devote special efforts to the gifted students in their classes. Also, teachers may not be trained to stimulate the higher thinking and productivity levels of gifted children. The child's verbal skills, large vocabulary, and ability and eagerness to question traditional facts and conclusions may be perceived as irritating by some teachers and fellow students. This can lead to social problems that require developing better social skills. Some schools, for a variety of reasons, divert their special-needs funding to those students who are struggling to maintain grade level standards, as opposed to appropriately challenging gifted kids.

If possible, schools should hire teachers who are trained to work with gifted students in a variety of fields. Often, gifted students are brought together for several hours a day to allow them to work with other gifted students and with a mentor. Independent study, advanced special classes, and taking advantage of resources outside the school (such as college courses) are other possibilities. Some gifted students prefer to go to schools that specialize in the field in which they excel, such as a performing arts school, a math and science school, or a school that emphasizes sports. Specialized summer camps are another option for uniquely talented kids.

If your school does not offer specific services for gifted children other than advanced courses, you may need to seek out extracurricular activities and situations for your gifted child.

The Gifted Underachiever

Despite their high intelligence and talents, some gifted children do not live up to their potential in the classroom. These are the gifted children who also have a learning disability. More boys than girls fall into this category. Approximately 10 percent of gifted children are delayed in reading by two or more grade levels, and approximately 30 percent of gifted children have a significant discrepancy between their potential, as measured by intelligence tests, and their achievement. Many gifted children also have dyslexia.

When an educational specialist diagnoses a gap or underachievement, she will look for signs like a significant discrepancy between the verbal and nonverbal portions of an IQ test, or between scores on an IQ test and a standardized achievement test. The assessment may also include aptitude testing, as well as emotional, behavioral, and family evaluations.

In some cases, parents may hold especially high or unrealistic expectations of a gifted child. These parents may have difficulty understanding why a child of superior intelligence or talent is underachieving. Gifted underachievers are especially prone to developing a poor self-concept. Talk with your school principal, a learning specialist, or a professional who works with gifted children to help an underachieving gifted child get back on track. Early recognition of the situation and appropriate intervention make for the best outcome.

~ 43 ~

School and Your Child's Health

The School as a Health Educator

Many parents are keenly interested in their children's basic academic education—reading, writing, and STEM (science, technology, engineering, and math) curricula—but are not nearly as conscientious in finding out about the other learning that goes on in the classroom. A comprehensive health education program is an important part of the curriculum in most school districts. For kindergarten through high school, it provides an introduction to the human body and to factors that prevent illness and promote or damage health.

The middle years of childhood are a time to adopt health behaviors that can have a positive lifelong impact. Health themes discussed in school include nutrition, disease prevention, physical growth and development, reproduction, mental health, drug and alcohol abuse prevention, consumer health, and safety (crossing streets, riding bikes, first aid, the Heimlich maneuver). The goal of this education is not only to increase your child's health knowledge and to create positive attitudes toward his own well-being but also to promote healthy behavior. Children are being taught life skills in addition to academic skills.

Your child will soon be approaching puberty and adolescence and facing many choices that can impact his health. These choices include risk-taking behavior; alcohol, tobacco, and other drug use; sexual behavior (abstinence, prevention of pregnancy, and sexually transmitted infections [STIs]); driving; and stress management. Most experts agree that education about issues like alcohol abuse is most effective if it begins at least two years before the behavior is likely to start. This means that children 7 and 8 years old are not too young to learn about the dangers of tobacco, alcohol, and other drugs, and that sexuality education also needs to be part of the experience of elementary-school-age children. At the same time, positive health behavior can also be learned during the middle years of childhood. Your child's well-being as an adult can be influenced by the lifelong exercise and nutrition habits that he adopts now.

Health education programs are most effective if parents are involved. Parents can complement and reinforce during conversations and activities at home what children are learning in school. The schools can provide basic information about implementing healthy decisions—for instance, how and why to say no to alcohol use. You should also educate your child and share your family's values, particu-

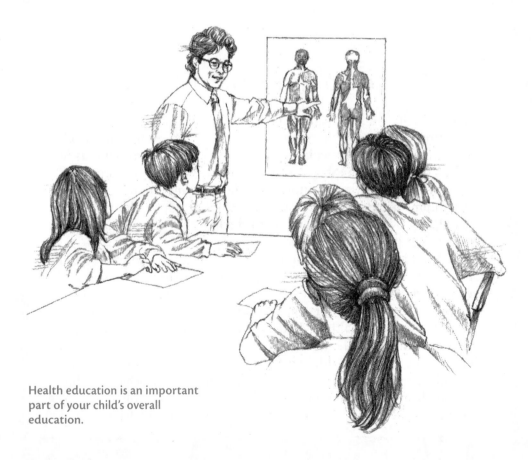

Health education is an important part of your child's overall education.

larly in matters of sexuality, STI prevention, and tobacco, alcohol, and other drug use.

Many parents feel ill-equipped to talk to their child about puberty, reproduction, sex, and sexually transmitted infections. Despite this, you need to recognize just how important your role is. With sexual topics—as well as with many other areas of health—you can build on the general information taught at school and, in a dialogue with your child, put it into a moral context. Remember, you are the expert on your child, your family, and your family's values. For more on talking to your child about these issues, see page 71.

Education seminars and education support groups for parents on issues of health and parenting may be part of the health promotion program at your school. If they are not offered, you should encourage their development. Many parents find it valuable to discuss mutual problems and share solutions with other parents.

As important as the content of a health curriculum may be, other factors are powerful in shaping your child's attitudes toward his well-being. Examine whether other aspects of the school day reinforce what your child is being taught in the classroom. For example, is the school cafeteria serving fresh, healthy meals that support the good nutritional decisions encouraged by you and the teachers? Is there a strong physical education program that emphasizes the value of fitness and offers each child thirty minutes of vigorous activity at least three times a week? Does the school district support staff wellness programs so that teachers can be actively involved in maintaining their own health and thus be more excited about conveying health information to their students? School fund-raisers should not just be sweets or snacks; non-food items should be considered as well.

In addition to school and home, your pediatrician is another health educator resource for you and your child. Since your child's doctor knows your family, he or

WHERE WE STAND

The American Academy of Pediatrics supports sexuality education in the schools, with content that is developmentally appropriate for specific age groups and that focuses on responsible sexual behavior and decision-making. The AAP believes that parents should participate in the development and the evaluation of the sexuality education curriculum. Qualified teachers should be assigned to teach these programs, and the curriculum should be revised and updated at regular intervals.

she can provide clear, personalized health information and advice. For instance, the pediatrician can talk with your child about the child's personal growth patterns during puberty and answer questions specific to your child's own developmental sequence and rate.

Dealing with Health Problems at School

There is wide variation in the health services offered by schools.

- In some schools there is a full-time certified school nurse who spends most of the day attending to the acute and chronic health needs of students. She handles acute health problems, administers medications, and performs health assessments and screenings as well as special procedures ordered by a child's physician; she also refers children to their physician for physical exams, diagnosis, and treatment. School nurses can play a central role in promoting a healthy and safe school environment as well.

- In some communities, a full-time school nurse is responsible for several schools and thus spends only a limited amount of time in each school. She is responsible for training other staff members (teachers, administrators, secretaries, health aides) to handle acute health situations when the nurse is not on-site.

- A full- or part-time nurse practitioner is available in some schools, working with consulting physicians, school nurses, social workers, or health educators in a school-based health center where routine medical care is

WHERE WE STAND

School nurses play a vital role in promoting school-age children's health and emotional well-being in the school setting. There is a wide range of school nurse resources across urban and rural areas, as well as across different regions of the country. Pediatricians and parents should recognize and support their communities' school nurses for kids' wellness and health. If a community does not have the resources and skills of a school nurse, steps should be taken to pursue adding this valuable asset to the school environment.

delivered in the school. This has been an important and successful way to provide care to students in areas where care has been limited because of a lack of healthcare providers, an absence of insurance, or transportation problems. The American Academy of Pediatrics believes that all children deserve a "medical home" and supports the implementation of school-based clinics, especially in areas where children do not have access to healthcare.

Acute Health Problems

Most illnesses and injuries that arise during school are minor (bumps, scrapes, headaches) and can be cared for by the school nurse. In many instances the child can return to class. Parents should be notified if a child has a head injury so they can monitor for concussive symptoms at home. When the problem is more serious, a parent will be called to come and take the child home. If the situation is extremely serious or life-threatening, the child will be transported by ambulance to the hospital emergency room or nearest physician. In many but not all schools, one or more staff members have been trained in CPR (cardiopulmonary resuscitation) and first aid. Parents should know how these situations are handled at their child's school. For more on how chronic health conditions are managed in school, see page 509.

Seeing the Nurse

Most students can go to the school's health office and speak with the nurse whenever they need to during the day, usually just by asking their teacher. If you would like your child to consult with the nurse, send a note to school with your child, or call the school early in the day. Let your child know the reason for the visit so that she will not be confused or surprised when she is called to the office.

Short-Term Health Problems

Sometimes your child may have a health condition that does not last long but still interferes with her functioning at school. This kind of problem should be brought to the attention of the school nurse, the teacher, or the principal. For instance:

- Hearing loss related to an ear infection could require a temporary change of seats to the front of the classroom.

■ Some infections—especially an ear infection, strep throat, bronchitis, and sinusitis—may necessitate the administration of medication for a week after your child is well enough to return to school. In most cases a medication can be prescribed that can be given before and after school and then at bedtime, thus not requiring it to be taken at school. Ask about your school's policy about medication before your child's first illness. Your school may require a written order from the doctor before it will administer the medication, including even acetaminophen, ibuprofen, and other over-the-counter medications, plus require that the medication be in its original, labeled container. It will be easier to take care of this during the visit to the doctor's office. Many school districts keep necessary forms available on the district website, and they are easily downloaded at home.

■ If your child has a readily visible problem—like a rash, conjunctivitis (pink-eye), or unusual bruises—that has already been evaluated by your pediatrician, let the school staff know about the doctor's diagnosis and treatment. School personnel will then not have to pursue further evaluation of your child, which might disrupt her classroom work and unnecessarily concern her.

■ If your child has an injury or illness that requires immobilization or limitations on physical activity, ask the school about alternative activities available during physical education classes and recess. When the child is unable to participate in PE for months or even years, a formal adaptive PE program—one that is appropriate and safe—must be designed for her. An IEP or 504 Plan (a plan that formally assures equal access to education and services), may need to be implemented in this case; for more information on IEPs, see page 473. When you obtain a note from the physician, ask that the note delineate what specific activities the child can or cannot do. For example, a student recovering from a broken arm can still walk laps around the school track during PE class.

Chronic Health Conditions and Food Allergies

If your child has a chronic health condition or food allergy, you need to ensure that he receives proper medical care and supervision at school, that he can participate fully in the educational program, and that steps have been taken to ensure safety in case of emergency, such as if an allergenic food has been accidentally ingested. Make certain the school nurse and your child's teacher have enough information to understand how your child's health problem affects him and how it may influence his school performance.

When to Keep Your Child Home from School

If your child is not feeling well, your pediatrician is the best person to consult about whether she can go to school. Common sense, concern for your child's well-being, and the possibility of infecting classmates should all contribute to the decision about whether your child should stay home.

As a general guideline, keep her home if:

1. She has had a fever above 101 degrees Fahrenheit within the past twenty-four hours.

2. She has had episodes of vomiting or diarrhea within the past twenty-four hours.

3. She is not well enough to participate in class.

If your child has been ill but is feeling better, yet has still awakened with a minor problem, such as a runny nose or slight headache, you can send her to school if none of the circumstances listed above is present. Make sure the school and your child have a phone number where you can be reached during the day if more serious symptoms develop and she needs to return home.

Talk with school personnel about what steps they should take if your child develops symptoms at school. These guidelines should be written in the form of an individual health plan that the school should follow, based on directions from you and your pediatrician. Specifically, asthma action plan forms and food allergy action plan forms should be completed by the family and physician and kept on file at the school so that all involved parties know what to do in case of an emergency. These forms are often found on the school district website and can be easily downloaded; food allergy action plan forms are also found at the Food Allergy Research and Education (FARE) website at www.foodallergy.org. When the school staff is familiar with this plan and the health problem, they will be better able to make sure your child's activities are not restricted unnecessarily. If your child does experience an issue, the school staff will be able to provide immediate and appropriate attention. Be certain the school has emergency numbers to reach both you and your child's doctor during the day.

When your child needs to take medication at school, it should be kept in a locked cabinet. In some schools, inhalers for older children with asthma may be carried and self-administered under well-defined guidelines. Medication should be administered in a private place to help your child avoid feeling self-conscious. If this is not happening—for instance, if your child is required to take his medication in a busy school office and feels uncomfortable doing so—you or your child should consult with the school nurse or principal to identify an alternative plan. Additionally, speak with your child's teachers and the school nurse to determine what steps need to take place in the event of a school field trip.

If major changes occur in the status of your child's condition, including modification of his medication schedule, let the school know, particularly if it is relevant to his school functioning and routines. During this time of change, since your child spends so many hours a day at school, the teacher and school nurse can often provide you with helpful feedback on how your child is progressing.

When you switch schools or if a new illness develops, the nurse may find it helpful to talk directly to your child's doctor. For this conversation to occur, you may have to sign a release-of-information form, which the school nurse will send to the doctor prior to their discussion of your child.

Sometimes, with both the child's and parent's permission, a disease like diabetes can be explained to the child's class so that his classmates will become more knowledgeable and supportive of their fellow student in an open and comfortable way. A similar kind of class education about seizure disorders can make the situation less uncomfortable for a student with frequent seizures and minimize the disruption if he should have a seizure in class. Elementary school children are frequently quite accepting and supportive in these circumstances.

WHERE WE STAND

Food allergy affects roughly 4 percent of all school-age kids in the United States, and is the most common cause of anaphylaxis, a life-threatening allergic reaction. Schools must recognize the need to reduce the risk of the allergen in the child's environment, as well as have protocols in place to recognize and treat an allergic reaction in a timely fashion. Pediatricians will work with the child and her family to diagnose a food allergy, prescribe the necessary autoinjectable epinephrine, educate the child and family on how to store and use the medication, and work with the family to reduce risks in the home, school, and outside environments. In addition parents, pediatricians, and schools should work together to develop written action plans to reduce risks and clearly outline necessary steps should there be an allergic reaction, whether mild or life-threatening. For more on food allergies, see page 542.

Children with chronic health conditions should still participate in all educational trips and other activities. If special arrangements need to be made to accommodate your child, such as autoinjectable epinephrine, special food, or transportation of essential medical equipment, communicate with school staff as to the best ways to achieve this. At each parent-teacher conference, make sure that your child's educational program is not being adversely affected by his condition.

For further information, see Part VII, "Chronic Health Problems," as well as the comments on specific diseases that may require special considerations at school.

Health Screenings in School

In most schools, children in the middle years are routinely screened for a number of common physical conditions. Hearing and vision tests are two of the most frequent evaluations; these are important because difficulties with these senses are often subtle, and neither parents, teachers, nor children may even recognize that a problem exists. While most difficulties with hearing or vision should have been identified prior to entering school, some may have been missed and others develop later. A child who has difficulty reading the blackboard may not know that she is seeing differently than anyone else. Nevertheless, even mild deficiencies of sight can significantly affect a child's ability to learn.

In some states these screening tests are mandated by law and may also include dental checks, scoliosis evaluations, blood pressure readings, and height and weight measurements. In school districts in which nurses are available for more thorough assessments, testing for tuberculosis and even physical exams may be conducted.

If the school notifies you that these screenings have identified a potential issue in your child, have her checked by your pediatrician. In the meantime, the school nurse should be able to tell you what the school's findings may mean, and whether there is any urgency in obtaining an evaluation by your doctor. In some cases, you may be able to wait until your child's next well-child visit for a repeat screening or a more comprehensive evaluation.

Sometimes your child's pediatrician will find that the suspected abnormality is not serious after all. Even so, this does not mean that the screening was inaccurate. Screening tests are designed to identify children who *may* have a problem, but a more thorough examination by a doctor is always necessary to determine the extent and severity of the condition.

Other Health Problems at School

When potentially contagious health problems appear at school, the health of your child must be considered along with the health of other children and school staff. Some health disorders are of particular concern in schools. Problems like head lice can spread from one child to another rather easily and thus can become mini-epidemics in classrooms. Additional common conditions seen in school-age children, such as colds, sore throats (including strep), diarrhea, fifth disease, and impetigo, are dealt with in more detail in Part VIII, "Medical, Mental Health, and Behavior Issues."

Head Lice

Head lice are quite common in school-age children, but usually cause more emotional upset than is warranted. Head lice do not discriminate between "clean" and "dirty" heads—in fact, they often prefer freshly shampooed hair, as it is easier for them to attach to. While efforts are required to eradicate head lice, the lice do not carry disease or cause illness.

Head lice are extremely small, about the size of a sesame seed, and do not fly. An individual is called a "louse." Head lice cannot survive long away from a human's scalp, as they feed on blood from the scalp. Eggs are attached to hair shafts, usually within a couple of inches of the scalp. Eggs and shell casings are called "nits" and do not easily brush off, which is a helpful way to tell the difference between nits and dandruff, which is easily brushed away.

When should you suspect lice? Your child may complain of an itchy scalp, although lice may be present for weeks or months without causing an itch. Lice often prefer the warmer locations at the back of the head near the neckline or behind the ears.

Lice are contagious and can be spread by close contact with a friend or classmate, almost always by head-to-head contact, but also by shared hats, hairbrushes, or other items that touch the head.

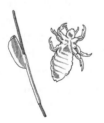

This is what an individual louse looks like. Eggs are attached to the hair strand a couple of inches off the scalp.

Head Lice Checks

To inspect your child's head for lice:

- Have your child sit in a brightly lit room.

- Working by sections, examine the scalp itself as well as the three inches of hair closest to the scalp. Make sure to part the hair, especially if the child has thick hair.

- Look for nits and live lice. Often only nits are visible; the presence of nits alone still indicates the child has head lice. Differentiate between nits and dandruff by the fact that nits adhere to the hair shaft and are not easily brushed away.

- Use a nit comb (a fine-toothed comb) to comb the nits out of wet hair, working through small sections at a time. Wipe the comb on a wet paper towel after each comb-through, examining scalp, comb, and paper towel throughout the process.

Lice can be difficult to treat. Your doctor may prescribe a treatment or recommend a nonprescription anti-lice shampoo or rinse containing a substance called pyrethrins. Follow the instructions carefully. Your child will need to scrub in the shampoo, working up a good lather, and then rinse thoroughly. This treatment can often take care of both the lice and their eggs, although a second application may be required several days later. Do not treat longer than the manufacturer or your physician recommends. Unfortunately, many lice have developed resistance to most pesticide medications in common use.

Although lice move quickly away from any disturbance in dry hair, when they are thoroughly wetted their mobility is much reduced. Fine-tooth combing after ordinary shampooing is a simple way to lift out lice. Repeating this process every three to four days for two weeks is usually effective in ridding a child of head lice. Combing your child's hair with a fine-tooth comb can also remove some nits, as can pulling them off with your fingernails. Be sure to wash the comb thoroughly or soak it in anti-lice shampoo before anyone else uses it. Any bedding, pillowcases, or stuffed animals that have come into contact with an infected child's head should either be washed and run through a hot dryer or, for items such as hairbands, barrettes, and hairbrushes, stored in a plastic bag for two weeks to allow any remaining lice eggs to hatch and die before reuse. Extensive home vacuuming and upholstery treatment are typically not required.

The presence of lice does not mean that your child has poor hygiene habits. Anyone can get lice, even if she bathes or shampoos every day. As a preventive measure, discourage your child from sharing combs, brushes, towels, or hats with friends.

WHERE WE STAND

Some schools have "no-nit" policies stating that students who still have nits in their hair cannot return to school. The AAP and the National Association of School Nurses discourage such policies and believe a child should not miss school because of head lice. Head lice do not put your child at risk for any serious health problems. If your child has head lice, work quickly to treat your child to prevent the head lice from spreading. Most parents and schools now recognize that head lice can happen to anyone and do not pose an emergency situation.

PART VII

Chronic Health

Problems

~ 44 ~

If Your Child Has a Chronic Health Condition

AS A CHILD matures, parents have the privilege to bear witness to the evolution of the child's developing skills, interests, and values. Mothers and fathers, as the years pass, learn with experience as well as trial and error how best to raise their children. Parents are their child's most devoted advocate and guide through life, helping her develop skills, tools, and resilience to empower herself to navigate the array of obstacles that inevitably come with life.

All children will experience minor, short-lived illnesses. For some children, however, illnesses or health impairments are not self-limited but are a chronic health condition. These children may have a serious physical disability, such as spina bifida, a genetic syndrome, or an injury-related disability; a sensory deficit, such as blindness or deafness; or a chronic condition, such as asthma, epilepsy, diabetes, or a life-threatening food allergy.

Children with *special healthcare needs* are defined as those who have or are at increased risk for a chronic physical, developmental, behavioral, or emotional condition and who also require health and related services of a type or amount beyond that required by most children. Based on this definition, about 15 percent of children have a special healthcare need. Most of these conditions are neither life-threatening nor severely limiting in terms of activity. However, children with *medical complexity* are a subset of children with special healthcare needs, and are defined as those who have multiple chronic conditions that often require the care of an array of community- and hospital-based providers.

Most children with chronic health conditions do well in school, develop appropriately, and achieve their goals in much the same way that other children do. Most are healthy children who happen to have a chronic health condition. While their illness may create certain challenges, with the support of their parents, school, and medical home, most lead effective and exciting lives and grow up to become productive adults.

Parents' Initial Reactions

When you first learn that your child has a disability or a chronic condition—perhaps it is discovered during pregnancy, or perhaps it develops after the child is born—the news is often unexpected and can seem devastating. Many families experience a sense of powerlessness at the prospect of dealing with an unexpected illness and facing a future filled with unknowns.

As a first step to coping with your child's special needs, find out as much as you can about his condition and its care. The more information parents and children have, the less frightening the present and future will seem. Knowledge is empowering. It can help you and your child feel more in control of the condition you both must face. Information will also help you guide your child—and serve as her advocate—through the potentially complicated medical care system. Ask your medical team for preferred books on the subject and for information about national organizations, websites, and support groups. Another important aspect of dealing with your child's illness is being connected to parents who are dealing with diagnoses and experiences similar to those you and your child are facing. You may be able to access resources and parent organizations locally or nationally for more information.

The type of information you convey to your child should be appropriate for your child's age. You can gauge this best by listening to her questions. Studies show, for instance, that kindergarten-age children typically view illness as quite magical: one child, when asked, "How do you get better from an asthma attack?" simply responded, "Don't wheeze." Young children who have diabetes may sometimes attribute their illness to eating too much candy. Some children believe they have become ill and been hospitalized as punishment for disobeying their mother or father. Before the age of 9, children tend to believe that germs cause all illness. Beginning at about ages 10 to 12, children begin to grasp the complex mechanisms that can contribute to disease. These older children may be capable of understanding more straightforward information about their disorder.

Remember that as children grow up, their ability to understand information and assume responsibility for their own care increases. Every year or so, someone should check out what the child understands about his illness, fill in the gaps, and correct misperceptions. All too often, the explanations stop at the time of diagnosis. Your primary care pediatrician can assist you with addressing the transition to adult-oriented care and systems, as this process should start by age 12. There are multiple resources and tools to help you and your child prepare for this transition into adulthood, self-care, and awareness.

The Medical Home

Your pediatrician should be accessible, trustworthy, knowledgeable, and relatable, as well as someone who can coordinate your child's treatment with other healthcare providers. You are choosing a professional partner for a relationship that may last many years.

The concept of a "medical home" is a good idea for all kids, but especially those with a chronic medical condition. A medical home provides a partnership among the child, her family, the primary care pediatrician, and all the supports and resources outside of the medical arena necessary to care for your child. Within a medical home, your primary care doctor knows your child's health history, listens to your child's and your concerns, understands your child's strengths, helps to develop a care plan when needed, and respects your family's culture and traditions.

Your pediatrician can help you and your child access and coordinate specialty care, other healthcare and educational services, in- and out-of-home care, family support, therapists, community partners, mental health services, and other public and private community services that are important to the overall well-being of you and your child.

Work with a pediatrician who is not only well informed about your child and his condition but also familiar with your other children and the family. Look to her for guidance when selecting other healthcare professionals and specialists who will work with you and your child. If you feel you would like a different primary care provider, ask for a recommendation. (See Chapter 1, "Maintaining Your Child's Health," or Chapter 17, "Seeking Professional Help.")

Convenient care clinics or emergency rooms are meant for urgent medical needs; they cannot and do not provide ongoing "big picture" care for your child over the long term, so they are not satisfactory substitutes for the comprehensive care of the medical home. Your primary care pediatrician will serve as somewhat of an air traffic controller, coordinating care among your specialists, therapists, and other ancillary staff, as well as recognizing trouble areas that may need to be addressed.

What Do You Need to Know?

When your child is diagnosed with a chronic condition, you will want to inform yourself thoroughly about it. Here are some questions to pursue through reading and talking with your child's pediatrician and other health-care providers.

- Is this going to be a lifelong illness, or may your child outgrow it?

- What is the expected course of the illness, and what is the usual regimen of medication, diet, and other treatments required?

- How can you explain the condition to your child appropriately?

- Will the illness require expensive treatment, frequent disruptions of school or vacations, and restrictions of activities?

- In what ways is the illness likely to alter your family's daily routines?

- Who are the best specialists available to care for a child with this condition?

- Will your child need special supports in school to deal with this condition?

- Will this affect your child's ability to learn and live independently?

- Who and where are the specialists in your geographic region who treat this condition?

- What are the currently accepted ways of caring for this illness?

- Are there any controversies in the area?

- Which of the costs associated with this condition are covered by your health insurance?

- What additional funding is available for children with this condition?

- What parenting books specific to the medical condition and other literature should you read? What are good age-appropriate, kid-friendly books regarding the condition for your child to read?

- Are there local or national parent groups or advocacy groups?

- Are there local groups for children with this or related conditions? Are there groups for siblings of children with chronic conditions?

Many children with chronic health conditions have special healthcare needs and require care from multiple pediatric specialists such as allergists, neurologists, rheumatologists, hematologists, endocrinologists, or surgical specialists. Whenever possible, a child with special healthcare needs should receive specialty care or consultation from a pediatric specialist, rather than an adult medicine specialist. Many will also benefit from services provided by occupational therapists, physical therapists, speech and language therapists, or mental health professionals. Sometimes the various health professionals involved with your child's care will offer conflicting advice, leaving you uncertain which professional's advice to follow. Parents are also often uncertain about which health professional to turn to with a specific concern or question.

You should have one professional you can call upon to coordinate your child's care and to help make sense of any conflicting advice. Care coordination and the integration of the necessary services and supports should start with your goals and wants for your child. At every step of the way, you and your child should be informing the process and what would work best for your child. If you are comfortable with your child's pediatrician in this role, then explore how to establish open communication and collaboration with this physician most effectively. In some instances it may make sense to have a medical specialist play this role. Parents should seek assistance from professionals who are knowledgeable about their child's illness, are aware of common side effects and consequences of treatment, and know about the natural course of the illness and about long-term effects of medical interventions. Such a person can anticipate or at least identify common problems at an early stage. A clear understanding of how best to reach this individual (for instance, the best times to call with nonemergency concerns, how to set up conferences or extended appointments for extensive discussions, how to

WHERE WE STAND

The American Academy of Pediatrics supports the concept of the "medical home." Children should have access to primary care physicians who can coordinate and facilitate the child's pediatric care needs. Mutual trust and responsibility between the child, family, and physician within the medical home will foster compassionate, effective care of the child. In contrast to the medical home, emergency departments and urgent/convenient care clinics, which may be needed at times, are not as effective in care coordination, and are more costly.

reach him or her for emergencies, whom to turn to when he or she is unavailable) will greatly improve your child's care.

Care planning is important for children with chronic conditions. A care plan includes salient medical, therapeutic, mental, medication, equipment, and educational needs in one repository. A care plan is typically maintained by your child's medical home, updated regularly with relevant information, easily accessible, and informed by your and your child's goals and needs. Healthcare teams and families

Questions to Ask Your Medical Insurance Company

- Does your child's primary care physician belong to the insurance company's provider network? What is the out-of-network coverage?

- Can families choose their primary and specialty providers?

- Does your child's physician have any financial incentives to limit your access to care?

- Are pediatric specialists available through the insurance company?

- Do benefits include enabling services: transportation, care coordination, home care, or experimental medications or treatments?

- How is healthcare paid for while traveling out of town?

- Does the insurance company have a case manager unit that assists families with special healthcare needs?

- Is medical equipment covered by the insurance?

- Until what age is the child covered with this insurance?

- Is a specialty hospital part of the network?

- If you disagree with a benefit decision, what recourse do you have to resolve your grievance?

- Are there limitations on the amount of services a child can use in a year? In a lifetime?

- What will you pay for each visit and prescription?

- Does the plan provide family-centered care?

should develop a shared, written plan of care with the support of a high-level, team-based care coordinator.

Consider yourself, your child, and to some extent the rest of the family as partners with the physician or physicians, sharing the responsibility for your child's well-being. Even when you feel your child is under the best of care, continue to serve as your child's strongest advocate: ask questions, air concerns, and inquire about available alternatives to formal recommendations. You and your child should participate in making plans and decisions as much as possible.

Parents and professionals sometimes get so wrapped up in a child's chronic health problem that they forget his other healthcare needs. Remember that routine health issues such as immunizations, dental care, injury prevention, good nutrition, and regular exercise are as important for your child as they are for children without a chronic condition. At times routine immunization is even more important for a child with chronic health conditions: for example, a child with persistent asthma should obtain the seasonal influenza vaccine every fall, as influenza can lead to concerning complications for any child with an underlying respiratory condition.

Helping Your Child with a Chronic Health Condition

The Stress of Chronic Health Needs

Stress is part of life. It motivates us to problem-solve, but it can also interfere with life's joys and accomplishments. Children with chronic health conditions often deal with more stress than other children. They may have to adjust to frequent appointments with healthcare professionals, missed days at school, bringing separate food to friends' birthday parties, hospitalizations, or surgeries.

A child with kidney disease who requires dialysis three times a week faces predictable and repeated periods of stress. A child with cancer, who must undergo repeated chemotherapy, copes with the fears and anxieties of each approaching treatment. A child with epilepsy may feel apprehensive about the possibility of having another seizure.

Listen to your child. Whether she is feeling sadness, frustration, or rage, it is helpful for her to express her emotions. She should feel that she can share her thoughts and fears without your overreacting or becoming upset. Ask how she is feeling. Be available and supportive. Listen to what your child says, but also try to hear what is left unspoken. Remind yourself that sometimes the best thing for a parent to do is simply listen so that the child feels heard; all too often, parents are eager to chime in with suggestions and possible solutions, yet at times the child just needs us to listen without judgment or troubleshooting.

- Inform your child about what lies ahead as honestly and as age-appropriately as you can. Anxiety is often based on the unknown or on inaccurate presumptions about the future. Find out what your child does and does not know. Explain exactly what will happen during an upcoming doctor's appointment or hospital visit; if you are unable to answer all your child's questions, both of you should talk to the doctor. Do not expose a child to a frightening procedure unless she has been informed of it beforehand.

- Find a support group (local or national, online or in-person) for your child's condition. This can be helpful for both adults and children for peer support. For example, FARE (Food Allergy Research and Education) has newsletters for children with articles written by other kids living the same experience, as well as teen-specific newsletters. Support groups help both the child and family feel less isolated and learn from others' experiences. Additionally, it is a wonderful life lesson for your child to connect with and offer her experiences and support to another child with a new diagnosis.

- A "rehearsal" can help children cope with frightening situations. Many hospitals can now arrange for children to take a kid-friendly tour of the surgery floors or spend time in the children's ward *before* they undergo surgery or other procedures. These visits are geared toward children and can familiarize children with the hospital setting and what to expect.

- Connecting your child with other children with similar chronic health conditions can often be helpful if offered at the right time. Reach out to other families to learn more about what support options are in your community. For example, GiGi's Playhouse (gigisplayhouse.org) is a nationwide network of Down syndrome achievement centers with programs, information, and connections for not only the affected child but parents and siblings as well. Look into summer camps specifically focused on your child's condition; for example, there are many camps specifically for kids with asthma or type 1 diabetes.

- In a balanced manner, speak openly about the condition so that your child feels comfortable talking about her condition.

- Emphasize your child's strengths—the things she can do well.

- Help your child feel that she can be in control of some aspects of her situation. Try to find choices that can be given to her, such as which arm to have blood drawn from or when a procedure will occur.

■ Look into your medical center's child life services for child and family support and additional resources. Ask your pediatrician for recommendations for a professional counselor if you think it might help your child.

Common Issues Faced by Children with Chronic Illnesses

■ Accepting limitations caused by the health condition

■ Anger

■ Anxiety

■ Embarrassment; feeling "different" from peers

■ Fear

■ Feelings of inadequacy

■ Frustration

■ Guilt

■ Inappropriate reactions or expectations of family members, other children, and professionals

■ Pain

■ Problems with self-esteem

■ Restriction of activities

■ Sadness

■ School absences

■ School difficulties

■ Sense of powerlessness

■ Social isolation

■ Stress

Maintaining and Building Self-Esteem

Children with different types of special healthcare needs share similar life experiences and problems, regardless of their particular condition. For example, they often are anxious about medical treatments and hospitalizations. They may be absent from school more frequently and, as a result, have academic challenges. If your child misses school regularly due to chemotherapy, for example, or has longer hospitalizations or periods when he cannot attend school, most school districts can arrange home tutoring to supplement the missed days. Ask your school district if such options are available. A chronic health condition may prevent a child from participating in some school and social activities, either because of physical disabilities or from a simple lack of energy. These situations can challenge self-esteem and confidence.

If there are visible signs of the health condition—such as the loss of hair from chemotherapy, weight gain due to medications (such as corticosteroids), or congenital conditions or injuries—children may retreat from social situations. They may avoid contact even with friends. Talk with your healthcare team regarding these issues. Healthcare professionals welcome the opportunity to educate the community: your specialist could come into the classroom (or even speak at a school assembly) regarding the condition to demystify it for your child's peers as well as teachers and school staff.

Children with chronic conditions, as well as their siblings and parents, can experience a sense of pride and accomplishment as they overcome their disabilities and fears and succeed in their endeavors. Early success in overcoming adversity can yield lifelong inner strength, resilience, and the ability to master subsequent challenges. There are many ways in which children can achieve a strong sense of self-esteem and pride. Try to identify activities that can bring your child pleasure and a feeling of mastery, and then help facilitate his participation in these activities. Children limited in their ability to take part in certain competitive sports often gain considerable satisfaction from participating in noncompetitive sports. Or they may find a lot of enjoyment by becoming knowledgeable about a particular sport.

Many children derive pride and pleasure from various crafts and creative activities such as drawing, painting, writing poetry or fiction, or learning to play a musical instrument. Collecting records, books, stamps, coins, or baseball cards can be great fun and instill feelings of expertise and mastery. Children may also enjoy and feel pride through reading or academic achievement.

A child with a chronic illness can feel angry at times if the condition places restrictions on physical activity. This is a healthy and normal response; you need to help your child accept his limitations, and then find alternatives in which he can find a passion and shine. All children get a boost in self-esteem from a sense of accomplishment. Explore the options for activities in your community until you find one that is attractive to your child and in which he can succeed.

Throughout this process, monitor siblings' emotional status as well as how the relationship between you and the child's other parent is faring. If you feel you need additional support in these areas, speak with your pediatrician.

Leading a "Normal" Life

Children with a chronic health condition or special healthcare needs should lead as normal or typical a life as possible, both at home and at school. Unnecessary restriction of activities can reduce your child's enjoyment of life and interfere with friendships and social activities. A "normal" life for a child with a chronic health problem means more than controlling the illness and minimizing hospital visits. It also includes developing realistic expectations, keeping up with schoolwork, forming friendships, and participating in the same activities as other children her age whenever possible.

If your child has epilepsy, do not discourage her from camping because of your fear that she will have a seizure, but do make arrangements to have her cared for if a seizure should occur. If your child has a heart problem, do not prohibit him from playing Little League baseball if his doctor says it's okay for him to participate; be sure the coach and the team members know about the condition and the precautions appropriate for it.

All parents want to protect their children from pain and disappointment. Parents of children with chronic health conditions may worry about extra risks to their children and may want to protect them from experiencing pain and frustration. At the same time, the goal is for kids to grow up to become self-sufficient and competent adults. To that end, you need to encourage your child to be as independent as is reasonably possible during childhood.

As part of this process, continue to give your child the information she needs about her illness—both the positives and the negatives. These conversations will evolve as the years pass, since your child will be growing in maturity. This will permit her to face the condition realistically and begin to master it as fully as possible. Keep in mind, however, that children differ in their ability to understand their health problems and to see ahead toward what they can do in the future. Answer questions fully and ensure that your child understands your explanations. Expect and encourage more questions as your child's capacity to understand and reason increases.

As children enter school age, they spend an increasing amount of time away from their home and family. A chronic health condition, however, can interfere with their widening social networks and activities. A second-grader with a peanut allergy needs to remember not to trade lunchbox items with classmates. The child with diabetes who is embarrassed about dietary restrictions or the child with asthma who becomes upset by her wheezing while playing may isolate herself from friends.

Other problems can arise. As kids mature through middle childhood, they will increasingly seek mastery and control over their activities and social environment. However, the child with a chronic health condition may feel powerless over her own body and well-being. While friends are learning to assert their autonomy and independence, children with chronic conditions may be restricted and unable to keep up with their peers. Some chronic conditions remain relatively unchanged over time. Others may remit or progress, requiring the child and family to adapt to changing symptoms, altered functional ability, and varying treatment plans. Even a seemingly stable illness has different meanings for and impacts on the child as she develops. A physical limitation or stigma that had apparently little importance in first grade may become a more significant issue at puberty.

Children's capacity for independence varies from illness to illness and from child to child, and will steadily increase with maturity. If your child has diabetes, you will need to test her blood sugar levels and make sure insulin injections are given regularly during her younger years. If she requires a special diet, you will need to supervise food choices and eating habits closely. At the same time, watch for signals from her that she is able to assume greater responsibility for herself, and help her take on more of the management of the illness little by little as she grows up. Children who exhibit good responsibility for their self-care can transition to an insulin pump sooner.

Some children may go through phases where they avoid accepting more independence. Families may inadvertently foster dependency because they find it easier to maintain responsibility for their child's care, rather than teaching the child to perform certain tasks and relying on her to do so. Also, these children, like most children, may enjoy being the object of their parents' special attention. They may relish having certain tasks performed for them, and may resist taking responsibility.

It is critical to help your child come to terms with her health condition and accept appropriate responsibility for caring for herself. Do not deprive your child of the important and rewarding experience of mastering day-to-day tasks; it can instill pride, self-esteem, and self-confidence that can prepare her for adult life. Praise her efforts at assuming responsibility, and applaud yourself for having the wisdom and courage to let her take these very important steps.

Discuss with your doctor your concerns and the limitations you think are reasonable for your child. Using your physician's input, develop some guidelines for sensible restrictions while also encouraging your child to participate in a diversity of activities. Parents need to recognize their children's changing needs and to plan for them. It is also important for parents to be educated and up to date about their child's health condition and about new treatments and their effects. If your child or your family is in need of greater mental health support and resources, speak with your pediatrician.

Addressing Your Child's Fears
Strategies to Consider

Even with the calming reassurance of a parent or a physician, some children still become anxious about upcoming treatments and surgery. Their hearts may race; they may start to perspire; they may cry frequently and uncontrollably. But while recognizing and accepting your child's feelings, reassure him about his safety and outcomes.

During medical procedures, deep breathing exercises can help children to relax. You may also be able to help by encouraging your child to shift his attention away from the therapy, concentrating instead on more pleasant thoughts—perhaps a recent music recital, a hike, or something else he enjoys. Many children's hospitals employ child life staff whose purpose is to help children feel comfortable in an age-appropriate way; reach out to your healthcare professionals to take advantage of these opportunities.

Children can be taught relaxation and self-hypnosis techniques, and can benefit greatly from learning these skills. They take time and practice to learn, and must be mastered well before a procedure or hospitalization is scheduled. Ask your physician where you and your child can learn these techniques. Meditation and child-friendly yoga are other options.

Pain Management

For many children with a chronic condition or special healthcare needs, pain is their greatest fear. In your discussions about a procedure, if your child asks, "Is it going to hurt?" you and your doctor should give a direct, honest answer.

When kids (and adults) hurt—or even when they just anticipate discomfort—they often function less well than usual in their day-to-day lives. Their schoolwork and self-image may be impacted. With some diseases—juvenile idiopathic arthritis, for instance—some pain may be inevitable. With other conditions, such as migraine headaches, an increase in pain is a signal to touch base with the healthcare team to determine if the child's management should be adjusted. With medications and techniques, pain can often be controlled. Many children's hospitals now have dedicated staff for pain management; ask your healthcare team for more information.

Much of the pain children experience is caused by procedures and treatment, and so part of the treatment plan should include steps to prevent pain. Anxiety can heighten a child's experience of pain. Whenever possible, parents should be present with their child during painful or frightening procedures. Topical anesthetics applied in advance can reduce and often prevent pain caused by injections or spinal taps. Systemic medicines are available for more severe pain. For children of all ages, there are ways to judge the severity of pain, and these measures can be used to help decide when, what, and how much pain medication to use.

In some cases, children can use patient-controlled analgesia (PCA), a system that allows the child to control how much medication she receives. The old fear about children with chronic health conditions such as cancer or sickle cell anemia becoming addicted to pain medication is a myth. If your child is in pain, tell your doctor and jointly develop a plan to manage that discomfort. No child should experience pain unnecessarily.

There are a variety of ways to help control pain. Some treatments using positive imagery, distraction, or hypnosis are quite effective. Some medical centers have pain clinics specializing in pain management. Often they will use a combination of approaches such as medication, relaxation techniques, and electrical stimulation. None of the common chronic health problems of childhood should be accompanied by worsening pain. If your child's pain is increasing, there is the possibility that the disease is progressing or the child is developing a complication. Inform her physician promptly about such changes.

Dealing with Emotional Problems
and Depression

Feelings of sadness, depression, or being overwhelmed may come and go for both you and your child. This is normal and appropriate, and indicates a healthy response. As tumultuous as these times can be, most kids and their families emerge with few if any long-term behavioral problems or lasting psychological scars. In fact, the majority of children manage their situation well, despite riding an emotional roller coaster on occasion. Children are often more resilient than adults predict. Researchers believe that the likelihood of emotional and behavioral problems associated with chronic health conditions has been decreasing because parents, school staffs, and healthcare providers are learning more effective ways to help children and their parents meet their psychological needs.

Nevertheless, children who have a chronic health condition often feel "different," socially isolated, and restricted in their activities. They may have school problems and feel overprotected. They may experience recurrent fear and pain. When these emotional difficulties are not dealt with, they can lead to anxiety, sadness, withdrawal, rebelliousness, or decreased interest in school.

School-age children rarely state that they are sad or depressed. Instead, they may withdraw from friends and family or exhibit rebellious or angry behavior. They may do poorly in school. They may interfere with their medical treatments, perhaps by refusing to take medication as scheduled. They might experiment with alcohol, drugs, or early sexual activity. Or they may run away from home or contemplate suicide.

Make an ongoing effort to discuss with your child what he is experiencing. Do you think he is displaying signs of despair and hopelessness related to his condition and future? Encourage him to talk about these feelings with you or with another trusted adult. Some parents are hesitant to discuss feelings about the disease with their child, in an effort to protect the child from emotional hurt. Most experts, however, disagree with that point of view. Children can usually adjust much better to an unpleasant truth than to the perception that their parents are upset and hiding something from them. If parents and children do not talk openly, the opportunities for misinterpretation are high. A child's imagination can run wild, and fears may emerge or be exaggerated.

It is best to make a commitment to be as communicative as possible. Remind your child that he is not going through this alone and that you will remain a constant source of love and support. Many studies show that the key to a child's resilience is a relationship with a caring, loving, accessible adult—someone the child can count on and trust.

If you are concerned about how your child is faring with these stresses, talk to your physician. If your child is exhibiting concerning behavior, if he refuses to take his medication, if he is withdrawn, or if his schoolwork has deteriorated, your doctor may recommend some counseling for the child or the entire family. (For more information, see Chapter 49, "Behavior and Emotional Issues.") Similarly, monitor the emotional health of your other children, and pay attention to your own emotional health and your relationship with the child's other parent. If your family needs additional emotional support or resources, be proactive and reach out to your medical team.

~ 45 ~

School Issues for Children with Chronic Health Conditions

SCHOOL IS MORE than a place to acquire knowledge and skills. It is also a place where children meet new friends, discover how to interact with other children and adults, experience success and failure, and learn about themselves. Children acquire many important social skills, expectations, and behaviors in school, including sharing, empathy, understanding rules, and dealing with peer pressure. During the school years, children yearn to be accepted by their peers.

Social Difficulties

A chronic health condition can present a special challenge for your child as she relates to other children. A child with a visible disability or one who receives special treatment may be singled out by classmates because of those differences. Middle childhood is a hard time of life for all children to feel that they are different in their appearance or their capacity to keep up with classmates. A condition that requires medication, frequent absences from school, rest periods, or special equipment, such as braces or eye patches, can make children feel like outsiders.

However, children who differ in health, race, religion, family, and a

WHERE WE STAND

The pediatrician has a critical role in supporting the health and well-being of children and adolescents in school environments. It is estimated that 15 percent of children in the United States have a disability. The Individuals with Disabilities Education Act entitles every affected child in the United States from infancy to young adulthood to a free appropriate public education through Early Intervention and special education services. These services bolster development and learning of children with various disabilities. The pediatrician should work with families and schools to ensure that every child in need receives the Early Intervention and special education services to which he or she is entitled. School nurses mitigate long-term impacts of chronic health conditions on children by coordinating the interests of families, educational institutions, healthcare providers, public health services, insurance companies, and community agencies.

Children with disabilities have been entitled to a free appropriate public education since 1975, when the U.S. Congress mandated public special educational services for those with special needs through the Education for All Handicapped Children Act, later renamed the Individuals with Disabilities Education Act (IDEA). IDEA has undergone several reauthorizations and amendments by Congress since its initial adoption, most recently in 2004.

myriad of other circumstances can discover that they have more similarities than differences. One of the goals for your child's school experience is that she learns to accept and be accepted by others, regardless of differences. Bear in mind that while feeling different can be traumatic, most children are quite resilient. They and their families not only usually learn to accept their limitations but also find creative alternatives to problems that initially may have seemed overwhelming. These children—when assisted and supported by family, friends, and professionals— can develop into stronger individuals.

On the academic side, children with chronic health conditions and typical intelligence should demonstrate classroom achievement just as high as that of their peers. That said, children with chronic conditions are at risk for low student engagement, more exposure to bullying, disruptive behaviors, poor grades, and below-average performance on standardized achievement tests. This may occur for a number of reasons. Their physical limitations may impact their performance, or their medication may impair their alertness or make them irritable. If their illness causes them frustration, they may have emotional or behavioral problems that can interfere with schoolwork.

With diseases such as sickle cell anemia, asthma, cystic fibrosis, and diabetes, children may frequently miss several days of school at a time, a period that may not be long enough to qualify for home tutoring. Hospitalizations may also keep them away from the classroom. In situations such as these, your child could be at a disadvantage. If she falls behind her classmates because she is absent from school too much, she may become frustrated and her motivation may falter. She might also become anxious about having to catch up on missed assignments. This anxiety can lead her to avoid school, even when she is physically able to attend. (See "School Avoidance" on page 562.)

Most of these issues, however, can be dealt with successfully by working with the teacher, the school nurse, the pediatrician, or a child psychologist. If your child has a health problem that is likely to interrupt her regular attendance at school, plan ahead. Meet with her teacher at the start of each school year to discuss how best to keep your child up to date on her work. Plan how homework will be sent home and thereby prevent your child from slipping too far behind. Interruption of attendance can also be addressed more formally either in a 504 Plan or Individualized Education Plan in order to provide the needed supports to the child, even if she doesn't have a documented learning impairment. Since your child may have frequent doctors' appointments, discuss with your child's physician the importance of scheduling them after school hours whenever possible so as to avoid missing class.

Keep your child's teacher and school nurse updated about her health condition so that you and your pediatrician can work with the school to prevent unnecessary disruptions of your child's academic progress. However, be cautious about requesting preferential treatment for your child at school. If her teacher frequently excuses her from homework or exams, your child may become overly dependent on this kind of special attention. The teacher may also underestimate the child's real capacity for learning and therefore have lower expectations. Most school districts provide home tutoring for long or intermittent but frequent absences; this usually requires a statement of necessity from your child's pediatrician or primary physician and should be based on a careful assessment of the benefits and risks for your child.

Serving as a Child Advocate

Your child's school should be a place where both his academic needs and his health-related needs can be met. Federal statutes mandate that every child is entitled to an appropriate public education in the least restrictive environment possible. They require local school districts to develop and implement programs to evaluate and place children with special healthcare needs or disabilities into appropriate programs, aimed at providing them with full educational opportunities. Special classes or schools are acceptable only when the severity and nature of the handicap prevent children from attending a regular class or school.

Some chronic health conditions or their treatments may lead to cognitive and learning problems. These biological effects can interfere with a child's ability to be successful in school. Parents need to be aware of their potential problems, inform the school, and advocate to have a child-study team convened to evaluate the need for special education services. For children with chronic health conditions, the special education category is "physical impairment or other health impairment." This classification allows children to have Individualized Educational Programs (IEPs) developed that address the specific needs associated with their illness. It is critical to address this issue because many of the cognitive impairments are subtle, and children's performance on standardized assessments does not follow patterns typical of children with other types of learning problems. School personnel will need to be provided with information about these issues in order to make appropriate plans for your child.

As a parent of a child with a chronic health condition, you are your child's strongest advocate; familiarize yourself with federal, state, and local laws so you can be sure that your child is receiving all the routine and special services he is entitled to. Parents can also seek support through their local protection and advocacy agency to support their child's educational rights. If your child needs speech therapy, psychological counseling, or physical therapy, for instance, the school must make them available. He also may be eligible for home tutoring. You should monitor your child's educational experience to be sure that it is allowing him to make the most of his potential, providing appropriate programs without overprotecting or overly restricting him. School personnel should also be careful not to push your child too hard, which is likely to make school more frustrating than fulfilling.

Your child's teacher or school nurse should be prepared to manage any health problems your child may encounter during the school day. It may be advisable for you or your child's doctor to speak with the school nurse or other school personnel to give them specific information about your child's condition and what to do in the event of a problem during the school day. They should know how to respond to a seizure or an asthma attack, for example, with updated action plan forms on hand where applicable, and should be aware of activities that may lead to a complication of an existing condition. Coordination of care among home, your child's physician, and the school nurse allows development of an Individualized Health Plan (IHP) that can serve to improve both health and academic outcomes.

Some parents are hesitant to give school personnel information about their child's medical condition, but keep in mind that the school staff will work with you and your child more effectively if they have complete information. Teachers and school nurses often can identify problems early and help solve them, and they can recognize your child's achievements in managing the illness. Work toward assisting school personnel in becoming advocates for your child, and keep the lines of communication open. If school personnel do not have accurate information to work with, they may start making erroneous assumptions, which can lead to mismanagement of your child's condition or inappropriate academic expectations.

Classmates should also be told about your child's health condition in order to avoid their exaggerating or misinterpreting the severity and danger of the illness and the limits it places on your child. Some children may be frightened about a diagnosis like leukemia or diabetes. They may not know how to relate to your child; they may be concerned that they will "catch" the disease. If those anxieties are not dealt with effectively, your child may find himself isolated from his classmates.

To avoid this kind of problem, you might suggest that your pediatrician or

What Does the School Need to Know?

If you have a school-age child with special health needs, make sure the school has a written document outlining a healthcare and emergency plan. This document should contain the following information:

- A brief medical history
- The child's special needs
- Medications or procedures required during school
- Medications or procedures required outside of school hours
- Special dietary requirements
- Transportation needs
- Possible problems, special precautions
- Important personnel (e.g., pediatrician, hospital)
- Action plans, where applicable; emergency plans and procedures (including whom to contact)

school nurse visit your child's classroom. Also, some families have become involved in school curriculum committees and parent-teacher associations to help educate both parents and students about their child's chronic condition. A number of school systems have created programs in which students are taught about peers' chronic illnesses, health conditions, and disabilities.

Teachers are a valuable source of observations of your child. They can let you know about changes in behavior, signs of anxiety or distractibility, and how your child relates to his classmates, as well as updating you on his academic performance.

If Your Child's Educational Rights Are Denied

By law, your child is entitled to an education that will help her develop to her full potential. That means providing her, if indicated, with additional services that will assist in both educational programs and extracurricular events.

Sometimes, however, schools do not meet their legal obligations. There may be insufficient sensitivity to your child's special needs in the classroom, or too little flexibility in school policies. Your child may be excluded from activities like field trips, or denied help in making up assignments after periods of absence. State or local protection and advocacy agencies can be instrumental in negotiating with the local education agency to ensure that a student's rights are not being violated.

Here are some steps you can take if you feel your child's needs are not being met.

- Ask that the teacher and other school staff meet with your child's pediatrician to create guidelines to help your child succeed at school, taking into account health-related and other issues. These guidelines should specify the obligations of the school toward your child.

- If the school does not cooperate, there are procedures—spelled out by every school district—through which you can appeal and try to rectify the situation. Ask the school for a written copy of these guidelines for resolving complaints.

- If you still are not satisfied, contact the local board of education, or the regional office of the United States Department of Education.

Returning to School

When a child begins a new school year, or is about to return to the classroom after a prolonged absence, he might be anxious and fabricate reasons or exhibit behavior to postpone that return. "What are my friends going to think?" he may ask tearfully. "Why do I have to go to school at all?"

Parents can help ease the transition. Try preparing him for what he might encounter at school with some rehearsal or role-playing, deciding together how to respond to insensitive questions or teasing. Help your child develop some appropriate responses to what he is likely to encounter. This type of preparation will help him deal with these situations more confidently.

Physicians, psychologists, and social workers can provide assistance in this process. Other children with long-term illnesses who have made successful transitions back to school after a prolonged absence can also be a useful resource, as can their parents. Child and parent support groups are available in many communities.

Hiding or Revealing the Condition

Some parents urge their children to hide their illness or medication from friends, believing this will protect them from ridicule or insensitive questions. That advice, however, gives a child the message that she has a shameful problem that has to be kept secret. Ultimately, circumstances often arise that make it apparent to other children that a child has special health needs. Try gently to encourage your child to disclose information to her peers in settings she finds comfortable. A best friend—even just one trusted confidant—can greatly ease the isolation felt by a child with a chronic medical condition.

As your child becomes more comfortable and secure with close friends and important school personnel, encourage her to talk with them about her condition. She should go into as much detail as she feels comfortable with; remind her that it is neither necessary nor beneficial to share every personal piece of information indiscriminately. A school nurse or a favorite teacher might be able to assist in this process.

~ 46 ~

The Family's Adjustment to a Chronic Health Condition

Dealing with Your Own Feelings

Parents often experience an array of emotions as they come to terms with their child's medical condition. Immediately after the diagnosis has been made, many mothers and fathers enter a mourning period, grieving over the "loss" of their healthy child. They must cope with the shock and the pain and accept the new reality of having a child with a chronic health condition. Parents may initially be in denial of the diagnosis. Eventually, families begin to find ways to accept their child's illness, despite periodically feeling sad, resentful, anxious, and angry.

Guilt is common among parents, who often feel that they must have somehow caused the condition. Self-blame is particularly prevalent when the condition was present at birth, when there is a genetic basis, or when the cause is not known. Guilt can be an excruciating and disabling emotion, adding to the stress within the family and sometimes making it difficult for parents to be supportive of their children and each other. If guilt or other emotional difficulties are interfering with your parenting abilities or the quality of your family life, you may benefit from professional counseling.

Other adjustments may be necessary as well. There can be considerable financial cost associated with a child's chronic medical condition. As medical bills mount with frequent doctor visits, medications, hospitalizations, and outpatient services, worries over finances can intensify.

Many parents find it to be difficult to discipline their child who has been diagnosed with a chronic medical condition. However, all children need and benefit from having clear limits and consistent expectations. Without effective discipline, children may become overly dependent, have lower self-esteem, and begin to have behavioral and social problems. Parents should establish a consistent set of expectations, adjusting them as needed for acute episodes as the child's health fluctuates. They should provide an environment that encourages independence and self-confidence.

Sometimes a parent may have to give up a career or education to become the primary caretaker at home; this is particularly true when the child requires a great deal of assistance with daily activities. A parent may have to change jobs, or take on a second job, to increase the family income. These adjustments are sometimes

Common Feelings of Parents of Children with Chronic Illnesses

Negative	Positive
Anger	Achievement
Anxiety	Closeness
Embarrassment	Joy
Frustration	Love
Grief	Mastery
Guilt	Pride
Isolation	Self-confidence
Powerlessness	Self-esteem
Resentment	Strength
Sadness	Usefulness

complicated when a new job necessitates switching health insurance policies, causing a situation in which medical bills associated with the child's chronic health condition (referred to as a *preexisting condition*) are not covered. The family might also have to move, relocating closer to the medical services the child needs.

Several state and federal programs are available to help families with the costs of managing chronic illness. Your physician or the social worker at your medical center should be able to refer you to the proper agencies for help.

Strains on the Parents' Partnership

Every family is a balanced system. After learning of a child's chronic medical condition, families understandably experience some loss of equilibrium that threatens their stability. The stress of a serious illness can cause severe disruptions, particularly if each parent attempts to deal with his or her fears and frustrations alone.

In some instances, mothers and fathers may become consumed with the care of their ill child, at the expense of nearly everything else in their lives. In these situations, parents may find themselves almost constantly investigating new options, reading about alternative treatments, and pondering the future: Is there a better medication for my child? Is it worth getting another doctor's opinion? Can I be doing more?

As a parent, you might sometimes feel that the demands upon you are unending, from trips to the doctor's office to the preparation of special meals. You may feel fatigued, finding it a challenge to recoup your energy. If anything gets sacrificed, it is often time spent with your partner, or time for your own personal interests and pursuits.

On the other hand, a child's chronic medical condition can have positive effects on families. A child with health problems may bring parents and other family members closer together. Families—especially those who communicate openly—may be strengthened by experiences associated with managing their child's health condition. In many cases, the family's management of a child's chronic condition may provide them with a sense of cohesiveness, mission, mastery, and pride.

Physicians, psychologists, social workers, family therapists, and parents of other children with chronic illnesses are invaluable resources for working through family difficulties. Ask for help. You should not expect or attempt to solve all family problems associated with your child's condition by yourself. Isolation is a preventable side effect of caring for a child with a chronic health condition.

Avoid Burnout

For your own physical and psychological health, you need to take periodic breaks from the day-to-day routine now and then. That means finding time to devote to your partner and to yourself, including recreational activities. To maintain your own health, you need to achieve balance by pursuing activities that are not strictly child-oriented. Some mothers and fathers, however, have difficulty taking time off. Without breaks to regroup, the tasks of parenting can become oppressive, and your child's chronic illness may come to feel like an enormous burden in your life.

If you need to find someone with medical sophistication to watch your child while you are gone, ask your doctor or local hospital staff for suggestions. Many parents work out arrangements with other families who have children with the same disorder. Enlist the help of relatives and friends. Teach family members to participate in the caregiving, and then use their assistance to take some time for yourself. If cost is a concern, brainstorm creative solutions such as trading sitting services with another trusted family.

The local social services agency or public health department may provide respite services to families caring at home for children with severe and demanding illnesses. These agencies often supply other types of support as well, such as loans of medical equipment or transportation to doctors' appointments. Your doctor may be able to help you make the proper connections with social workers who are aware of available services and resources in the community.

It is not a sign of weakness or lack of love if you need to take time off, or if you let doctors, friends, or family know that you are depressed, anxious, or worried about becoming burned out.

Siblings of Children with Chronic Health Needs

Parents are not the only ones who must adjust to a child's illness. Life changes for the entire family. Parents need to pay extra attention to the affected child, and brothers and sisters may feel neglected. They might also have difficulty learning to live with the stresses of having a sibling with a chronic health issue.

Some children experience guilt that *they* are not sick ("Why him and not me?"). As part of the magical thinking of young childhood, they may wonder whether an evil thought they have had about a sibling might have caused his condition. They may feel anxious about becoming sick themselves, or they may sometimes wish they were sick too, so they could become the center of the family's attention. They might feel angry if they are asked to assume more household chores than their affected sibling, or guilty when they resent the additional responsibility. They may become self-conscious when strangers stare at their brother or sister in a wheelchair, or when other children tease their sibling because she looks different.

Be aware that while attending to the needs of your child with a chronic medical condition, siblings can participate in the family and feel pride and love in helping their brother or sister with his or her health problem. The presence of a family member with a chronic illness provides opportunities for increased empathy, responsibility, adaptability, problem-solving, and creativity.

Establish balance between the needs of your affected child and those of your other children. Spending time with each child individually, one-on-one, helps. Develop a special, unique relationship with each one of your children. Also, keep in mind that siblings need to have honest information about the illness and to have their questions listened to and answered. (On family meetings, see page 268.)

A hospital stay can be challenging for a sibling of a child with health condi-

Are Your Other Children Having Trouble?

When there is a child with a chronic health condition in your family, your other children may be affected. Warning signs indicating that the siblings of your affected child may need some extra attention include:

- Anxiety
- Depression
- Withdrawal from usual interests and activities
- Anger
- Disinterest in friends and social circles
- Poor school performance
- Pressure on self to overachieve
- Rebellion
- Loss of interest in activities that once brought pleasure, such as sports or music lessons
- Blaming herself for her sibling's illness
- Attention-seeking behavior

tions. Look into available resources for longer-term hospital stays—for example, the Ronald McDonald Houses, which offer apartment-style accommodations for families of children undergoing treatments or needing a longer hospital stay.

Developing Resilience

Living with a chronic medical condition can teach both adults and children much about themselves, those around them, and what really matters in life. Adults and children can learn about their strengths and limitations, and they can learn new ways to solve problems and to be resilient. These are lessons that can serve them well for the rest of their lives.

In the months and years ahead, continue to reassess your goals for your child and your family. Be willing to make changes that serve both your child with the chronic health condition and everyone else in the family. As much as possible, involve your child in these decisions, particularly when they affect him.

No family knows from the outset how it will adapt to the reality of a child with a chronic health problem. There is no right way or wrong way to adjust; rather, every family should strive for its own balance. Many factors will influence this process, including the course of the condition and the resources available to the family. While all families with chronic health issues struggle through challenging times, many also develop a resilience, a creativity, and a closeness they did not always have.

Family Support and Advocacy Groups

Social isolation is common in families who have a child with a chronic condition. Children with chronic medical conditions may try to shelter themselves from other children, or the condition itself may limit or alter their social interactions. Parents may also have fewer social contacts than in the past because of the time required to care for the child, because friends and relatives sometimes find it hard to cope with a childhood cancer or other serious illness, or because of the parents' own sadness about the condition.

This kind of seclusion can be emotionally painful. You need contact with other adults, including those undergoing similar experiences. Ask your child's physician, a social worker, or the staff at your child's school if they can put you in touch with parents of other children with chronic health problems. There are hundreds of organizations across the country that help parents create support networks. The internet has brought together families dealing with even the rarest conditions, and online social networking groups can lead to "in real life" friendships and support.

Connecting with other families similarly affected by medical conditions will provide opportunities to share information and emotional comfort. Parents often find it useful to discuss their common concerns—for example, locating good healthcare professionals, identifying competent sitters, and resolving school issues. While family and friends serve to support an affected family, parents may find they develop deeper bonds with their "newer" friends who are similarly affected by a chronic medical condition.

Your child with a chronic health problem can also benefit from participation in a support group for children with chronic conditions. If a group like this is not available in your community, work with other parents to put one together. Some communities also have support groups for siblings and grandparents, who can benefit from information-sharing and emotional support as well. GiGi's Playhouse (gigisplay house.org) is an example of a national network of Down syndrome achievement centers with programming that benefits every member of the family and provides connections with other families undergoing similar experiences.

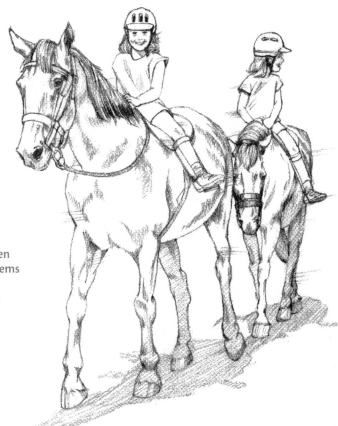

Summer camps for children with chronic health problems can be very beneficial for children who feel isolated by their condition.

Summer camps, some run by nonprofit organizations, are available for children with chronic health conditions. They can be beneficial for children who feel isolated by their disease. These camps can also help children increase their ability to care for themselves and their medical needs; for example, a child with type 1 diabetes can gain more independence tracking her sugar levels.

PART VIII

Medical, Mental Health, and Behavior Issues

~ 47 ~

Abdominal Issues and Gastrointestinal Tract

Abdominal Pain

Abdominal pain occurs quite frequently in children; thankfully, most of the time, it is not a sign of a serious condition, and often clears up on its own without special treatment. That being said, it is important for parents and caregivers to recognize worrisome signs that require further evaluation by the pediatrician. Abdominal pain can be influenced by both physical and emotional issues (for example, anxiety before an important test). *Acute* abdominal pain is when new pain comes on suddenly, as opposed to *chronic* abdominal pain, which can come and go, and last for weeks to months.

Acute Abdominal Pain

Look for symptoms associated with the abdominal pain for clues as to a possible cause. For example, if your child has diarrhea or vomiting along with the pain, think of gastroenteritis; for more on this, see page 535. If your child has had continuous pain for at least three hours, and it began near her navel and is now toward her lower right abdomen, think about appendicitis; for more on this, see page 529. If your child also has a sore throat and headache, a virus or strep throat could be the cause; for more on this, see page 595.

Other body systems besides the abdomen can be involved and give clues as to the cause. For example, if your child has painful swelling in the groin or testicles, the cause could be a torsion (twisting) of the testicles or a strangulated hernia, cutting off necessary blood flow; call your pediatrician in this case (for more on hernias, see page 533). If the abdominal pain is accompanied by fever, urinary accidents, increased urination, or pain with urination, a urinary tract infection may be the problem; for more on this, see page 621. Any vomiting of greenish material could signal an intestinal blockage, and the pediatrician should be called.

Call your pediatrician if your child has continuous abdominal pain for three or more hours, has pain along with swelling in his groin or testicles, vomits greenish material, or passes blood in his vomit or stools. Don't force a child with abdominal pain to eat, but make sure he has plenty of clear fluids to drink as tolerated. Don't give a pain reliever to your child unless your pediatrician says it's okay.

Chronic Abdominal Pain

Chronic abdominal pain is quite common in children, but thankfully not usually serious. Unlike acute pain, chronic pain lasts for a week or more and comes and goes. Often the stomachaches of chronic abdominal pain disappear within 1 or 2 hours. In many cases, no physical cause is found and the symptom is described as functional pain (i.e., nonspecific pain, most often related to stress). The pattern and location of symptoms may reveal the reason for the pain (e.g., school phobia or emotional upset with transitions). As long as your child's growth and physical examination are normal, his pain isn't limited to a specific site, and he has no associated symptoms, a stomachache is unlikely to signal a serious condition that would require immediate treatment. Even when no cause is found, your child's pain is real, and his distress requires attention.

Constipation is a common cause of chronic abdominal pain in school-age children, particularly pain located in the lower part of the abdomen. Bowel problems are more likely to occur when children don't drink enough water or eat enough fresh fruits, vegetables, and whole grains. For more information on constipation, see page 530.

Emotional upset in school-age children sometimes causes recurrent abdominal pain that has no other obvious cause. The first clue is pain that tends to come and go over a period of more than a week, often associated with activity that is stressful or unpleasant. In addition, kids with emotionally related abdominal pain have *no* associated findings or complaints (such as fever, vomiting, diarrhea, coughing, lethargy or weakness, urinary tract symptoms, sore throat, or flu-like symptoms). There also may be a family history of this type of illness. Your child probably will act either quieter or louder than usual and have trouble expressing her thoughts or feelings. If this type of behavior occurs with your child, try to determine if there's something troubling her at home, at school, or in connection with siblings, relatives, or friends. Have there been recent difficult transitions such as the loss of a close friend or a pet? Has there been a death of a family member, or a divorce or separation?

Your pediatrician can suggest ways to help your child talk about her troubles. For example, for younger children she may advise you to use toys or games to help the child act out her problems. If you need additional assistance, the pediatrician may refer you to a child therapist, psychologist, or psychiatrist.

Bloating, cramping, and diarrhea after certain foods may indicate a food intolerance. Pain associated with milk, ice cream, or other dairy products may indicate lactose intolerance. Pain with foods containing wheat, especially in conjunction with poor weight gain, may indicate celiac disease; talk with your pediatrician to determine what testing is needed (for more on celiac disease, see opposite). Abdominal pain associated with bloody stools could be a sign of an inflammatory bowel disease.

Call your pediatrician if your child has severe pain that does not improve with time, pain that wakes your child from sleep, decreased appetite and weight loss, severe vomiting, or blood in stools, urine, or vomit.

Appendicitis

Appendicitis is an infection or inflammation of the appendix. The appendix is a worm-shaped attachment located where the large and small intestines join together, in the lower right side of the abdomen. A classic scenario for appendicitis includes abdominal pain that starts near the navel and then migrates to the right lower side, fever, and lack of appetite that only worsens as time passes; however, children may not exhibit all these symptoms. If a medical evaluation is concerning for appendicitis, ultrasound and blood tests may help make the diagnosis. If appendicitis is suspected, the appendix should be surgically removed as soon as possible. Otherwise, the appendix may burst, causing peritonitis, a dangerous infection that spreads throughout the abdomen. Children typically do quite well after an appendectomy, especially if the signs of appendicitis are caught early.

Celiac Disease

Children with gluten enteropathy or celiac disease cannot tolerate gliadin, a protein constituent of gluten, which is found in many grains. Foods containing wheat, barley, rye, buckwheat, or millet can cause celiac symptoms. Affected children may gain weight poorly. They often have chronic diarrhea, although some may be constipated. They may vomit or have pale or foul-smelling stools. Celiac disease is increasingly common, affecting about 1 in 300 children and possibly as many as 1 in 80, but it can be difficult to diagnose. It can present either in infancy or later in childhood. It tends to run in families and is most common in those of European and Middle Eastern descent.

The only treatment for celiac disease is strict avoidance of cereals, pasta, breads, and baked goods made with grains containing gluten. Children often can tell if they accidently ate gluten by a return of their symptoms—for example, intestinal inflammation. Your pediatrician will provide dietary advice and refer you to a dietitian for nutritional guidance. Many grocery stores and bakeries now sell gluten-free products (from breads to pasta) that can be built into a healthy eating plan, and many of these products include the term "gluten free" on their packaging. Also, because celiac disease symptoms are often similar to those of other medical conditions, your doctor may recommend diagnostic tests, such as blood tests to look for high levels of particular antibodies (specialized proteins in the immune system) or a biopsy that takes a tissue sample from the small intestine through a thin tube (endoscope). Because celiac disease can be a serious disorder and is a lifelong condition, diagnostic confirmation is necessary. Because this condition tends to occur in families, the family members of a child with celiac disease may decide to be tested as well, especially if there are unexplained medical problems.

Constipation

A child's bowel habits can vary depending on his diet and fluid intake, as well as his daily schedule. A child may not necessarily stool every day; even if he has a bowel movement every second or third day, as long as it is soft (the consistency of soft-serve ice cream), he is not constipated. Conversely, a different child may have many bowel movements a day, yet if there is difficulty passing the stool, or if it has a hard consistency (e.g., small "rabbit pellets"), that child is constipated. It is possible for a child to pass a small stool each day yet retain a buildup of backed-up stool in the colon. Any child with infrequent, painful, large, hard, or dry stools should be evaluated for constipation. Accidental soiling between bowel movements or the presence of blood is also of concern.

Often a cycle can form that worsens the constipation: the child works hard to pass a painful, hard stool, and this experience causes the child to consciously hold in future stools to avoid pain, which makes the problem worse. Children who experienced constipation as infants or when toilet training may be more likely to experience constipation during the school years. Some kids prefer to avoid stooling outside of the home, which can exacerbate constipation. An overscheduled child rushing to school and then to many after-school activities may simply not have sufficient quiet time to "listen" to his body and use the toilet at appropriate times.

If constipation has been going on

for a while, the retained stool can stretch out the rectum, which results in a loss of the ability to feel the urge to defecate, as well as a less effective coordination of muscles during the defecation process. Soiling (encopresis) occurs when liquid stool leaks around the retained stool blockage; often these children don't even realize they are leaking until after the fact. Encopresis looks like diarrhea or soiling of the underwear. These children in particular should undergo treatment with a physician and possibly a pediatric gastroenterologist. For more on encopresis, see page 534.

Mild or occasional constipation can be helped by drinking more water and increasing high-fiber foods in the diet. Prunes, apricots, plums, mango, peas, beans, broccoli, and whole-grain products are good choices. Be mindful to cut back on constipating foods such as excessive milk, rice, bananas, or low-fiber cereals. A regular toilet routine, such as making it a daily habit to visit the bathroom after breakfast or dinner, can help your child stool regularly, as food in the stomach can help stimulate the bowels to move. Similarly, regular exercise and playing outdoors can help maintain a regular bowel pattern.

In more severe cases of constipation, your pediatrician may prescribe stool softeners, a laxative, or an enema. Although these medications are sold over the counter, consult with your physician before using any of them, in order to determine the safest plan for your child.

Diarrhea

All children at various times experience looser stools and diarrhea, possibly to the point of frequent, watery stools. The cause can be dietary, such as drinking too much sugar-containing juice; infectious, such as a viral, bacterial, or parasitic cause; or food poisoning. For diarrhea that occurs with vomiting, see page 535.

Usually diarrhea goes away on its own without specific treatment. In these cases parents and caregivers should provide supportive care to the child, ensuring proper fluids and hydration. Initially a simple diet of banana, rice, applesauce, and toast may be warranted, and an electrolyte solution is an option if there is associated vomiting, but usually the child can return to a normal diet as soon as possible. A day or so of an altered appetite is usually not harmful to a typically developing child.

Kids should be reminded to always wash hands with soap and water after using the toilet. If diarrhea lasts more than two weeks, consult with your pediatrician. Sports drinks have a lot of added sugar, which can make diarrhea worse. Call your physician if you see signs of dehydration, such as no urination for six hours, dark urine, refusal to drink, dry mouth, and lack of energy. Pediatricians do not recommend over-the-counter antidiarrheal medications.

Food Poisoning and Food Contamination

Food poisoning and food contamination are quite common occurrences, and can be particularly harmful to younger children. Food poisoning should be considered if more than one person in your family develops the sudden onset of cramping, nausea, vomiting, or diarrhea after eating the same food. Preparing your food at home instead of eating out at restaurants means a greater likelihood that the food has been stored and prepared properly. When cooking at home, wash hands with hot water and soap both before and while preparing food; ensure that sponges and dish towels are sanitized regularly and replaced frequently; avoid mixing cutting boards for meats and produce; and refrigerate prepared food promptly.

Hepatitis

Hepatitis is a general term that refers to inflammation of the liver, which can be caused by infections, toxins, medications, and metabolic diseases. There are five hepatitis viruses that can cause infectious hepatitis; for two of them there is a safe and effective vaccine to prevent illness and complications.

Hepatitis A is contracted by eating or drinking contaminated food or water, or by close contact with someone with the virus. The virus can be shed in the stool as early as a couple weeks before showing signs of the infection. The virus is of particular concern in daycares and for international travelers, but domestic outbreaks occur as well. There is a vaccine for hepatitis A; two doses are recommended at 12 and 18 months.

Hepatitis B is spread by the blood and body fluids (saliva, semen) of an infected person. The virus can be spread by saliva from a kiss, sexual contact, or non-sterilized needles used in drug use, tattoos, or body piercing. An infected pregnant mother can transmit the infection to her baby during delivery. There is a vaccine to prevent hepatitis B infection; three doses are recommended, to be given shortly after birth, at 1 month of age, and between 6 and 9 months of age. Vaccination in infancy is important to prevent the increased probability of cancer from long-standing hepatitis B and liver cirrhosis.

Hepatitis C infections are transmitted by transfusions with contaminated blood, although donated blood is routinely tested. Hepatitis D is transmitted in similar ways as hepatitis B; it causes inflammation only in people who already have hepatitis B. Hepatitis E is rare in the United States.

Regardless of the virus type, hepatitis symptoms are similar, including flu-like symptoms (fever, nausea, vomiting, appetite loss, fatigue) and jaundice, a yellowing of the skin and whites of the eyes. Stools can turn clay-colored and urine may be dark orange.

Unfortunately, it can be difficult to tell if a child is infected, as often they do not show symptoms. If your child has any symptoms or has been in contact with a known case of hepatitis, call your pediatrician, who will evaluate your child and possibly order blood tests. If a diagnosis is confirmed, treatment is mainly supportive, including rest and hydration. Avoid acetaminophen, as it is cleared from the body by the liver, which may not be fully functioning.

Inguinal Hernia

Inguinal hernias occur more commonly in boys and appear as a small bulge in the groin (where the abdomen meets the thigh). An inguinal hernia results when a small opening in the abdominal wall allows abdominal contents (i.e., intestine) to pass through the opening. This type of hernia can run in families, and is different from the type of hernia adults can develop by lifting heavy objects.

Usually a hernia is painless and is found by either a parent or the pediatrician. As school-age children typically no longer require diaper changes, educate your child to monitor himself when bathing, and to inform you if he notices new bumps in his privates, even if the bump does not hurt. Inguinal hernias typically need to be repaired surgically, and usually are not an emergency unless a section of intestine is stuck in the opening (called an incarcerated, or trapped, hernia). If the area is swollen and painful, an urgent repair is needed, so call your pediatrician immediately. Often the opposite side of the abdomen should be corrected as well, since the same abdominal wall de-

fect may be present on both sides; both can be done at the same time, preventing the need for future surgery for the same reason.

Malabsorption

Malabsorption occurs when the body is unable to absorb nutrients from ingested food into the bloodstream; the nutrients are then passed on in the stool instead. This may occur if the intestinal wall is damaged by infection with a virus, bacteria, or parasite. Malabsorption occurs commonly in healthy children for a day or so after recovering from gastroenteritis (stomach flu; for more on this, see page 535). Usually the intestinal lining heals quickly and the symptoms do not last long.

However, if symptoms persist for longer than a couple of weeks, including abdominal pain, vomiting, frequent and loose foul-smelling stools, weight loss, skin rashes, or an increase in skin bruises, contact your pediatrician. Your doctor may ask you to keep a food log documenting what kinds of foods are eaten and when, with any resulting symptoms. Testing including stool samples may be needed, and possibly consultation with a pediatric gastroenterologist. Treatment is focused on the reason for the malabsorption.

Reye Syndrome

Reye syndrome is a rare but serious illness in children that affects the brain and liver. It is strongly associated with using aspirin during viral infection, specifically varicella (chicken pox) or influenza (respiratory flu). Signs include a worsening of symptoms (instead of slow recovery from the virus) leading to fatigue or even delirium. If you are concerned about your child, call your pediatrician or take your child to the nearest emergency department.

Thankfully, for decades pediatricians have warned families and the general public about the use of aspirin in children, and the number of cases of Reye syndrome has decreased. However, the warning remains just as important: do not give aspirin or any medications containing aspirin to your child, especially when he is infected with a virus such as chicken pox or influenza. Instead, use acetaminophen or ibuprofen if needed.

Soiling and Encopresis

Encopresis refers to the passing of stools into the underwear, beyond the stage of normal toilet training. Encopresis can create anxiety and embarrassment for children and their families. Encopresis is not a disease but rather a symptom of a complex relationship between the body and psychological and environmental stresses. Boys with encopresis outnumber girls, although the reasons for this greater prevalence among males is not known. The condition is not related to social class, family size, the child's position in the family, or the age of the parents.

When encopresis occurs, it begins with stool retention in the colon. As the intestinal walls and the nerves within them stretch to accommodate the retained stool, nerve sensations in the area diminish. The intestines progressively lose their ability to contract and squeeze the stools out of the body. These children find it increasingly difficult to have a normal bowel movement. Most of these children are chronically constipated. (For more on constipation, see page 530.) With time, these retained stools become harder, larger, and much more difficult and painful to pass, which further discourages these children from passing the stools. Eventually liquid stool can begin to seep around the impacted mass, passing through the anus and staining the underwear. At other times, semi-formed or partial bowel movements may pass into the underwear, and because of the decreased sensation, the child may not be aware of it.

Many parents are astonished that their child with encopresis may not even be conscious of the odor emanating from the stool in his pants. When this odor is constant, the smelling centers of the brain may become accustomed to it, and thus the child actually is no longer aware of it. While your child may not be bothered by the smell, the people around him may not be sympathetic to his problem. Exasperated parents often place great pressure on their child to change this behavior—something the child may be incapable of without help from a pediatrician.

Encopresis is a chronic and complex but solvable problem. However, the longer it exists, the more difficult it is to treat. The child should be taught how the bowel works, and that he can strengthen the muscles and nerves that control bowel function. Parents should not blame the child and make him feel guilty, since that contributes to lower self-esteem and makes him feel less competent to solve the problem.

When encopresis is occurring in a school-age child, a physician experienced in encopresis treatment and interested in working with the child *and* the family should be involved. The treatment goals are to establish regular bowel habits in the child, reduce stool retention, restore normal physiological control over bowel function, and defuse conflicts and reduce concerns within the family brought on by the child's symptoms. To accomplish these goals, attention will be focused not only on the physical basis of encopresis but also on its behavioral and psychological components and consequences.

In the initial phase of medical care, the intestinal tract often needs to be "cleaned out." For the first week or two the child may need enemas or strong laxatives to empty the intestinal tract so it can shrink to a more normal size. The maintenance phase of management involves scheduling regular times to use the toilet (typically following meals) in conjunction with daily laxatives. Proper diet is important, too, with sufficient fluids and high-fiber foods. These steps will keep the stool soft and prevent constipation. These interventions should be done only under the supervision of the child's physician. The maintenance phase will usually last two to three months or longer.

Parents often use a behavior modification or reward system that encourages the child's proper toilet habits. He might receive a star or sticker on a chart for each day he goes without soiling, and a special small toy after collecting a week's worth of stickers. This approach works best for a child who truly wishes to solve the problem and is fully cooperative in that effort. Children with encopresis may have occasional relapses and failures during and after treatment; these are actually quite normal, particularly in the early phases. Ultimate success may take months or even years.

Vomiting

In children, vomiting is a common response to various events or stimuli, including illness, ingestion of toxic substances, or emotional stress brought about by pressure at school or tension at home. At times a child may cough so much (because of an infection or respiratory wheezing) that she gags and then subsequently vomits. An isolated vomiting episode is not a cause for concern. Vomiting that happens again and again, however, may be a sign that your child needs medical attention, especially if she also has abdominal pain, fever, or headache.

If the vomiting is associated with a head injury, if the child is more irritable or drowsy than expected, or if the child also has headache or fever, call your pediatrician to rule out complications from the head injury or meningitis.

Most often, a viral infection of the

stomach (gastritis), intestines (enteritis), or both (gastroenteritis) is the cause of vomiting. These symptoms can last from a few days to a week. Because it is usually a viral illness, antibiotics are not effective as a treatment. In fact, medication given by mouth can sometimes aggravate an already upset stomach.

Much of the care should be directed at preventing dehydration (excessive fluid loss) due to diarrhea and vomiting. Make sure your child drinks adequate fluids—in small quantities, but frequently. It is usually safe to allow the child to select the liquids she would prefer. Commercially prepared hydration solutions are a good choice for the child in the middle years if only one liquid is preferred.

If drinking liquids aggravates vomiting, reduce the intake to frequent spoonfuls or have the child suck on small ice chips or ice pops. Children of this age are usually good judges of whether they can tolerate eating and drinking. Notify your doctor if the vomiting continues for longer than six hours, if abdominal pain and fever are present, or if your child has not urinated in longer than six hours.

Your child's appetite will likely be decreased. Allow the child to eat what she wants. Good choices include bland foods such as toast, bananas, oatmeal, cooked rice, and crackers. A normal diet can be reintroduced as soon as your child is hungry, usually about twenty-four hours after the last vomiting episode. Keep your child home from school for as long as the vomiting continues and until she is able to control her bowels without the risk of an accident.

Sometimes, severe abdominal pain accompanies viral infections of the stomach and intestines. Call your pediatrician at once if this discomfort occurs, so that other, more serious problems, particularly appendicitis, can be ruled out.

~ 48 ~

Allergies

Anaphylaxis

Anaphylaxis is a life-threatening allergic reaction. The symptoms of anaphylaxis can progress quickly; parents and caregivers should be able to recognize early signs and symptoms of this medical emergency, and take action immediately if suspected. Autoinjectable epinephrine should be administered as quickly as possible, and 911 should be called so that treatment can be continued at a hospital.

Anaphylaxis can be triggered by foods, insect stings, or medications. The most common foods that can trigger this overreaction of the immune system are peanuts, tree nuts (such as walnuts, almonds, pecans, cashews), shellfish (such as shrimp, lobster), fish (such as cod, salmon), eggs, cow's milk, and soy. Insect stings that can cause anaphylaxis include bees, wasps, hornets, yellow jackets, and fire ants. Any medication has the potential to cause a severe allergic reaction; however, most commonly, antibiotics and seizure medications are the culprits.

Recognizing early symptoms of anaphylaxis in a child can be lifesaving. The most dangerous anaphylaxis symptoms are restricted breathing (airway) and low blood pressure; before it gets to this stage, look for the following symptoms. If two or more organ systems are involved, epinephrine should be given.

- **Skin:** itching, swelling, hives, redness

- **Nose:** sneezing, stuffy or runny nose

- **Mouth:** swelling of lips or tongue, itching

- **Throat:** progressive tightness, difficulty swallowing, itching, hoarseness

- **Chest:** shortness of breath, coughing, wheezing, chest pain, tightness

- **Heart:** weak pulse, passing out, shock

- **Gastrointestinal tract:** vomiting, diarrhea, cramping

- **Neurologic:** dizziness, fainting, an "ominous" feeling that you are about to die

The main treatment for anaphylaxis is epinephrine, which essentially reverses this dangerous progression of symptoms. Parents need to know that a secondary reaction can occur after successfully reversing the first episode, which is why seeking medical attention is very important. Epinephrine is injected into the muscle of the outer part of the thigh. If the child is not noticeably better quickly, another injection should be given within five to twenty minutes.

Any child who has a known food or insect sting allergy, or anyone who has ever experienced anaphylaxis before (even if the cause was not determined), should have autoinjectable epinephrine readily available. School-age children should be taught about their condition and how to give themselves epinephrine if needed. The dose will be prescribed by your pediatrician, based on your child's weight. The child should have at least two doses of autoinjectable epinephrine with him at all times (including in the school setting, along with a written emergency action plan) due to the chance of a second wave of symptoms after the first has been successfully stopped. For more on administering autoinjectable epinephrine, as well as allergy and anaphylaxis emergency care plans, see "Food Allergy," page 542.

Asthma

Asthma (also referred to as "reactive airway disease" in younger children) is a common chronic medical condition in children. For kids who have asthma, the smaller airways in their lungs become inflamed and periodically tighten up. Airway constriction and inflammation can vary over time and can be impacted by the season of year, viruses and infections, and exposure to certain trigger irritants. For some kids, asthma requires medications and lifestyle modifications; for others, asthma, if not controlled properly with preventative steps, may mean hospital stays and could be life-threatening. Asthma tends to run in families with allergic conditions.

Some children's asthma worsens with colds and upper respiratory viral infections; allergen exposure, such as to dust and dust mites, cockroaches, mice, pets such as cats or dogs, or mold; change in weather or season; or exposure to secondhand cigarette smoke. The resulting inflammation in the smaller airways can lead to narrowing, and the child will cough, wheeze, feel short of breath, have chest tightness, and may describe a sensation of "trying to breathe through a straw."

Any child who experiences recurrent symptoms of coughing, wheezing, or chest tightness, or any asthma symptoms more than twice a week, needs an evaluation by the pediatrician. Medica-

Asthma Management at School

During the school year, kids spend a significant part of their day at school. Good communication among the child, family, and school will help take proper care of your child's asthma and make adjustments as needed. An *asthma action plan* is a helpful tool to inform school staff about how severe your child's asthma is, what medications are necessary, how to manage symptoms, and what steps to take in case symptoms are worsening. Schools also need medication permission forms; as the child grows older and more independent, she will then be able to carry and self-administer her own inhaler. There should be plans in place for after-school activities and field trips.

It may be necessary for the child to use her inhaler before physical education classes; as the child gets older and has demonstrated increased maturity and good decision-making skills, consider allowing her to carry her own inhaler so she doesn't need to take an extra trip to the nurse's office. The family and school should also watch for medication side effects or missing an excessive amount of school due to asthma symptoms or doctor visits.

Kids with asthma absolutely can and should participate in physical exercise and activities. Exercise obtained through free play at recess, physical education classes, and organized athletics not only is healthy for the body and promotes good lung function but also boosts emotional health. If your child has wheezing issues related to exercise, this could be a clue that her management needs to be adjusted. Some kids feel awkward about using their inhaler in front of classmates; troubleshoot and role-play different scenarios to help your child feel more comfortable and empowered. Asthma symptoms are quite common, and your child should be reassured that there are likely other students who are experiencing similar scenarios.

tions and reducing exposure to allergens through environmental modifications are two ways to reduce airway inflammation. The child, family, and pediatrician should work together to form a plan to reduce the severity and frequency of asthma symptoms.

Inhaled medications for asthma target the lungs specifically, reducing side effects for your child. There are two general categories of asthma medications: controllers and relievers. *Controllers* control inflammation in the lungs and are used daily to prevent symptoms and exacerbations. Controllers may take days to as long as two weeks to really start working. *Relievers* are used as needed to provide quick relief of symptoms. Children with asthma may be on only a reliever if their symptoms don't occur very frequently. Children who have more frequent symptoms are put on a controller to prevent the frequent symptoms, and then use their reliever medication for "breakthrough" symptoms.

Inhaled medications include both controller and reliever medications and can be delivered by a metered dose inhaler (also known as a pump or dry powder inhaler) or by a nebulizer (machine). A *metered-dose inhaler (MDI)* is pressed to release a puff of medication that is immediately inhaled into the lungs. MDIs usually have a "countdown" counter so you can tell how many puffs are left. A spacer device attaches to the MDI to help properly coordinate inhalation of the puff of medication. Both quick-acting and preventative medications can be given via an inhaler. A *nebulizer*, often used with younger kids, aerosolizes liquid medication into a mist that is inhaled through a mouthpiece or mask. As with the MDI, both quick-relief medications and preventative inhaled steroids can be administered with a nebulizer.

As children get older, it is important to monitor their technique with self-administering medications to ensure that they are receiving the appropriate dose of medication.

Eczema (Atopic Dermatitis)

Eczema, also known as atopic dermatitis, is a common recurrent skin condition that causes flare-ups of dry, irritated, and itchy skin. Most children who have eczema will show signs of this condition before their first birthday. Many kids do improve with time over the school years, although they may continue to have dry or sensitive skin in general. Eczema often runs in families, along with other allergic or sensitive tendencies such as seasonal allergies or asthma. The main treatment goal is clear, comfortable skin, but just as important is preventing skin infections. The skin serves an important function as a barrier, and eczema can result in small openings in this barrier, allowing infection to cause further skin problems. Minimizing eczema symptoms not only helps your child's comfort level but will prevent further skin complications.

A key to managing eczema is to understand that eczema is a chronic skin condition, meaning the symptoms can worsen and get better, but the underlying condition remains. When the skin is more irritated, this is called a flare or exacerbation, and when skin is improved or completely clear, it is called a remission. Each child may experience eczema differently, but common symptoms include itchy, irritated, dry patches and rashes. Common locations are the inner folds of the elbows and knees as well as the neck. Hands and feet can also be involved. Viral illnesses "rev up" the immune system and can trigger an eczema flare-up.

Prevention of eczema, as well as recognizing early signs of a flare-up, can help keep symptoms under control. Use a daily fragrance-free moisturizer; an ointment or cream may help more than a simple lotion by virtue of being thicker. A daily bath can be a hydrating step; make sure the bath is not too hot and not too long (which can strip the skin of its natural oils), pat dry with a towel (don't rub), and *immediately* after the bath apply moisturizer or medication to the damp skin to lock the moisture into the outer layers of the skin. Prevent flare-ups by using soft clothing (100 percent cotton fabrics are a good choice), choosing gentle body cleaners and laundry detergents, and avoiding prolonged, hot baths. Trim or file fingernails to minimize the itch-scratch cycle. For some kids with persistent eczema, food or environmental allergies (such as pets or dust mites) may play a role. Evaluating for these allergens and avoiding them can improve eczema.

There are both over-the-counter and prescription medications that can be used in case of a flare-up. The medication may be adjusted depending on how severe the flare-up is and the involved location of the body. Topical (meaning applied to the skin) steroid medications calm the inflammation and itch and come in a wide range of strengths; milder versions are sold over the counter (such as hydrocortisone 1 percent ointment), and stronger versions can be prescribed. More severe eczema can be tamed with a stronger ointment; as time passes and the child is feeling better, the strength of steroid can be dialed back to a milder strength or discontinued. Some children benefit from an over-the-counter oral antihistamine to relieve the itch-scratch cycle; older-generation antihistamines can wear off quickly and cause drowsiness, but there are also newer-generation antihistamines that are longer-acting and non-sedating.

If prevention and over-the-counter treatments are not working, the next step to care for eczema is prescription medications. Topical steroids have six different classes of strengths; your pediatrician will prescribe an ointment that is strong enough to improve the eczema while minimizing side effects. Once the skin is improving, the strength of steroid can be reduced. A side effect of steroids is lightening of the skin (hypopigmentation) or thinning of the skin where used. There are also steroid-free medicines called immunomodulators, a relatively newer group of medications.

With prevention, early detection of flare-ups, and good treatment, you and your child can manage this fluctuating, ongoing skin issue. If you feel your child's eczema is not adequately controlled, speak with your pediatrician.

Food Allergy

Food allergies, like allergic conditions in general, are increasingly common in children and are the focus of ongoing research. For people with food allergies, the body's immune system reacts to proteins found in certain foods. Food allergy reactions typically occur within a short time of eating the specific food. While some food allergy reactions can be mild, others can be life-threatening.

Food allergy symptoms can include skin issues such as hives (raised itchy areas that look like mosquito bites and can come and go), an itchy rash consistent with eczema (atopic dermatitis), or swelling. The respiratory system can be involved; breathing issues, sneezing, wheezing, and a tightening of the throat may occur. Abdominal symptoms including nausea, vomiting, or diarrhea may be involved, as well as systemic symptoms such as circulation problems, pale skin, dizziness or light-headedness, or even loss of consciousness. If two or more organ systems are involved, this may be a life-threatening reaction known as anaphylaxis and requires emergency medical attention (for more on anaphylaxis, see page 537).

Any food can cause a food allergy, but most food allergies are caused by peanuts, tree nuts (walnuts, cashews, almonds, etc.), eggs, cow's milk, soy, wheat, fish (tuna, salmon, etc.), or shellfish (shrimp, lobster, etc.). Meat, fruits, vegetables, grains, or seeds such as sesame can also be the culprit of a food allergy. The most severe reactions are often caused by peanuts, tree nuts, or seafood. Egg, milk, wheat, and soy allergies are often outgrown by kindergarten, although these and other allergies can persist through adulthood. Nut and seafood allergies are often lifelong. Never attempt a food challenge at home; your allergy specialist can determine the safest way to determine if a food allergy has been outgrown.

Some reactions to certain foods are the result of a food *intolerance* or sensitivity; these are different from a true allergy, as these reactions do not include the immune system. For example, lactose intolerance is caused by a lack of an enzyme, lactase, which helps digest lactose, a milk sugar, causing symptoms such as loose stools, stomachaches, and bloating. Similarly, diarrhea from too much juice containing excessive sugar, skin irritation from acidic foods (pizza sauce, tomato products, orange juice), medication side effects, reactions to food dyes or preservatives, and food poisoning are not food allergies.

An *allergy and anaphylaxis emergency plan* is a written plan that should be shared among the family, physician, and school, so that all parties can take appropriate action in case a food allergy reaction is suspected. The plan is individualized for the child, lists symptoms, and explains when the use of auto-injectable epinephrine is warranted. For more on managing food allergies in the school setting, see page 484.

Hives

Hives, also known as urticaria, are red, itchy, raised bumps that look like mosquito bites. The hives may occur head to toe, or may be focused in a single area such as the face. Even with head-to-toe hives lasting longer than a single day, a hallmark of this rash is that no one individual spot lasts longer than twenty-four hours. The hives can appear and disappear in a matter of hours, so it can be helpful to take cellphone pictures of the rash to show your pediatrician.

Hives are most commonly caused by the body's immune response to an infection such as a simple viral illness, but at times there will be no identifiable trigger. Food allergies (see page 542), medication, or insect bites or stings may also cause hives, but hives from these exposures are much less common than hives associated with a viral illness or hives without an identifiable trigger.

Over-the-counter oral antihistamines (both the newer, longer-acting, non-sedating type as well as the older, shorter-acting, sedating type) can help reduce the itch of hives. Some kids will need to take antihistamines for longer than just one day; if this is the case, consult with your pediatrician. If other system symptoms are present such as wheezing, seek emergency medical attention.

Insect Bites and Stings

Insect stings, especially from bees, hornets, wasps, and yellow jackets, can cause pain, swelling, itching, and redness at (and possibly surrounding) the sting site. For some people, an allergic reaction to the insect's venom can trigger symptoms beyond a local skin reaction; they may develop anaphylaxis, a life-threatening reaction (for more on this, see page 537). Any insect bite or sting, even from a mosquito, breaks through the skin barrier and has the potential to become infected. If you note that the location of the bite is becoming more swollen, red, or painful over the following day or so (instead of improving), see your pediatrician to rule out a skin infection at the sting site.

If your child is stung by a bee, carefully remove the stinger from the skin as quickly as possible to prevent further venom from entering the body. Use the edge of a credit card to scrape away the stinger without releasing further venom from the sac. After removing the stinger, apply an ice pack to relieve pain and minimize swelling. Oral antihistamines or an over-the-counter hydrocortisone ointment can relieve the itch.

If your child has difficulty breathing or becomes dizzy with cool, clammy skin, these could be early signs of anaphylaxis; call 911 and give autoinjectable epinephrine as soon as possible. If your child has received multiple stings or develops hives in a different body part than where the sting is located, call your pediatrician.

An allergy specialist may suggest allergy shots (desensitization) for a child who has severe reactions to stings; with desensitization, increasing amounts of the insect's venom are given over time so the body learns to "accept" it.

Seasonal Allergies, Hay Fever, and Environmental Allergies

When the seasons of spring, summer, or fall arrive, many school-age children develop a runny nose and sneezing, or itchy and puffy eyes. Seasonal allergies may run in the family. Although some allergies may be season-specific, other environmental allergies may be present year-round. For some children, allergies may be just a temporary nuisance, but for other children, symptoms may interfere with daily activities and school attendance, as well as lead to complications such as ear and sinus infections or respiratory wheezing.

Allergy symptoms occur when the body's immune system reacts to certain substances (allergens), and typically develop over a child's first few years of life. Signs of seasonal allergies include cold (upper respiratory infection) symptoms lasting more than a week around the same time each year, including runny nose, sneezing, congestion, throat clearing (which can look like a nagging cough in younger children, especially when waking up for the day), nose rubbing, or itchy eyes. Usually colds don't cause itchy symptoms, but allergies do. Also indicative of allergies are respiratory symptoms such as coughing and wheezing, or skin symptoms such as eczema-like red itchy rashes in the creases of the skin, elbows, and knees (for more on eczema, see page 540).

Not everyone with allergies has asthma; however a majority of kids with asthma also have allergies. Allergies can trigger asthma; for more on this, see page 538. Environmental allergies can be caused by dust mites, mold, animal dander from furry pets (cats, dogs, guinea pigs, gerbils, rabbits, etc.), cockroaches, and mice.

Allergy symptoms can be prevented by minimizing exposure to the allergen(s) to which your child is allergic. Using an air conditioner and keeping the windows closed can help reduce pollen exposure. Cover mattresses, box springs, and pillows in zip-up allergy covers to reduce dust mite exposure. Wash linens regularly to minimize dust mites as well.

Discuss your child's allergy symptoms with your pediatrician. Over-the-counter antihistamines and allergy nasal sprays may be helpful. If the symptoms are severe enough to interfere with daily activities or school attendance, or are leading to complications such as ear and sinus infections or asthma exacerbations, your pediatrician may refer you to a pediatric allergy specialist for additional evaluation and treatment.

~ 49 ~

Behavior and Emotional Issues

Anger or Aggression

A child displaying aggression is one who hits, yells, bites, bullies, demands, or destroys. Although aggression is a part of human nature, most people learn to manage and control their aggressive impulses and modify them into appropriate and socially acceptable activities. Aggression is particularly likely during times of stress, threat of trauma, anger, rage, and frustration. A key task of early childhood is to develop skills to manage aggression and replace it with more socially acceptable responses.

By the time most children reach school age, their coping skills are advancing and their range of social skills is broadening, so they can generally remain calm and cooperative even in the face of stressful or unpleasant circumstances. Such appropriate behavior does not prevent them from competing and striving toward competence.

Some elementary school children have not yet mastered the skills needed to manage their aggression effectively. Their behavior ranges from hitting to throwing to having tantrums. By kindergarten, children whose aggressive behavior is a threat to their peers and to themselves should receive professional help. Other children, usually between ages 6 and 9, occasionally regress and exhibit aggressive behavior when they are under extreme stress or have a history of trauma. Boys have more problems with aggression than girls; this is due to a combination of factors, including the innate aggressive tendencies of boys, the ways that our society encourages and accepts more aggressive behavior from them, and the fact that boys may not be as comfortable using words to let others know how they feel.

Socially immature children may express their negative and hostile feelings in destructive ways. They may throw objects, turn over furniture, break lamps, or kick walls. These behaviors are usually triggered by frustration, anger, or humiliation. Some children who have failed to receive sufficient positive attention for their more socially desirable behavior develop a habit of resorting to negative behaviors to get parental attention.

Sometimes these children exhibit even more serious antisocial behavior—so-called *conduct disorders*—such as setting fires, being cruel to animals, hurting other people (physically or emotionally), or lying habitually. As children grow older, this pattern may evolve to include vandalism and truancy and is often associated with alcohol and other substance use. These kinds of worrisome behaviors occur only rarely in some children, but they have serious implications for later functioning, and their presence should prompt an evaluation by a specialist in child behavior and emotional problems.

Anxiety

Anxiety is a common reaction to the stresses of life, and all children feel anxiety at some point. A case of the jitters isn't necessarily harmful; in fact, at times it can push us to pay close attention and perform our best. Most of the time, stressful situations start up a flurry of brain and hormonal activity in what is called the fight-or-flight response. Body systems get ready to meet the challenge, and a person feels more alert, focused, and energetic. In other situations, however, the response can be to freeze and not do anything, or shut down.

An *anxiety disorder*, by contrast, can interfere with a child's daily life, interactions with her family, and school attendance and success. It is a condition that often runs in families. The anxiety may be too much for a child to handle and at times terrifying, or it may be mild but persistent, often with no clear cause. Anxiety is one of the most common mental health conditions among all age groups.

If your child's worries or fears are getting in the way of daily activities or school attendance, your family should take a closer look at the situation. There are many kid-friendly, age-appropriate books for kids of different ages to learn more about their anxious feelings as well as help them know they are not alone; from time to time, *all* people have these feelings. These books also can help children learn to identify early signs of an episode and empower themselves with tools to combat the anxiety.

Discuss the situation with your pediatrician. Age-appropriate counseling with an objective of helping your child learn skills and tools to manage his anxiety may be appropriate, depending on the situation.

Anxiety and depression often go hand in hand. For more information on stress, see page 565; for depression, see page 549.

Fears and Phobias

From time to time, every child experiences fear. As children grow and explore the world around them, having new experiences and confronting new challenges, anxieties are almost an unavoidable part of growing up. A fear of darkness, particularly being left alone in the dark, is a common fear in this age group. So is a fear of animals, such as large barking dogs. Some children are afraid of fires, high places, or thunderstorms. Others, conscious of media images, are concerned about war or terrorism. If there has been a recent serious illness or death in the family, they may become anxious about the health of those around them.

In middle childhood, fears wax and wane. Most are mild, but even when they intensify, they generally subside on their own after a while. Sometimes, however, these fears can become so extreme, persistent, and focused that they develop into phobias. Phobias—which are strong and irrational fears—can become persistent and debilitating, significantly influencing and interfering with a child's usual daily activities. For instance, a 6-year-old child's phobia about dogs might make him so panicky that he refuses to go outdoors at all because there could be a dog there. A 10-year-old child might become so terrified about news reports of a serial killer that he insists on sleeping with his parents at night. Media usage and exposure can lead to a child's increased fears, especially if the child is viewing films or online videos that are not age-appropriate. Screen films ahead of time or use parent information websites such as commonsensemedia.org to learn why a film earned a PG-13 rating, for example.

Some children in this age group develop phobias about the people they meet in their everyday lives. This severe shyness can keep them from making friends at school and relating to most adults, especially strangers. They might consciously avoid social situations like birthday parties or Scout meetings, and they often find it difficult to converse comfortably with anyone except their immediate family.

Separation anxiety is also common in this age group. Sometimes this fear can intensify when the family moves to a new neighborhood or children are placed in a child care setting where they feel uncomfortable. These children might become afraid of going to summer camp or even attending school. (See "School Avoidance" on page 562.) Their phobias can cause physical symptoms like headaches or stomach pains. At about age 6 or 7, as children develop an understanding about death, the normal worry about the possible death of family members—or even their own death—can intensify.

Since fears are a normal part of life and often are a response to a real or at least perceived threat in the child's environment, parents should be reassuring and supportive. Talking with their children, parents should acknowledge, though not increase or reinforce, their children's concerns. Point out what is already being done to protect the child, and involve the child in identifying additional steps that could be taken. Such simple, sensitive, and straightforward parenting can resolve or at least manage most childhood fears. When realistic reassurances are not successful, the child's fear may be a phobia.

Fortunately, most phobias are quite treatable. If your child's anxieties persist and interfere with her enjoyment of day-to-day life, she might benefit from some professional help from a psychiatrist or psychologist who specializes in treating phobias. As part of the treatment plan for phobias, many therapists suggest exposing your child to the source of her anxiety in small, non-threatening doses. Under a therapist's guidance a child who is afraid of dogs might begin by talking about this fear and by looking at photographs or a videotape of dogs. Next, she might observe a live dog from behind the safety of a window. Then, with a parent or a therapist at her side, she might spend a few minutes in the same room with a friendly, gentle puppy. Eventually she will find herself able to pet the dog. Over time she will expose herself to situations with larger, unfamiliar dogs.

This gradual process is called *desensitization*, meaning that your child will become a little less sensitive to the source of her fear each time she confronts it. Ultimately, the child will no longer feel the need to avoid the situation that has been the basis of her phobia. While this process sounds like common sense and as though it would be easy to carry out, it should be done only under the supervision of a professional. Sometimes psychotherapy can also help children become more self-assured and less fearful. Breathing and relaxation exercises can assist children in stressful circumstances too.

Behavior therapy is the first line of treatment. In rarer cases where behavioral therapy isn't helping enough, your doctor may recommend medications as a component of the treatment program in addition to the behavioral therapy. These drugs may include antidepressants, which are designed to ease the anxiety and panic that often underlie these problems.

- Talk with your child about his anxieties, and be sympathetic. Explain to him that many children have fears, but with your support he can learn to put them behind him.

- Monitor your child's media usage, including frightening images in movies, online videos, and violent videogames. Ensure media are age-appropriate: commonsensemedia.org has detailed information for parents, including why a particular film earned a PG-13 rating, for example.

- Do not belittle or ridicule your child's fears, particularly in front of his peers.

■ Do not try to coerce your child into being brave. It will take time for him to confront and gradually overcome his anxieties. You can, however, encourage (but not force) him to progressively come face-to-face with whatever he fears. If he is afraid of darkness, hold his hand as you spend a few seconds together in a dark room. If he is fearful of water, accompany him as he wades into a children's pool, with the water reaching up to his knees. Praise every small success, and the next step will be easier. Focus most of your attention on what he has accomplished, not on the anxiety itself.

■ Practice breathing and relaxation exercises, mindfulness, and meditation.

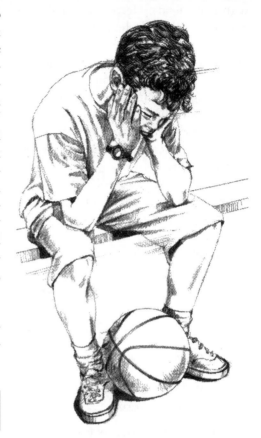

Depression

Everyone feels sad or blue once in a while. However, when that sadness persists for weeks or interferes with a child's daily activities and relationships with others, then it becomes the emotional disorder known as depression. Depression is a condition in which an individual feels discouraged and hopeless for at least two weeks.

In the United States, it is estimated that up to 3 percent of children and up to 8 percent of adolescents suffer from depression. Estimates of lifetime prevalence are significantly higher, at 18–20 percent, and depression often runs in families. Highly stressful events such as physical or sexual abuse or the loss of a family member or close friend may contribute to depression. Additional stressful events such as family discord, school failure, bullying, or difficulty with peers can also produce depressive symptoms. Sometimes it is not possible to identify a cause of depression.

In middle childhood most children will not label themselves as depressed. Instead, they might use words like "sad" or "bored." In many cases they will not even speak of feeling any different from the way they did before. As a parent, you need to be sensitive to the signs of childhood depression. A depressed child may spend more time alone in her room and stop playing with her friends. Her grades at school may noticeably decline. She may become more quiet and less talkative than usual; she may eat slowly or lose her appetite altogether. She may have trouble falling or staying asleep, become fatigued easily, and stop showing concern about her grooming and dress. She may complain of headaches, stomachaches, or chest pains.

Often a depressed child's symptoms are more subtle than you might expect. For instance, she might make less eye contact than in the past. Her mood and behavior may turn from being good-natured to irritable and angry. She may become harder to get along with, and fights and arguments with siblings and parents might become more of a problem.

Monitor your child's media usage. All too often depressed children regress into electronic devices, perhaps reaching out to strangers on the internet. Too much media can also add to depressed feelings. Parents are wise to be aware of their child's online activities in any situation, but especially if their children are showing signs of depression. Physical activity, especially when

Is Your Child Depressed?

Here are some signs to look for:

- Does your child cry more often than in the past?

- Does he complain of feeling blue or empty inside?

- When things do not go your child's way, does he tend to view his life as hopeless?

- Does he have difficulty keeping his attention focused on his homework?

- Has your child had difficulty falling asleep at bedtime, or does he awaken in the middle of the night and have trouble going back to sleep?

- Is he using media, social networks, or texting to a concerning degree?

- Does your child have a limited number of activities he enjoys, or has he lost his enthusiasm for the activities that used to occupy his time?

- Does he spend more time alone, away from friends and family?

- Has your child gained or lost weight in recent weeks?

- Does he seem more fatigued and tired than in the past?

- Does he talk about hurting himself?

outdoors, can boost endorphins and help lift a child out of a depressed mood.

If you suspect that your child is depressed, you need to get her professional attention as early as possible. If treatment is delayed or avoided, the child's functioning in everyday life will continue to erode, as will her self-esteem, her schoolwork, and her relationships with friends and family. Also, the longer the depression persists, the more difficult it may be to treat.

If you suspect depression in your child, talk to your pediatrician. Before referring you to a child mental health professional, he or she will rule out medical conditions whose symptoms can cause or mimic those of depression. The therapist will also speak extensively to both you and your child, reviewing her history to determine your child's moods and feelings. Without careful evaluation, children with depression may be misdiagnosed as having a conduct disorder or an attention deficit disorder.

Once the diagnosis of depression has been made, treatment can begin. Psychotherapy (talk therapy or cognitive behavioral therapy) is often part of the treatment program, during which your child will be encouraged to discuss and to play out what is occurring in her life. She will be asked to describe her anxieties, sadness, and other emotions. If there are particular negative events that she is dwelling on, the therapist will try to help her resolve them. While achieving a better understanding of her own life situation, your child will

be able to relate in more positive ways to the people around her.

Throughout the treatment process, the therapist will also involve you as much as possible, scheduling regular conferences with you and her other parent and suggesting ways to help your child meet her own needs and adjust to the world around her. You might also be asked to participate in family therapy, in which you, your child, and her siblings together will explore how all of you can function more positively as a family unit. At home, you should make sure you spend time with your child apart from other family members. Provide her with special times to talk with you about the day's events. Let her know that you are available to discuss any problems or concerns she may have.

Sometimes your doctor may recommend not only psychotherapy for your child but also medication as part of the treatment regimen. Particularly when the depression is severe—with major weight loss, sleep problems, and school difficulties—medication may be advisable. Some of the same drugs used to treat depression are also used to treat anxiety and obsessive-compulsive disorders.

Occasionally, during times of anger and upset, children in middle childhood may make a concerning statement such as "I'm going to kill myself." This statement is a clear message of an unhappy child, and parents need to be sure that they talk with their child and bring him to the pediatrician to determine if the child needs to be evaluated further. There is an increasing trend of suicide attempts among children in middle school. Sadly, online information about suicide, as well as popularization of suicide in the media in general, underscores the importance of monitoring your child's online activities, phone, and media usage.

Children who do attempt suicide often first display warning signs, including withdrawal, sadness, excessive media usage, loss of appetite, and sleep disturbances. There may be multiple factors contributing to the situation. Poor grades, the end of a romantic relationship, or the suicide of a friend or classmate can prompt children to consider killing themselves to reduce the psychological pain they are feeling. Substance use and mental illness increase a child's risk of suicide. Impulsivity may be the greatest component of risk of suicide for some adolescents.

If you sense that your child is troubled, talk with him about it. Listen and share feelings. Do not hesitate to use the word "suicide." Despite the myth that talking about suicide might give your child the idea of killing himself, that will not happen. Instead, your concern will show your child that you care about him and his well-being and are willing to help him with his problems. You should obtain professional help for a seriously troubled child. If your pediatrician has developed a good relationship with your child over the years, he or she may be the best person for your child to talk to in the beginning. The doctor might then refer your child to a clinical social worker, child psychia-

trist, or child psychologist. If a child is truly suicidal and cannot be constantly monitored by the family, he may need to be hospitalized

Disasters and Terrorism

Between the internet, television, and other media, global information is more accessible than ever before—disasters and acts of terrorism, such as school shootings or the impact of a tornado, receive immediate and plentiful coverage. After any disaster, parents often are struggling to understand the event themselves, and then must discuss the event with their children. For school-age children, the age of the child is important. A kindergartener or first-grader will have a different understanding of such events than a fifth- or sixth-grader will have. Key to all ages is to help the child adjust to and cope with the upsetting information. An overall theme of these conversations should be that despite scary events occurring, the family members love and support one another. Emphasize that law enforcement, medical personnel, and the community are trying to work together to help others as well as keep the community safe and prevent this from happening again.

A good starting point is to ask kids what they already know or have heard. Even if you feel your family doesn't watch too much television, classmates and friends will talk on the bus and at recess. Keep the conversation straightforward and ask your child what questions she has. Overly graphic information and images should be avoided, especially for younger children. Shielding your school-age child from the event may not help and may even cause more concern; even if you don't receive a daily print newspaper, newsstands are available in town and, even more accessible, social media and other apps will have images and updates. Your child will understand the information better with assistance from and discussions with a parent.

Follow your child's cues; some children move on from bad news relatively quickly, and others may show difficulty coping, which can manifest as sleep problems (such as trouble falling asleep), physical complaints (such as headaches), behavior changes, or emotional troubles. Even if your child tells you he doesn't want to talk about it, let him know he can come to you if and when the time comes that he does want to talk. If you are unsure if your child needs extra help, and he is showing troublesome signs such as difficulty with school, discuss this with your child's pediatrician.

Kids need relationships with parents and caregivers in which they feel accepted for their feelings, listened to, and supported. You will not have a perfect response for a senseless tragedy. Listen to your child, answer questions simply and directly in an age-appropriate manner, minimize excessive exposure to the event, and provide reassurance. Some older kids benefit from directing their attention to how to help others after the event has occurred.

Eating Disorders

The media bombards society with images of the "perfect" physique, yet this perfection is often unattainable—for example, magazine cover images are very often heavily edited, even after hours are spent on the model's hair and makeup. Awareness of body size begins as early as preschool age, and the drive for thinness can intensify with age. The results can have both physical and psychological repercussions, including potentially serious disordered eating.

Disordered eating is an unhealthy

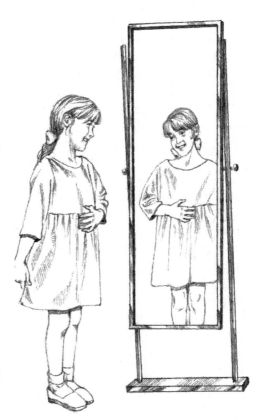

preoccupation with food and one's body. It includes compulsive eating, anorexia nervosa, bulimia, and, most commonly, dieting and restrictive eating. During the middle years, children ages 10 to 12 are at greatest risk. More girls and women are affected by eating disorders than males, although the number of boys affected is on the rise.

Anorexia nervosa is characterized by self-induced starvation, a troubling degree of weight loss, and a distorted body image fueled by an intense fear of being overweight. Anorexia is more common in girls than in boys, but can occur in either sex. The child's body image is unrealistic and distorted to the point that she complains of looking fat, even when it is obvious to others that she is severely underweight. *Bulimia* is a different condition but is characterized by some of the same activities. It is often referred to as the binge/purge syndrome. A binge is a period of voracious eating, while at the same time having a fear of not being able to stop. Following a binge, purging is common. Children with this condition try to rid their bodies of food, either by self-induced vomiting (sticking a finger or an object such as a toothbrush down the throat) or by abusing laxatives or diuretics. Most children with bulimia feel ashamed of their bingeing and purging, and they become skilled at keeping it a secret from friends and family. The strong emotional compulsion to maintain the binge/purge cycle, as well as their success at disguising their problem, makes bulimia difficult to detect and treat. *Dieting* and *restrictive eating* are characterized by a disturbing preoccupation with the need to lose weight. These children weigh themselves frequently, engage in fad diets, and are unreasonably restrictive about food intake. This behavior pattern is unrelated to whether the child is over, under, or at a healthy body weight. The restrictive-eating child may initially appear only to be a picky eater, cutting out certain foods—refusing to eat bread, for example. Since these children still have normal appetites, their eating behavior is a way of exerting control in one area of their lives.

Beyond a preoccupation with weight and dieting, psychological factors may be involved in these eating disorders. Children with disordered eating tend to be perfectionists and set unrealistically high goals for themselves, both academically and socially. These children may struggle with a sense of having lost control of their lives because of family stress, emotional turmoil, or social pressure. Their self-imposed starvation—however destructive—may be the only part of their lives that they feel they can control. With media access and the internet, children can often find information online to fuel the cycle, underscoring the need for parents to monitor children's online activities.

Eating disorders have complex causes within the child's or adolescent's experiences in her family and the society in which she is raised. There is no certain way to prevent these disorders, but focusing on a child's personal and social strengths rather than on appearance and popularity is a good place to start. Eating disorders may be especially difficult to detect in the middle-years child and younger adolescent. For a 10- to 12-year-old child, the symptoms of the disorder may be much more subtle than in an adolescent. Failure to gain appropriate weight, rather than weight loss, may be the only physical sign of a problem.

If you are concerned that your child has disordered eating, talk with your pediatrician. Even with professional intervention, cures are difficult and relapses are common. There are medical risks with resuming regular food intake after a period of relative starvation, for which the child should be closely monitored. The earlier the problem is identified and treatment starts, the better the chances of success. Eating disorders are complex, and the best treatment programs are multidimensional, with medical, psychiatric, and nutritional components. Medications might be prescribed, especially to help the child cope with depression or anxiety. Hospitalization or residential treatment may be required, particularly for patients who have lost large amounts of weight or developed serious complications. Counseling and emotional support are essential components of the treatment program.

Habits

From time to time children can exhibit repetitive behavior and habits—fingernail biting, thumb-sucking, nose picking, and twirling the hair. Children often resort to these repetitive activities during times of tension, idleness, fatigue, or boredom. Many of the habits begin during the preschool years and continue as the child grows to school age, or they reappear at various intervals. Children are frequently unaware of the behavior in which they are engaging and are not using these habits to defy their parents. The repetitive nature of these habits suggests that they serve to soothe or calm the brain. Even in adulthood many people cling to some of these self-comforting traits during times of stress: sucking on pencil tips or their fingers, pulling their earlobes, fingering their hair.

Some self-comforting habits—such as thumb-sucking and body rocking—begin in infancy and gradually fade in middle childhood. During these middle years, most thumb-suckers will confine their sucking to the privacy of their home, at bedtime, while watching TV, or when they are upset. Often, this behavior is accompanied by other vestiges of earlier years, such as cuddling with a blanket. As children mature and develop greater self-control and self-understanding, their thumb-sucking usually disappears, most often by ages 6 to 8. Also, with increases in peer pressure, children tend to assume greater mastery over their behavior.

Similarly, a small number of middle-years children exhibit the normal behavior of rocking themselves to sleep in bed. They may curl into a knee-to-chest position and rock with such vigor that the bed shakes and even bangs the walls until they are fast asleep. A few children roll their head back and forth, at times banging into the wall. Still others sit up and rock. As unsettling as parents may find these habits, children may exhibit them every night in order to settle into sleep. The rhythmic motion seems necessary to soothe or calm the central nervous system in the transition from wakefulness to sleep.

Fingernail biting, cuticle picking, hair twirling, and nose picking are also very common habits of childhood, developing between ages 3 and 6. This behavior may continue throughout middle childhood and perhaps longer. Like other self-comforting habits, they are tension reducers and seem to be outside of consciousness or awareness. Masturbation is also common; for more on this, see page 117.

The frequency and intensity of these habits tend to ebb and flow, often without apparent explanation or parental intervention. Some observers have noted that the child who bites his fingernails or picks his cuticles often causes bleeding or pain; perhaps this natural consequence plays a role in the eventual disappearance of the habit. In any case, these habits frequently fade with time.

As a first step in the simple management of your child's self-comforting habits, ignore them. Most commonly, they will disappear with time. When you call attention to them with harsh words, ridicule, or punishment, the tension that the habit presumably relieves will increase, and the habit will actually get worse. Punishment is not an effective way to eradicate habits. Although it may be difficult, try to withhold your negative comments and wait for the habit to pass.

If your child sucks her thumb or bites her fingernails, she may be interested in overcoming the habit and thus will cooperate with your own efforts toward that goal. Try using these techniques:

- When you notice that your child is not doing the behavior for extended periods, reward her in some agreed-upon way.

Common Childhood Habits

Here are some of the most common self-comforting habits of middle childhood that concern parents.

- Thumb-sucking
- Body rocking
- Head banging
- Fingernail biting
- Cuticle picking
- Hair twirling
- Masturbating

- Use over-the-counter agents, such as bitter-tasting compounds that can be brushed onto the fingers or the cuticles, to remind your child when she begins to bite or suck her thumb. This approach has a relatively low rate of success, but it is simple and, with your child's cooperation, may be an effective strategy. The dentist can recommend a mouth guard for thumb-suckers.

- Positive reinforcement is the most successful way to produce a change in behavior. Accentuate and reward the new behavior you want to see adopted. Star charts and daily rewards are helpful. (For a complete discussion on this subject, see Chapter 15, "Your Child's Behavior and Discipline.")

In more persistent cases—for example, a child who picks at her skin to the point of repetitive scabbing and scarring, or hair-pulling to the point of bald patches on the scalp—counseling may be recommended. Discuss with your pediatrician to see if a referral is warranted.

Further along the spectrum of childhood habits and anxiety is OCD, or obsessive-compulsive disorder. A small number of children are preoccupied with repetitive thoughts or actions that, to the outsider, seem illogical. These recurring ideas (obsessions) and repeated actions (compulsions) are uncontrollable, and can upset their lives and ultimately disrupt the normal functioning of their families. In about one-third to one-half of all affected individuals, obsessive-compulsive disorder begins in childhood or adolescence.

Children with obsessive-compulsive behavior may excessively wash their hands or brush their teeth. They may be driven to check things repeatedly, making sure they have packed their homework assignments or their lunch in the morning. They may repeat certain rituals, perhaps entering and exiting a room a particular number of times. They may arrange and rearrange a table setting meticulously, or become concerned with germs, dirt, crime, violence, disease, or death in an overly dramatic manner. Most children and adults display similar behavior from time to time; however, with OCD these habits interfere with activities of daily living and relationships.

Even at a young age, these children often recognize that their behavior is unusual. However, if they attempt to control it, they are usually overcome with anxiety and revert to their peculiar rituals for relief. Knowing that their behavior is not normal, they often try to hide it from family and friends. Many children have these unusual behaviors for many months before they are discovered. Researchers investigating the causes of obsessive-compulsive disorder describe it as a neurobiological disturbance that seems to run in families. If your child is exhibiting compulsive behavior, talk with your pediatrician, who may refer you to a child mental health professional. Behavioral therapy or medication may be recommended.

Attention Deficit Hyperactivity Disorder (ADHD)

Attention deficit hyperactivity disorder (ADHD) is a developmental condition that affects the behavior, attention, and learning of children. Children affected by ADHD are easily distracted and have trouble concentrating. They may be impulsive and seem to act without thinking, touching objects that are off-limits or running into the street to chase a ball without apparent regard for their own safety. They may not cope well with frustration and can have dramatic mood swings. At school they may be fidgety and brimming with energy, finding it difficult to sit still, jumping out of their seat constantly, unable to control their perpetual motion. They often have difficulty with sequencing and organizational skills. Others who cannot concentrate may sit quietly, daydreaming and appearing "spaced out." For affected children, the classroom may pose a challenge; in the process, their self-esteem may suffer, despite the fact that they are as bright as their peers.

Since all children have these traits some of the time, the diagnosis usually requires that the symptoms be present for at least six months by age 7, be evident in various situations and in more than one environment (e.g., home and school), and be more intense than usually seen in other children of the same age and gender.

Roughly 10 percent of school-age children have ADHD, and boys outnumber girls. Some researchers believe that children with ADHD have abnormally low levels and imbalances of certain neurotransmitters, the chemicals that convey messages between brain cells. Other studies suggest that various parts of the brain may be functioning differently than in the majority of children. Learning at school can be hard for children with ADHD. Children with ADHD are at risk for learning difficulties, including learning disabilities or difficulties with organization and completing tasks. Some have trouble reading or doing math calculations, but this doesn't mean they are less intelligent than other children. Children who have difficulties with language and memory have problems with schoolwork that are increased when ADHD characteristics like distractibility and impulsiveness are present.

A child's ADHD can affect his family in many ways. Normal family routines may be hard to maintain because the child's behavior has been so disorganized and unpredictable, often for a number of years. Parents may not be able to comfortably plan outings or other family events, not knowing what their child's behavior or activity level is likely to be. Children with ADHD frequently become overexcited in stimulating environments. They may also exhibit angry and resistant behavior toward their parents or have low self-esteem. This may be the result of the child's exasperation at failing to meet his parents' expectations or manage day-to-day tasks due to ADHD symptoms. School performance also suffers, and teachers complain to parents, who also must struggle with their child's difficulties with peers, including conflicts and inappropriate behavior.

ADHD Diagnosis

If you suspect ADHD in your child, discuss it with your pediatrician. Unfortunately, there are no specific medical or blood tests that can make the diagnosis. Instead, the diagnosis is made by a complete evaluation of a child's health, combining information obtained from a history and a physical examination, the observations of parents, teachers, and others collected through standardized questionnaires, and psychological testing, if needed.

During these evaluations your pediatrician will rule out other conditions whose symptoms can sometimes mimic ADHD. Poor concentration, poor self-control, and overactivity can be signs of many other conditions, including

Does Your Child Have ADHD?

Only a physician or mental health professional can properly diagnose attention deficit hyperactivity disorder. If your school-age child exhibits several of the following symptoms, which are associated with ADHD, and they are interfering with his ability to achieve academically and socially, as well as diminishing his motivation and self-esteem, have him evaluated by a physician, child neurologist, child psychiatrist, child neuropsychologist, child psychologist, or pediatric specialist in child behavior and development.

Inattention	Hyperactivity-Impulsivity
■ Produces careless work at school	■ Squirms and fidgets
■ Exhibits an inability to pay attention	■ Has trouble with quiet activities
■ Does not seem to listen	■ Is restless
■ Is disorganized	■ Lacks patience
■ Avoids tasks requiring sustained effort	■ Displays uncontrollable energy
■ Loses things	■ Interrupts others
■ Is easily distracted	■ Has trouble waiting his turn
■ Is forgetful	

depression, anxiety, child abuse and neglect, family stress, poor sleep quality, sleep apnea, allergies, hearing and vision problems, seizures, or responses to medication. The doctor may suggest working with your child's school to arrange for further testing. Your pediatrician will want reports on how your child does at play, while doing homework, and while interacting both with you and with other children and adults.

During these evaluations your pediatrician will rule out other conditions, such as poor sleep quality or hearing problems, whose symptoms can sometimes mimic ADHD. In many cases, there is a strong family history of difficulty with attention, impulsivity, concentration, or learning difficulties. Often the child's mother, father, or another close relative has a history of similar struggles when they were young. Gathering this information is helpful for the pediatrician in this evaluation process.

ADHD Treatment

Although symptoms can be reduced, there are no cures and no easy solutions to ADHD and the problems it creates. That said, early diagnosis and treatment can decrease longer-term impacts of the condition. The disorder is chronic and requires ongoing management as well as great patience and persistence on the part of family, school, and the child himself. Treatment is always multidimensional, necessitating the cooperation of child, parents, pediatricians, teachers, and sometimes psychologists, psychiatrists, and social workers.

The majority of interventions for a child with ADHD involve behavioral and environmental modifications. Behavioral therapy, including a structured daily schedule with routines, consistency, and predictability, can be very helpful for an ADHD child. Regular, appropriate physical activity (both structured, such as formal sports programs, and unstructured, such as free play outdoors) are especially important for a child with ADHD. Establish consistency in the daily routine of eating, bathing, leaving for school, and going to sleep, and ensure that your child is sleeping enough. Reward him with praise for positive behavior and for adhering to rules. To keep him focused on the task at hand (for example, dressing in the morning), you may need to be present. Also, before going into situations with lots of stimulation (parties, large family gatherings, shopping centers), review with your child your expectations for his behavior.

A learning or educational specialist may work with your child's school staff to assist the teacher and school nurse in helping the child achieve academic success. As the teacher better understands the child's struggle, he or she may be better able to help him become organized. Simple environmental steps such as moving the child closer to the front of the classroom can be helpful. The teacher may establish a reward system for proper attention to the task at hand, while avoiding humiliating the child because of his inattention behaviors. Working in small groups is helpful, since ADHD children tend to become easily distracted by those around them.

Children diagnosed with ADHD are entitled to various supports from their school. Federal legislation specifies that under the category of "other health impaired" (OHI), a child may receive such assistance as preferential seating in the classroom, extended time on tests, reduced homework, and flexible teaching methods; this is usually referred to as "accommodations" and are covered under a formal 504 plan (a plan that formally ensures a child's educational access and accomodations). To receive such supports, a qualified pediatrician or other professional must make the ADHD diagnosis, and the child's teachers must confirm that the ADHD is having a significant impact on the child's learning. The child does *not* need to be on a prescription medication to qualify to take advantage of these resources.

Educational efforts and behavioral management, possibly in conjunction with medication, are all different aspects of a strategy to maximize the child's learning, emotional, and behavioral difficulties. For example, your doctor may recommend that your child participate in group therapy and social skills training for peer difficulties; individual psychotherapy for his struggles with low self-esteem, anxiety, or depression; parent training and parent support groups so that mothers and fathers can learn better management of their child's behavioral difficulties; and family therapy so the entire family can discuss the effect of ADHD on their relationships.

Your child's treatment plan must be individualized for her needs and include therapies for her behavioral, educational, social, and emotional difficulties. Medications remain an important component of treatment of ADHD, yet are only one aspect of the whole of a child's treatment plan. Your child's medication should be monitored and reevaluated regularly by her doctor to determine its effectiveness, what side effects (if any) may be present, whether dosage adjustments are necessary, and when it can be discontinued. It is important to make sure you understand potential side effects for any medication your child may be prescribed.

Some adolescents still have symptoms and continue to need medication or other treatments throughout their teenage years. Often, although the hyperactivity may have been resolved, problems with inattention and distractibility may persist. Particularly in middle school, when the demands for cognitive and organizational skills increase, these symptoms can interfere with academic achievement. In a portion of cases, classic ADHD signs such as impulsiveness, poor concentration, underachievement, and the resultant frustration continue into adulthood, although they may become less severe with time. ADHD is a true neurodevelopmental condition that, if unmanaged, can result in the impairment of a child's development and strain his relationships with others. With careful monitoring, family education, and environmental modifications, your child can achieve success both academically and socially.

School Avoidance

With the start of kindergarten, children begin to regularly spend a considerable amount of time away from the family. This time brings new experiences and personal challenges. Much of their time is spent at school—a place where pressures in the classroom and relationships with other children can be stressful. While some children naturally greet new situations with enthusiasm, others tend to retreat to the familiarity of their home. For some children, merely the idea of being at school, away from home and apart from their parents, causes great anxiety. Such children, especially when faced with situations they fear or with which they believe they cannot cope, may try to keep from returning to school.

This school avoidance—sometimes called school refusal or school phobia—is not uncommon and occurs in as many as 5 percent of children. These children may outright refuse to attend school or create reasons why they should not go. They may miss a lot of school, complaining of not feeling well, with vague, unexplainable symptoms. Many of these children have anxiety-related symptoms over which they have no conscious control. They may have headaches, stomachaches, hyperventilation, nausea, or dizziness. In general, more clear-cut symptoms like vomiting, diarrhea, fever, or weight loss—which are likely to have a physical basis—are uncommon. School refusal symptoms occur most often on school days and are usually absent on weekends. When

these children are examined by a doctor, no true illnesses are detected or diagnosed. However, since the type of symptoms these children complain of can be caused by a physical illness, a medical examination should usually be part of their evaluation.

Most often, school-avoiding children do not know precisely why they feel ill, and they may have difficulty saying what is causing their discomfort or upset. But when school-related anxiety is causing school avoidance, the symptoms may indicate emotional struggle with issues such as

- Fear of failure

- Increase in academic struggles

- Problems with other children (for example, being teased)

- Anxieties over toileting in a public bathroom

- The teacher's perceived "meanness"

- Online bullying outside of school hours

- Threats of physical harm (as from a school bully)

- Actual physical harm

For some children the school environment can increase preexisting tension. For example, if children tend to be overly conscientious and expect excellent performances from themselves, their fear of failure can gradually create overwhelming and paralyzing anxiety. In some cases, children have experienced the loss of a loved one through death, divorce, or moving to another locale. Especially when they are young, they may fear that in their absence from home another loss will occur.

In addition to the school environment itself, school avoidance may be related to a child's difficulty in separating from her parents and feeling safe while assuming more independence. These children tend to be unsure of themselves and less independent than most of their peers. They may be less socially involved. Some children who have a chronic medical condition or a disability may struggle more with entry to school and being away from the shelter and care of home.

As a first step, the management of school avoidance involves an examination by a pediatrician who can rule out physical illness and who can assist the parents in designing a plan of treatment. Once physical illness has been eliminated as a cause of the child's symptoms, the parents' efforts should be directed not only at understanding the pressures the child is experiencing but also at getting him back in school.

■ Talk with your child about the reasons why he does not want to go to school. Consider all the possibilities and state them. Be sympathetic, supportive, and understanding of why he is upset. Brainstorm together to help your child troubleshoot any stressful situations the two of you identify as causing his worries or symptoms.

■ Acknowledge that you understand your child's concerns, but insist on his immediate return to school. The longer he stays home, the more difficult his eventual return will be. Explain that he is in good health and his physical symptoms are probably due to concerns he has expressed to you— perhaps about grades, homework, relationships with teachers, anxieties over social pressure, or legitimate fears of violence at school. Let him know that school attendance is required by law. He will continue to exert some pressure upon you to let him stay home, but you must remain determined to get him back in school.

■ Discuss your child's school avoidance with the school staff, including his teacher, the principal, and the school nurse. Share with them your plans for his return to school and enlist their support and assistance.

■ Make a commitment to be extra firm on school mornings, when children complain most about their symptoms. Keep discussions about physical symptoms or anxieties to a minimum. For example, do not ask your child how he feels. If he is well enough to be up and around the house, then he is well enough to attend school. Err on the side of sending your child to school. Once your child begins to attend school regularly, his physical symptoms will hopefully disappear.

■ If your child's anxieties are severe, he might benefit from a stepwise return to school. For example, on day one he might get up in the morning and get dressed, and then you might drive him by the school so he can get some feel for it before you return home with him. On day two he might go to school for just half a day, or for only a class or two. On day three he can return for a full day of school.

- Your pediatrician might help ease your child's transition back to school by writing a note verifying that he had some symptoms that kept him from attending school, but though the symptoms might persist, he is now able to return to class.

- Request help from the school staff, especially the school nurse, who can help your child while he is at school. A school nurse or secretary can care for him if he becomes symptomatic, and encourage his return to the classroom.

- If a problem like a school bully or an unreasonable teacher is the cause of your child's anxiety, be an advocate for your child and discuss these problems with the school staff. The teacher or principal may need to make some changes to relieve the pressure on your child in the classroom or on the playground. Monitor your child's online activities, as internet bullying can occur at all hours outside of the classroom and impact your child's sense of security in the classroom.

- If your child stays home, be sure he is safe and comfortable, but he should not receive any special treatment. His symptoms should be treated with consideration and understanding. If his complaints warrant it, he should stay in bed. However, his day should not be a holiday. There should be no screen time privileges, no special snacks, and no visitors, and he should be supervised.

- Your child may need to see a physician when he has to stay home because of a physical illness. Reasons to remain home might include not just complaints of discomfort but recognizable symptoms: a temperature greater than 101 degrees Fahrenheit, vomiting, diarrhea, a rash, a hacking cough, an earache, or a toothache.

- Help your child develop independence by encouraging activities with other children outside the home, including clubs, sports activities, and socializing with friends or relatives.

While you might try to manage school refusal on your own, if your child's school avoidance lasts more than one week, you and your child may need professional assistance. If her school refusal persists, or if she has chronic or intermittent signs of separation difficulties when going to school—in combination with physical symptoms that are interfering with her functioning—your doctor may recommend a consultation with a child mental health professional.

Stress and Your Child

During the middle years of childhood, children experience rapid social, emotional, and intellectual growth, along with pressures to achieve, succeed, and conform. Some children adjust better to these challenges than others, and emotional and behavioral issues can develop from time to time.

In middle childhood, pressures may come from a number of sources—from within the child herself, as well as from parents, teachers, peers, the media, and the larger society in which the child lives. Pressure can take many forms, to which children must respond and adapt. Whether these are events of lasting consequence, such as the divorce of their parents, or merely a minor hassle, like losing their homework, these demands or stresses are a part of children's daily lives. The silver lining is that when a child is given opportunities to practice setbacks at younger ages, the child develops resilience and the tools needed to be an independent adult and handle future challenges. (For more on anxiety, see page 546.)

Children welcome some events and are able to adapt to them with relative ease. Other events are perceived as threats to their own or the family's daily routines or general sense of well-being, and these stresses are more troublesome. Most stress faced by children is in the middle, neither welcomed nor seriously harmful, but rather a part of accomplishing the tasks of childhood and learning about themselves.

Children may also worry about making friends, succeeding in school, dealing with peer pressure, or overcoming a physical injury or disability. Whatever its form, if stress is too intense or long-lasting, it can sometimes take a toll on children. Major events, especially those that forever change a child's family, such as the death of a parent, can have lasting effects on children's psychological health and well-being. Minor daily stresses can also have consequences. They can contribute to loss of sleep or appetite. Children may become irritable, or their school grades may suffer. Their behavior and their willingness to cooperate may change.

Children's temperaments vary, and thus they are quite different in their ability to cope with stress and daily hassles. Some are easygoing by nature and adjust easily to events and new situations. Others are thrown off balance by changes in their lives. All children improve in their ability to handle stress if they previously have succeeded in managing challenges, if they feel they have the ability to do so, if they have a strong sense of self-esteem, and if they have emotional support from family and friends. Children who have a clear sense of personal competence and who feel loved and supported generally do well.

A child's age and development will help determine how stressful a given situation may be. Changing teachers midyear may be a major event for a child in the first grade and merely an annoyance for a sixth-grader. How a child perceives and responds to stress depends in part on development, in part on experience, and in part on a child's individual temperament.

Children are sensitive not only to the changes around them but also to the feelings and reactions of their parents, even if those feelings are not communicated directly in words. If a parent loses a job, children will have to adjust to their family's financial crisis; they must deal not only with the obvious family budgetary changes but also with the changes in their parents' emotional state. Children may have to cope with a bully, a move to a new neighborhood, a parent's serious illness, or the disappointment of a poor sports performance. They might feel a constant, nagging pressure to dress the "right" way, or to achieve the high grades that can put them on a path toward the "right" college.

Middle-years children, compared to prior generations, have fewer social supports available. The change in family structure from the large, supportive, extended families (including both parents, aunts, uncles, and grandparents) of previous generations to the present high incidence of divorced families, single-parent families, and stepfamilies has altered the experience of childhood. Modern technology's continual presence of screens and electronic devices can interfere with communication between family members within the primary home.

Not all stress is a bad thing. Moderate amounts of pressure imposed by a teacher or a coach, for example, can motivate a child to keep her grades up in school or to participate more fully in athletic activities. Successfully managing stressful situations or events enhances a child's ability to cope in the future. Children are future adults, and through these experiences, they develop resilience and learn how to deal with life's inevitable bumps and hurdles. However, when the stress is continuous or particularly intense, it can take a toll on both the psyche and the body. Sudden stressful events will accelerate your child's breathing and heartbeat, constrict her blood vessels, increase her blood pressure and muscle tension, and perhaps cause stomach upset and headaches. As stress persists, she might be more susceptible to illness and experience fatigue, nightmares, teeth-grinding, insomnia, depression, and school failure.

The way children show they are overloaded and are having difficulty coping with stress is different at different stages of development. During the preschool years you may have noticed that under stress, your child regressed a little. Perhaps she had trouble separating from you, was especially clingy, or even temporarily lost some skills associated with growing up, such as toilet training. Young school-age children also openly act out their feelings; however, they may be more likely to internalize their stress. They might express stress through sadness, depression, or withdrawal. Other children will externalize stress by overactivity, anger, or creating conflicts. Parents should be attuned to these and other signs of overload.

Much of the stress in your child's life comes from outside the family and may be beyond your control. Yet many children may feel pressure because their parents, with the best of intentions, are overscheduling them with music lessons, sports activities, computer courses, and art classes. At first glance it might seem advantageous to expose your child to as many educational, cultural, and athletic experiences as possible. However, many children and their families are stressed by the multiple activities that fill children's free time. Overscheduled children with inadequate downtime can become exhausted. Parents should monitor the big picture several times a year to ensure that quality family time isn't being drained away by an excessive amount of extracurricular activities and athletics. When a child's entire day is structured for him,

he loses the opportunity to pursue his own passions and plan his own (screen-free) free time, which has consequences later on when he is expected to take increased ownership of his schedule and budget his time between school and other responsibilities.

You and your child together need to find a balance between structured and unstructured activities to allow for adequate physical activity, downtime, and well-being. Don't worry about his becoming bored; there are actually wonderful benefits from some unplanned time, when he can use his imagination, develop his own planning skills, and pursue interests of his own. As for his structured activities, limit them to those he truly enjoys. Solicit your

Signs of Overload

Although stress is a part of life and growing up, there are signs that stress is undermining your child's physical or psychological well-being.

- Your child develops physical symptoms like headaches and stomach pains.

- He seems restless, tired, and agitated.

- He appears depressed and is uncommunicative about how he feels.

- He gets irritable, becomes increasingly negative, and shows little excitement or pleasure in his activities.

- He seems less interested in an activity that was once extremely important to him and prefers to stay at home.

- His grades at school begin to fall, and he has less interest than usual in attending classes and doing homework.

- He exhibits antisocial behavior such as lying and stealing, forgets or refuses to do his chores, and seems much more dependent on you than in the past.

child's suggestions and opinions before making any plans for him. "Bored" kids should be sent outside to play, weather permitting. Some experts are concerned about excessive screen use inhibiting children's time outdoors appreciating and playing in nature. Simply playing outdoors in the fresh air releases endorphins (hormones triggering pleasant feelings), promotes physical activity, and relieves stress.

Your child may complain about losing interest in an organized program, or of feeling anxiety about his inability to perform as well as his peers or teammates. Explore the reasons for and realities of his complaints. There may be problems to resolve together, or it may be time to reevaluate participation in the current activity. As a general rule, it is appropriate to finish out a season instead of suddenly stopping or quitting, as a courtesy to the team and as a life lesson for the child.

When your child is facing a lot of stress, take the time to talk with her about the pressures she is feeling and the anxiety in her life. Put yourself in your child's place and imagine what she may be feeling. Talk about some of her behavior and displays of emotion you have noticed recently, which suggest to you that she may be struggling with some issues. Gradually, your efforts may help her put her feelings into words. (See Chapter 14, "Communicating with Your Child.") Help your child understand her own temperament (see page 131). Use guiding statements such as "I know you react pretty strongly to stress" or "You seem to prefer to take your time making decisions." This can help foster insight and help your child cope.

Together, you and your child should evaluate the situations or activities that are producing problems. Are there issues with friends that need to be resolved? Does she need to be reassured that, despite a divorce or other family disruption, she is still loved by both parents? Do you need to cut back her schedule of extracurricular activities or choose them more carefully? Clarify the problems together, and identify a number of possible solutions. Look at the influences that might be adding to the difficulty your child is having in adjusting to or managing the situation, and find ways in which she can change them.

Model healthy coping skills for your child. Avoid statements, even jokingly, such as "Mommy's stressed—she needs a drink!" This sends a message to your child that the answer to stress is a substance. Instead, say "Mommy is getting frustrated. Can you help me calm down by taking ten deep breaths with me?"

If your child seems to have too little free time, help her modify her schedule so she can relax and play. She will probably increase her creativity and devise her own forms of recreation. Encourage her to use her imagination and skills to create play and pleasure. Remember, your job is not to keep her entertained; in fact, most children enjoy playtime free of the frenetic pace and tension that usually accompany overscheduling.

Especially if you have multiple children, ensure that you have one-on-one time each day. Even a ten-minute conversation while in the car, chatting while playing catch in the backyard, or telling stories from your day while washing the dinner dishes together matters. It is often these conversations that occur while other things are happening that are the most insightful and productive, allowing you more insight into your child's world.

The idea of "mindfulness" has become increasingly popular, and is backed by research studies as a good way for kids and adults alike to combat the stress in our daily lives. Many mindfulness techniques use meditation practices such as breathing techniques to promote a calm state. A child and parent can sit together quietly, close their eyes, and count slow breaths together. If a child has difficulty sitting still, a movement-based meditation such as yoga is a way to maintain a body pose and take slow breaths.

If you feel you need additional help in the area of stress management, discuss this issue with your child's pediatrician. In some cases, when your child is coping especially poorly and the stress is interfering with her day-to-day functioning, the doctor might refer you to a mental health professional. Keep in mind that children under stress often have parents under stress, and some of the parents' anxiety can be transferred to the child. If you are undergoing a personal crisis—a divorce, for example—or have filled your child's day with activities because you yourself are over-committed, it may be time to make changes in your own life, easing the personal stress that might have an indirect impact on your child as well.

Stuttering

Stuttering or stammering (also called *dysfluency*) is a disorder of communication in which sounds or whole words are repeated as the child speaks, interrupting the flow of his communication. Sometimes these children make sounds that are prolonged, or their speech may actually stop momentarily.

Stuttering first becomes apparent during the preschool years. About 90 percent of children between the ages of 18 months and 4 years have some degree of dysfluency, which within a certain range is developmentally typical. This stuttering appears to be related to the development of language, perhaps occurring because the child's thought processes move much more rapidly than his ability to put those ideas into words. This type of stuttering disappears on its own, usually in just two to three months; it is helpful if the family does not draw too much attention to it, as this can exacerbate the issue.

At any age, children can develop stuttering as a manifestation of stress and social pressures. When a school-age child stutters, he can become more self-conscious, thus increasing his anxiety and making his speech dysfluency even worse. Pressure from teachers trying to be helpful or from peers can aggravate his stuttering too. In some cases, people who interact with a stuttering child—perhaps friends or relatives—notice the difficulties the child is having with his speech, feel uncomfortable, and change their behavior toward him. The child usually is aware that his speech patterns have produced this altered response, and thus he may become even more uncomfortable with the way he talks, perpetuating the stuttering. Some children try to deal with this by avoiding social contact and conversation.

If you have a child who stutters, you can help him by approaching the issue with some simple steps:

1. Encourage periods of conversation that your child will not find stressful.

2. Do not correct his speech.

3. Do not interrupt him.

4. Do not finish his sentences.

5. Do not ask him to repeat sentences or phrases.

6. Do not ask him to practice certain words or sounds.

7. Do not ask him to slow down his speech.

8. If he wishes, let him choose to avoid certain problematic words or sounds, finding alternative ones to use in their place.

9. If he finds it helpful, encourage him to pause, inhale a full breath, and then exhale while speaking.

10. Listen, offer encouragement, and provide support.

If your child's stuttering pattern continues, get professional help. When a stuttering problem begins during middle childhood, or if an earlier stuttering condition persists or resurfaces, ask your pediatrician for a referral to a specialist—most likely a speech and language therapist experienced in treating children with stuttering difficulties. Some children can also benefit from psychological counseling to address issues, like poor self-esteem, that may be contributing to the dysfluency.

You also should seek help if:

- Your child's stuttering becomes more severe.

- He becomes extremely self-conscious and fearful of communication.

- He develops new facial grimaces or tics.

The prognosis for children who stutter is excellent. About 80 percent outgrow their stuttering by adolescence. In a small number of individuals, however, it persists into adulthood, and they require continuous support and intervention.

Tics

Tics are rapid and repeated involuntary movements. Tics often affect the face and neck and take the form of eye blinking, shoulder shrugging, facial grimacing, neck twisting, throat clearing, sniffing, and dry coughs. Sometimes these movements occur frequently throughout the day; at other times, they occur only occasionally. Transient (meaning not long-lasting) tics occur in about 20 percent of school-age children, beginning most often between ages 7 and 9. Tics are irregular in their pattern, but they often appear suddenly after some type of physical or social stress, and they tend to increase when a child is tense, anxious, tired, or idle. Tics become less frequent when a child is able to relax, and are never present during sleep. Tics may run in families. School-age children who experience them may be embarrassed and teased by their peers.

Parents, under the false belief the child can control the tics, may urge their child to stop them, forgetting or unaware that the mannerisms are not under the child's conscious control. Sometimes they may feel that the child is purposely defying them as the tics continue. Fortunately, most tics disappear on their own within several months. They may last longer when parents create stress for the child by pressuring him to stop the repetitive movements.

Scolding your child or calling attention to her unusual mannerisms is not helpful, and usually makes it worse. Tics are best ignored. On the opposite end of the spectrum, since your child is likely to have questions about why her body is acting this peculiar way, silence about them might increase her anxiety. It is best to talk with her sensitively and supportively, letting her know there is nothing wrong with her and there is no reason to feel ashamed. Help her develop strategies for explaining the tics to friends who may ask about them.

Seek ways to decrease potential sources of stress and conflict in your child's life that seem to be playing a role in the tics. If she feels pressured or overscheduled, work with her to strategize priorities and lighten her commitments. Discuss with her other sources of stress

Types of Tic Disorders

Simple tics are single facial twitches that are persistent but do not change in character. By contrast, **multiple motor tic disorders** have ever-changing patterns of different visible physical tics.

The most severe tic disorder is **Tourette's syndrome**, which is characterized by multiple motor and vocal tics. The motor tics begin in the face but later involve all parts of the body. The vocal tics are vocalizations like snorts, coughs, or hiccups. This syndrome is often associated with learning disabilities, obsessive thoughts, hyperactivity, and attention deficit hyperactivity disorder.

and worry, and together find ways to deal with them. Sometimes tics may have started under times of stress or conflict but persist long after those situations seem to have passed. (See "Stress and Your Child" on page 565.)

In some situations, you and your child may benefit from some outside help or advice. Talk with your pediatrician in the following situations, as a referral to a neurologist who works with a therapist familiar with comprehensive behavioral intervention for tics (CBIT) or habit reversal training may be needed:

■ The tics interfere with schoolwork or friendships and cause your child embarrassment, anxiety, or emotional problems.

■ There are multiple tics or vocalizations, such as sniffs, snorts, throat clearing, chewing, and tongue thrusting. These may indicate the condition called Tourette's syndrome (see box on page 571).

■ The tics are intense and frequent.

■ The symptoms are present for longer than a year.

■ There is a strong family history of tic disorders, including Tourette's syndrome.

■ Your child is on medication for attention deficit hyperactivity disorder (ADHD); some of these medications have a side effect of increased tics and may need to be adjusted accordingly.

■ Your efforts to identify the source of your child's tension or your efforts to help her reduce the stress are unsuccessful.

~ 50 ~

Chest and Lungs

Flu/Influenza

The flu, or *influenza*, is an illness caused by a respiratory virus. Many people confuse the respiratory flu with stomach flu (or gastroenteritis; for more information, see "Vomiting" on page 535); however, respiratory flu and stomach flu are two completely different illnesses. The flu is spread by respiratory droplets scattered when an ill person coughs or sneezes. In addition, the virus can remain for some time on a contaminated hard surface such as a door handle; a child who touches that surface can then transmit the virus to his nose, mouth, or eye.

Flu season usually starts in autumn and ends in spring, although different parts of the country experience flu outbreaks at different times of the year. Sometimes flu cases emerge as early as November, and in some years as late as March or April. There are different strains or types of flu virus that can cause illness, and these change year to year, which is why yearly fall flu vaccination is recommended. The virus is most contagious in the first several days of the illness and the symptoms tend to be more pronounced in preschool- and school-age children.

Flu symptoms can last a week or more. Fevers above 100.4 degrees Fahrenheit, chills, body aches, headache, fatigue, sore throat, congestion, and a dry cough are all common symptoms. Vomiting and diarrhea may occur as well. Parents can tell flu symptoms apart from a common cold's symptoms by the severity and length of symptoms: typically the common cold has a lower fever, and not as much coughing or achiness. The flu can lead to complications such as ear infections or pneumonia (talk with your pediatrician if your child has symptoms such as ear pain or a cough that persist or worsen after the first few days). There can be serious complications or even death from the flu, but thankfully, due to the seasonal fall flu vaccine, these are uncommon. Children with underlying chronic medical conditions such as asthma or diabetes are at greater risk of complications.

Children with the flu need rest and fluids. Acetaminophen or ibuprofen can help a child with fever feel better, but do not give ibuprofen if your child is dehydrated or continuously vomiting. Never give aspirin to your child, as giving aspirin to a child with influenza is associated with Reye syndrome (for more on this, see page 533).

In the best of cases, the flu causes a week or more of missed school and work; in more severe cases, the flu can lead to bacterial complications, hospitalization, or even death. The best way to prevent you and your child from catching the flu is to get the seasonal fall flu vaccine every year. There is a new vaccine each year because there are different types of flu-causing viruses that shift and change globally over time. Vaccines are safe and effective. Kids should receive the yearly fall flu vaccine starting at 6 months of age. Younger kids, especially if it is their first time receiving the vaccine, may need another dose of the flu vaccine (a booster) four weeks after the first dose. Adults should also receive the yearly vaccine, especially if they live with younger children or someone at risk of flu complications.

While there is no cure for the influenza virus, there are prescription antiviral medications available that, if given early in the course of the illness, may help shorten the duration of flu symptoms. Call your pediatrician sooner rather than later if your child has asthma, diabetes, sickle cell anemia, or other underlying medical conditions and you suspect influenza.

Pneumonia

Pneumonia, an infection of the lung, can be caused by a virus (often following a viral upper respiratory infection) or bacteria. Kids with pneumonia do not necessarily need to spend the night in the hospital; in fact, most cases are successfully managed at home with comfort measures and other treatment as determined by your pediatrician to minimize the symptoms. Just as there are many different types of viruses that can cause the common cold, different viruses can spread to the chest and cause pneumonia, such as respiratory syncytial virus (RSV), influenza, parainfluenza, and adenovirus. Pneumonia can occur at any time of the year, but it is more common in fall, winter, and early spring.

A child can develop pneumonia either by contact with an infected person's saliva or mucus or as a complication of a viral infection such as a simple cold or the flu (respiratory influenza), after which bacteria then grow in the lungs. Children with immune disorders or a weaker immune system due to diabetes, sickle cell disease, or immunosuppressive drugs used to treat cancers or rheumatologic conditions may be more prone to developing pneumonia.

Signs of pneumonia include fever, fatigue, cough (which may or may not be productive), increased work of breathing, or chest pain (especially with coughing or taking a deep breath). Your child's pediatrician will examine your child's lungs with a stethoscope; the breath sounds typically are different from usual if a child has pneumonia. A chest X-ray is not always needed but may be helpful to further evaluate your child.

It can be difficult to tell the difference between viral and bacterial pneumonia. A viral pneumonia usually improves on its own after a few days, though a child may continue to cough for another month. Honey for children older than a year can help suppress a cough; codeine products are not recommended for children. A bacterial pneumonia will need an antibiotic; ensure your child takes the full course, even when symptoms are improving, so that the infection is fully treated. If your child seems to be worsening instead of improving, consult with your pediatrician.

Thankfully, the vaccines for pneumococcal and *Haemophilus influenza* type B, on the CDC schedule of recommended vaccines for all infants and young children, have reduced the incidence of pneumonia caused by these bacteria. There is an additional pneumococcal vaccine for older kids recommended if the child is at high risk for infections caused by pneumococcal bacteria, such as sickle cell anemia or heart disease.

~ 51 ~

Child Abuse

BY DEFINITION, CHILD abuse includes a number of forms of maltreatment by a parent, caregiver, or another person in a custodial role (e.g., clergy, coach, teacher), including physical abuse, physical or medical neglect, emotional abuse or neglect, and sexual abuse. Sadly, many children experience multiple types of abuse. For instance, a child who experiences repeated instances of emotional abuse might also be victimized by occasional, deliberate physical violence. Child physical abuse and neglect can inflict permanent damage on children and, in some severe cases, cause death. Several forms of abuse and neglect are now considered adverse childhood experiences with long-lasting health and emotional harms in adulthood.

Physical neglect includes inadequate food, clothing, or shelter. It can include supervisory neglect—in which a child receives little or no supervision in and around his home, for example—which can have tragic consequences if injuries occur. Even when it poses no immediate threat to a child's safety, prolonged or repeated neglect—in which his basic needs for clothing, nutrition, medical care, education, or shelter are not met—can have adverse physical, social, developmental, and emotional consequences.

Although reports of child abuse and neglect to child protection agencies have decreased over the years, self-report data suggest that it is highly prevalent. According to one study, at least one in seven children has experienced child abuse and/or neglect in the last year, and another study suggests as many as one in four children experiences some form of child abuse or neglect during childhood.

Most commonly, those who abuse or neglect children are the parents or caretakers of the child; if not a parent, then a close relative (such as an uncle or an older brother or sister) or a member of the household. The presence of an unrelated male in the home—the mother's boyfriend, for example—is a known risk for abuse. A number of factors can contribute to a parent abusing his or her child. Stress and pressures on the family, both internal and external, can take a toll. When parents are feeling financial strain, job stress, or marital problems, their anger and frustration may make them more prone to strike out at their child. At certain times of the day—perhaps in the early evening after a hard day at work—parents may find it particularly difficult to control their tempers when children misbehave or merely try their patience. Other violence in the home or community violence can also raise the risk for abuse. Life stresses such as poverty, illness, and alcoholism increase the risk of abuse. Parents who are socially isolated, without adequate sources of emotional support or a helping hand with daily tasks and responsibilities, are more likely to lose control and abuse their children.

Alcohol and other drug use by parents is often a contributing factor in child abuse. By reducing inhibitions, alcohol consumption often allows anger to explode in a parent who is confronted by his or her child's misbehavior. Some drugs, such as methamphetamine, can increase agitation and thus can contribute to an abusive situation in the home. Drug or alcohol use can lead to parents being unable to adequately care for their children. Children with learning or behavioral problems—conditions that themselves place more stress on parents and create more conflict within the family—can be at higher risk for maltreatment.

Physical Abuse

Parents who were physically disciplined or physically abused themselves as children, or who were or are intimidated verbally and physically by adults around them, often resort to similar means when they discipline their own children. The use of force, especially violence toward other people, is often a learned behavior. Some abused children live in families experiencing other types of domestic violence, such as spousal abuse, which is also associated with child abuse.

If you suspect that a child you know is being abused—whether a relative, a child in the neighborhood, or your child's classmate—you have a responsibility to become involved. Teachers are often the first to see the changes in a child's physical appearance, emotional condition, and behavior—changes that might suggest a child is being hurt or is in a potentially unsafe home environment. In all states, teachers, physicians, dentists, and other professionals are legally obligated to report suspected cases of abuse, and for good reasons: to identify the child who needs help and to prevent further abuse from occurring.

Sometimes it's difficult to decide if a child has been abused, but there are some physical signs to consider. For instance, normal, active children will have bruises and bumps that come from everyday playing. However, these routine bruises tend to occur over bony areas such as knees, elbows, and shins. If you see a child who has injuries on other parts of the body—the stomach, the face, the ears, the buttocks, the mouth, or the thighs—this should raise suspicions. Black eyes, human bite marks, and burns are *not* symptoms of everyday play. Sometimes these injuries are on hidden or hard-to-see parts of the body, like the backs of the legs, the inner arms, or the back.

In the majority of child physical abuse cases, parents do not consciously intend to injure their children. Most abusive episodes arise when adults have difficulty coping with life situations and lose control. However, even if their intentions are not malicious, a parent who abuses a child may do it again, especially if his or her underlying stresses are not addressed. As a result, society

Signs of Physical Abuse

These indicators may suggest a child has been physically abused:

- The child has had repeated injuries that are unexplainable or unusual.

- He appears withdrawn, passive, and depressed, and he cries a lot.

- He is unusually aggressive, disruptive in the classroom, or destructive of his personal property and that of others. He throws toys across the room or becomes violent toward a pet.

- He seems overly tired and mentions that he has trouble sleeping and frequent nightmares.

- The child seems genuinely afraid of a parent or other caretaker.

- He appears hesitant to go home after school, as if he is fearful of something there.

- His parents seem to be isolated from other parents in the neighborhood, do not participate in school activities, and may have a drinking or other drug abuse problem. They appear preoccupied with their own lives at the expense of caring properly for their child.

- The parent is unwilling to talk about the child's injuries, or is noticeably anxious when he or she does so.

must intervene in order to protect the child and assist the family.

Once a case has been investigated by law enforcement and social agencies, they may institute various forms of services and treatment to help the family. However, the safety and protection of the child are the first priority, so children may at times need to be removed from their family and placed in a kinship or foster home, at least temporarily; at the same time, efforts are made to work with the parents to address underlying problems and teach them coping skills to ensure that episodes of abuse are not repeated.

If you have abused your own child or feel that such behavior may occur, talk with a trusted individual such as a supportive relative, physician, counselor, or clergyman. He or she may refer you to a professional or an agency where you can obtain help, including assistance in dealing with your own fears and guilt. Both parents and children may benefit from some guidance and counseling, individually and together, that can help break the cycle. Programs that specifically address domestic violence and provide shelter if needed are important resources as well. You will be guided toward dealing with your emotions without resorting to violence. You will have the opportunity to discuss your own parenting experiences and your current life stresses. You will be shown ways to cope effectively with stresses so that you do not fall into inflicting injuries upon your child. You have a responsibility to your child and to yourself to find ways to relate at home that are nonviolent, day after day.

If you feel that you are in the midst of a crisis, call your local chapter of Parents Anonymous (parentsanonymous .org) or a child abuse crisis hotline such as 800-4-A-CHILD (800-422-4453), which can provide you with some prompt advice and support. You will be guided through the next steps on getting help.

Emotional Abuse

Not all abuse is physical. Neglecting your child's needs for emotional support, love, and caring is also a form of abuse. Emotional abuse is one of the most pervasive and damaging forms of child abuse. Belittling, ridiculing, name-calling, and being disrespectful and unreasonably critical toward your child can have serious emotional consequences and long-term repercussions.

Similar to more violent forms of abuse, emotional abuse can impair your child's self-image and self-esteem and interfere with his ability to function well in society. He may have difficulty making friends and relating to peers. A child may avoid participating in activities with other children and avoid situations in which he's required to give and receive affection. An affected child may be prone to being aggressive and oppositional, may develop learning difficulties or hyperactivity, or may have physical health problems such as bedwetting or soiling. A child (most often a girl) might act "pseudomature," becoming a caretaker for adults and others in ways far beyond any role appropriate for her age and development. Emotional abuse, especially when it occurs over an extended period of time, can have a lifelong impact, affecting a child's happiness, relationships, and success. He may become somber, unable to enjoy himself, and prone to self-defeating behaviors. At the extreme, he can become self-destructive, engaging in self-mutilation and even attempting suicide.

As with other types of abuse, emotional abuse is often inflicted by parents who themselves were raised in an environment where they experienced emotional mistreatment by their own parents. Being made aware of the way they are treating their children is an important first step for these parents in bringing their abusive behavior to a halt. Often they are not conscious that their behavior is damaging; if they knew what they were doing and were more sensitive to their child's pain, they would probably want to do something to stop it.

Visiting a physician or a clergy member is a good way to start looking for help with emotional abuse. You might be referred to a mental health professional or to community organizations or churches that offer parenting classes aimed specifically at helping you talk to and problem-solve with your child.

Sexual Abuse

Sexual abuse is a difficult subject for most people to discuss. As frightening and offensive as the topic may be, sexual abuse is a serious and not infrequent problem. Millions of children are victims of this form of abuse. According to self-report studies from the U.S. Centers for Disease Control and Prevention, one out of five women and one out of ten men remember being sexually abused as children or adolescents.

Sexual abuse includes inappropriate sexual acts, behaviors, or sexual exploitation of a child for the sexual gratification of the abuser. It includes not only intercourse but also fondling the child's genitals, forcing the child to fondle an adult's genitals, mouth-to-genital contact, or rubbing the adult's genitals on the child. Other types of sexual abuse may also take place, even though they may not involve physical contact—for instance, an adult exposing his genitals to a child, showing pornographic pictures or video images to a child, sending inappropriate images electronically, or taking pictures of the child for sexual purposes.

In most cases the offender is known to the child, and often is an authority figure whom the child trusts. The abuser might be a parent, a stepparent, an adult relative such as an uncle, a family friend, a neighbor, a sitter, a teacher, a coach, an older sibling or stepsibling, or a cousin. While children usually understand who a "stranger" is, they may be caught off guard by the advances of someone they know and respect. The offender usually first manipulates the child using threats, bribes, or aggressive persuasion, encouraging or threatening the child to keep a secret, and convinces the child that she has no choice but to participate.

In many cases the sexual abuse involves more than just a single incident. Often it is a pattern of ongoing sexual contacts, frequently beginning in the early years and persisting into adolescence. Sometimes the abuse stops only when the maturing child is capable of extricating herself from the situation, often by reporting the incident to another child or adult. Even after the abuse has stopped, the psychological repercussions of the abuse can last a lifetime.

Preventing Sexual Abuse

Using a balanced approach, parents need to teach their children about appropriate sexual boundaries and behaviors, and empower them to take appropriate action if an inappropriate situation arises. It is important to teach kids that no matter who is making them feel uncomfortable—even if it is a trusted adult—the child must clearly and forcefully say "No" or "Stop" and walk or run away. Your child should know that she should always come to you if a sexual incident ever happens to her, no matter who the perpetrator is and no matter what kind of warning the offender has given her ("Don't tell anyone or I'll hurt you"). Make sure the child understands that she will *not* get into trouble for telling about such an incident. Ensure that your child knows the difference between different types of secrets (a birthday gift for a parent, which is not a harmful secret, as compared to a situation that makes the child feel uncomfortable). Remember that while girls are the usual victims of

sexual abuse, about 10 percent of victims are boys.

In addition:

■ Teach your child about the right to privacy. No one should ever touch body parts that are covered by a bathing suit. There is a difference between "good" touch and "bad" touch: a parent's loving hug is different from putting a hand on the child's buttocks or inner thigh. Just as importantly, nurture the idea of *consent* from as early as preschool age. If a child does not feel comfortable hugging an aunt at a family reunion, she has the right over her own body to make that determination, and parents should not force the child to hug anyone she does not want to. A child has the right to say no to anyone who tries to touch her. In addition, your child should respect other people's right to privacy.

■ Sit down with your child and explain various situations that might indicate that someone is making advances. For example, a molester might offer a child candy, money, pets, or toys. Have a special phrase or code word that your children know a trusted adult will use in case there is an emergency and the adult needs to pick your child up from school. A potential offender may ask the child for assistance, such as directions to a particular street or landmark, or help in finding a missing dog or cat. Make sure your child understands that if she encounters suspicious situations as these, she should run away and yell for help.

- Talk about peer pressure. Make safety plans with your children so that they know what to do if they are asked to use drugs or alcohol, smoke, touch someone sexually, steal, cheat, or bully.

- Tell your child that threats such as "If you tell your mother what we did, I'm going to kill her" are against the law, and that she should tell you immediately about them. Make sure your child knows it's okay to tell you about someone who makes her feel uncomfortable, no matter who that person may be.

- If your child is in a position to do door-to-door solicitation—perhaps selling cookies or collecting money for a newspaper route—an adult should go with her. Warn your child that she should never enter someone else's home unless an adult accompanies her.

- Investigate whether your child's school has a sexual abuse education and prevention program. If not, encourage the school board to institute one. Many religious institutions also run similar sexual abuse prevention programs.

- Monitor the activities at your child's child care facility or summer camp. Participate in these activities whenever possible. Listen carefully when your child tries to tell you something of a sexual nature, particularly if she seems to have difficulty talking about it. As much as possible, create an environment at home in which sexual topics can be discussed comfortably. (See page 108 for additional information on this issue.)

- In general, spend quality time with your child, so that she does not feel the need to seek the attention of other adults. Children from unhappy or broken homes tend to be the easiest targets for molesters, since these children may be eager for attention and affection.

- If you do not already know whom your child spends time with, find out. If your child spends time in isolated or remote places with adults or older children, investigate what might be going on there. Question the motives of adults who want to spend large amounts of time alone with your child.

When Sexual Abuse Occurs

Most victims of sexual abuse remain silent. Often feeling guilty or helpless, they do not run to tell their parent or another trusted adult. Sometimes, when the perpetrator is a family member, they believe that by telling someone, they may split their family apart. Or they may feel embarrassed by what has happened, or they may have been warned or somehow threatened by the offender to remain quiet. All the while, however, they may be emotionally devastated. They may withdraw from family and friends, stop participating in school activities, experience chronic anxiety and insomnia, and exhibit aggressive and self-destructive behavior. Sometimes a sexually abused child may eventually tell her friends what has occurred. Or she may say something to a parent that hints at the abuse without describing it clearly.

If your child comes to you and reveals that she has been sexually abused, take it seriously. *Too often, children are not believed, particularly if they implicate a family member as the perpetrator.* You need to listen to your child, gently and sensitively ask questions to obtain more information, and then take active steps to protect her. Contact a pediatrician, the local child protection service agency or social welfare bureau, or the police (sexual abuse is a violation of the law). If you don't intervene, the abuse might continue for many more months and even years; at

Signs of Sexual Abuse

Symptoms that could indicate that a child has been sexually abused include:

- She seems to be afraid of a particular person or place and being left alone with that individual.

- He overreacts to a question about someone's touching him.

- She suddenly seems more aware of and preoccupied with sexual conduct, words, and parts of the body that are beyond what the child can be expected to know or understand.

- His behavior changes dramatically in any number of ways. A younger child may regress to bed-wetting or soiling his underwear, or his eating habits might change. He may relate to peers differently, either by withdrawing or by becoming more aggressive. He might act up in school,

his motivation and concentration may suffer, and his grades may fall. He may appear fearful, frequently crying and clinging to his parent; alternatively, he may avoid normal family intimacy.

- She has unreasonable anxiety over a doctor's physical examination.

- He has inexplicable physical complaints, such as headaches, stomachaches, or genital itching or pain.

- She draws unusually frightening or sad pictures, using a lot of black and red colors.

- He masturbates excessively and tries to get other children to perform sexual acts.

the same time, the child will come to believe, correctly, that home is not safe and that you are not available to help.

Unfortunately, in most cases of sexual abuse physicians are unable to find physical evidence of the abuse. Even so, the child should be brought to medical attention, to be examined for physical signs of sexual abuse such as genital or anal changes. The physician might also find evidence of sexually transmitted infections such as gonorrhea or herpes.

In the days and weeks ahead, make sure your abused child understands that she is not responsible for the abuse, and let her know how brave she was to tell you what happened. Reassure her that this abuse will not occur again. Offer plenty of love and support. If you are dealing with anger of your own, she might think that some of it is directed toward her, so continually reassure her that you are not upset with her and are proud of her for telling you what has happened. Your child should be treated for any physical injuries, either internal or external, related to the abuse. Children and their families will need professional counseling to help them through this ordeal.

A number of factors will influence the psychological impact of sexual abuse upon a child, including:

- **The nature of the sexual activity, the frequency, and the use of force.** The more intrusive the abusive experience, the more difficult and confusing it will be for the child. Sexual victimization that happens over a long period is much more damaging than a onetime episode. It can lead to runaway behavior and sexual promiscuity, and it can interfere with relationships and intimacy later in life. Perhaps most significantly, the use or threatened use of force or bodily harm upon the child or her family members can significantly intensify the child's psychological trauma. She may react with feelings ranging from anxiety and fear to guilt and depression.

- **The age and developmental status of the child.** A younger child may have less difficulty with a brief sexual experience than an older one. This younger child may not fully comprehend what has happened to her, and more often, she may have been subjected to less force and coercion from the perpetrator. By contrast, an older child may understand more about the abusive experience and may feel more guilt, fear, and other emotions.

- **The relationship of the child and the abuser.** Although victimization by someone unknown to a child is upsetting, it may not be as bewildering as when a relative abuses a child sexually. The child may feel confusion about her relationship with the perpetrator and whether she can trust this individual again. The child also may feel more pressure not to disclose the abuse if a family member is involved.

- **The family's reaction.** If you are supportive of your child and convince her that she is not at fault and that she will be protected, the trauma can be minimized. If family members fail to act on the information they are given by the child, the abuse will likely persist, and the child's sense of trust and intimacy will be damaged.

A child who has experienced sexual abuse often requires professional help to minimize the chances of lasting psychological effects from the abuse. Your pediatrician should give you a referral to a counselor, as can the local child protection agency. In many communities there are sexual abuse support networks, treatment groups, and therapists who specialize in sexual victimization. All sexually abused children need an evaluation by a professional who is knowledgeable about the psychological consequences of abuse, and who can recommend treatment if it is needed. Families too can benefit from support and counseling to help them deal with their own feelings and more effectively provide emotional support for their child.

~ 52 ~

Chronic Conditions and Diseases

Anemia

Anemia is a condition in which the body has less than the optimal amount of red blood cells. It can cause an individual to feel weak and may cause paleness, or it may not cause any signs at all. Anemia is both preventable and treatable. Red blood cells have an important job: to carry hemoglobin, a protein that carries oxygen to different parts of the body. If the body doesn't produce enough red blood cells (for example, if there is not enough iron in the diet), destroys too many red blood cells (such as in sickle cell anemia), or loses red blood cells (through bleeding, which can occur from the intestines, or through menstruation), then the affected child may become anemic.

Even mild anemia can impact your child's energy levels and ability to learn. Usually a simple blood test called a blood count can diagnose anemia. Prevent anemia by ensuring a well-balanced diet with plenty of vitamins and minerals. If your family observes a specific diet, such as a vegan diet, speak with your pediatrician to determine if nutritional supplements are needed. A common cause of anemia in younger kids is too much milk; more than 2 cups a day of milk can fill up a child, reducing his intake of other, iron-rich foods. Good sources of iron include red meat, egg yolks, some green vegetables, beans, and raisins. Foods containing vitamin C can help the body absorb more iron.

Sickle Cell Anemia

Sickle cell anemia is a genetic condition in which the usual shape of red blood cells is altered, resulting in difficulty flowing normally through blood vessels. As a result, there can be episodes where blood flow is blocked, causing pain and a lack of oxygen. There are different types of sickle cell conditions, and affected children can also be at risk for infections. Children with sickle cell anemia have a more rapid turnover of red blood cells (the altered shape causes early destruction), which means that kids with sickle cell have a lower blood count than other kids. As a result of this, some children will require a blood transfusion.

Thankfully, all babies born at U.S. hospitals are now screened for both the sickle cell trait and sickle cell anemia. Newborn screenings allow infants with the condition to be identified before problems are seen, and treatments can prevent further complications. In addition to the pediatrician, a child with sickle cell anemia will be seen by a pediatric hematologist; some areas of the country also have comprehensive sickle cell centers.

Diabetes Mellitus

Insulin is an important hormone that helps the body properly move sugars from the bloodstream into the cells to be used for energy. When the body does not have enough insulin, or the body's cells are resistant to insulin, diabetes mellitus results. Diabetes can cause long-term damage to the heart, eyes, and other organs if not properly controlled.

Type 1 Diabetes

Type 1 diabetes affects about 1 in 400 children under the age of 20 years. It is a lifelong disease for which ongoing research is searching for a cure. The pancreas, the main organ involved in the progression of type 1 diabetes, is an important abdominal organ that produces the insulin needed for the body's cells to properly use sugars for energy. Within the pancreas there are beta cells, which produce insulin; in type 1 diabetes, the immune system attacks the beta cells with antibodies. Without insulin, sugars (glucose) build up in the bloodstream. Thankfully, insulin is available as a medication to treat type 1 diabetes.

Symptoms of type 1 diabetes are caused by two factors: a lack of energy resulting from the bloodstream's sugar not being usable, and dehydration caused by the sugar pulling out water as it is lost in the urine. Children may show increased thirst and urination, hunger associated with weight loss, fatigue, irritability or not feeling like their usual selves, vision changes, nausea, vomiting, abdominal pain, rapid breathing, or loss of consciousness, if levels have gotten dangerously high.

Blood and urine tests can help determine the diagnosis of diabetes. Some children require an initial hospital stay to stabilize their condition, control sugar levels, and begin the educational process of learning how to treat diabetes. Blood sugars will be checked frequently with a finger stick and a home glucose meter, and insulin is given through an injection every day. Older children who have demonstrated good responsibility in their diabetes self-care may be advanced to an insulin pump, which administers insulin through a catheter instead. Equally important as checking blood sugar and administering insulin are healthy food choices and physical activity. A pediatric endocrinologist, as well as a diabetes educator and a dietician, will work together as part of the healthcare team to better manage your child's diabetes.

Type 2 Diabetes

Kids who develop type 2 diabetes do not make enough insulin (see above), and the body's cells do not use insulin very well (termed *insulin resistance*). Children who have an elevated body mass index (BMI) or concerning weight-to-height ratio are at risk for developing type 2 diabetes. Lifestyle changes, including a proper diet and regular physical activity, are important to not only prevent type 2 diabetes

but also treat it (for more on nutrition, see Chapter 3; for more on activity, see Chapter 4). Minimize family screen time and ensure a minimum of an hour of fun, vigorous physical activity every day. Similar to type 1 diabetes, sugars will be checked on a regular basis, and medications may be required. Your pediatrician may involve a pediatric endocrinologist in your child's care.

HIV Infection and AIDS

HIV (human immunodeficiency virus) is the virus that causes AIDS (acquired immunodeficiency syndrome). Current guidelines promote checking all pregnant mothers for HIV (by means of a blood test) in order to determine which infants may be at risk of infection. Prevention, as well as early detection and treatment, can keep kids healthy. HIV impacts the body's immune system; if undetected, the virus can be spread to others and will cause problems in the body over time. HIV can be spread by sexual contact with both males and females, by contact with infected blood, from pregnant mother to developing or breastfeeding baby, or through blood products (which today are all routinely screened for HIV). There are medicines that can reduce HIV's impact; however, there is no current cure for HIV or AIDS.

Older school-age children should have conversations with their families about abstinence (the best way to prevent any sexually transmitted infection, or STI) and condom use, as well as the fact that other forms of birth control do not prevent HIV and other STIs. Other risky behaviors such as drug use (especially with shared needles) should be discussed with your older child. Anyone involved in these risky behaviors should be checked for HIV with a blood test. For more information on having conversations with your children on sex, see page 110. For conversations about substance abuse, see page 95.

~ 53 ~

Ears, Nose, and Throat

Colds/Upper Respiratory Infections

The common cold (also known as an upper respiratory infection) is typically caused by any one of a number of viruses. Sneezing and coughing spread the virus, either through direct person-to-person contact or indirectly when viral particles are picked up from a surface such as a door handle, for example, then transferred to that person's nose or mouth. Symptoms include runny nose or congestion, sneezing, cough, possible fever, and sore throat. For a school-age child, symptoms should be improving after seven days or so.

Usually a typical cold can be cared for at home, unless there is a concern for complications such as ear or sinus infections. If your child is having trouble breathing or has ear pain, or if the congestion or cough lasts longer than two weeks, call your pediatrician. There is no cure for the common cold; antibiotics work against *bacteria*, not viruses. The best care is supportive care, encouraging fluids (clear is best) and lots of rest. Single-ingredient acetaminophen or ibuprofen (avoid multi-ingredient cold medications) can be helpful if there is a fever. Always dose these medications by your child's weight and age. Over-the-counter decongestants usually don't work very well, are pricey, cause side effects, and are not recommended for children under the age of 6. Honey for kids older than 12 months can be helpful for a cough: 1 teaspoon for children ages 6 to 11 years, and 2 teaspoons for children 12 years and older. If honey is given at bedtime, make sure you brush your child's teeth afterward. Remember that it's not safe to give honey to babies younger than 1 year. Saline (salt water) sprays can help relieve congestion, as can a cool-mist humidifier or vaporizer in the bedroom in which your child is sleeping. This helps moisten the air and may help clear your child's nasal passages. Be sure to clean the humidifier or vaporizer often, as recommended by the manufacturer.

It's important to teach your kids to wash their hands regularly and to cough and sneeze away from others either into a tissue or into the inside of her elbow. To help kids remember this, many people call it the "cough pocket" or "sneeze pocket." This can help minimize the spread of the virus to others.

Ear Piercing

Ears may be pierced for cosmetic reasons at any age, and during the middle years of childhood, some kids will ask to have their ears pierced. If the piercing is performed carefully and cared for conscientiously, there is little risk, no matter what the age of the child. However, as a general guideline, postpone the piercing until your child is mature enough to take care of the pierced site herself.

For the actual piercing procedure, have a doctor, nurse, or experienced technician perform it using sterile techniques. Rubbing alcohol or other disinfectants should be used to minimize the chances of an infection. At the time of the piercing, a round, gold-post earring should be inserted; some piercing instruments themselves can put the gold posts in place at the same time, thus avoiding any additional probing that can increase the chance of infection. The gold in the posts will reduce the risk of an allergic reaction and inflammation in the area.

After the piercing, apply rubbing alcohol or an antibiotic ointment to the area two times a day for a few days; these applications will cut down the chances of infection and hasten the healing process. The earring should not be removed for four to six weeks, but should be gently rotated each day. If the area of piercing becomes red or tender, an infection may be developing, and you should seek medical attention promptly.

Middle Ear Infections

Middle ear infections, which doctors call *otitis media*, are less common during middle childhood than at younger ages. When an ear is infected, the eustachian tube—the narrow passage connecting the middle ear (the small chamber behind the eardrum) to the back of the nose—becomes blocked. During healthy periods this tube is able to open and close and keeps the space behind the eardrum free of fluid; during a cold or other respiratory infection, or in children with allergies, this tube can become blocked, fluid begins to accumulate in the middle ear, and bacteria start to grow there. As this occurs, pressure on the eardrum increases. Hearing sometimes can be temporarily reduced, and at the same time the pressure on the eardrum can cause pain.

Your pediatrician will examine your child's ears with an instrument called an otoscope, and will look for inflammation and fluid behind the eardrums. If your child is uncomfortable, acetaminophen or ibuprofen can help ease the pain. Sometimes, using a heating pad or a warm towel over the ear can also make your child feel better. Antibiotics are not always necessary; for an otherwise healthy child, watchful waiting is often recommended. By waiting, medication side effects such as rashes and diarrhea can be avoided, as well as addressing the larger concern of antibiotic resistance. If your child is very irritable, has severe pain, has persistent fevers, or develops ear drainage, antibiotics may be given.

Occasionally, when a child has repeated ear infections with persistent middle ear fluid, and/or there are concerns about a child's ability to hear properly, the doctor may suggest a referral to an ear specialist to determine if inserting small drainage tubes (tympanostomy tubes) through the eardrum to help remove the trapped fluid is needed. Some doctors may also suggest surgical removal of the adenoids (an adenoidectomy) if they are blocking the child's eustachian tube.

Ear infections are not contagious.

Your child can safely return to school after the pain and fever subside. However, he should continue taking the antibiotics as prescribed until the pills or liquid are used up.

Sinusitis

A sinus infection (sinusitis) can be caused by viruses, allergies, or bacteria. The lining of the sinuses (air-filled spaces within the facial bones) become inflamed, often following a common cold. The common cold can be distinguished from the complication of a bacterial infection of the sinuses by the time course of the symptoms; colds typically improve after seven days with minimal fevers, and a sinus infection should be suspected if congestion, cough, or other symptoms persist past two to three weeks. A headache behind or around the eyes, or fever longer than two days, are also signs of a bacterial sinus infection. If your pediatrician suspects a sinus infection caused by bacteria, she may prescribe an antibiotic medication. Symptoms should improve after two days of the medication, and the entire course should be completed so that the infection does not return. For symptomatic relief, the methods used for the common cold may be helpful (see "Colds/Upper Respiratory Infections," page 591). A warm washcloth on the face can help relieve headache, and acetaminophen or ibuprofen may help too.

Herpes Simplex/Cold Sores

Cold sores are oozing blisters that can erupt on any part of the body, although they tend to occur most often on or near the lips or inside the mouth. The herpes simplex virus, which can be transmitted from child to child or from parent to child, often through saliva, is responsible for these sores.

The first time your child has a herpes simplex infection, the lesions will typically spread throughout his mouth. Thereafter, the virus itself changes character and lies dormant within the nerve, occasionally reactivating in response to any of a number of triggers, including sunlight, cold, heat, fever, and stress. Just before these new blisters emerge, your child may feel an itching or tingling sensation in the area.

There are antiviral drugs that are effective against herpes simplex virus; these drugs are used for severe infections and for infections in children whose immune systems are not normal. Although these drugs can relieve symptoms and shorten the duration of the illness, they are not cures and do not prevent recurrences. Most children do not need antiviral therapy; topical therapy is not very helpful, and oral therapy must be started very early to be effective. The only therapy needed in most cases of cold sores is symptomatic relief. Many doctors recommend that children keep cold sores moist with lip balm or petroleum jelly in order to help relieve discomfort. These sores will eventually form scabs and heal, disappearing after seven to fourteen days. Until they are gone, discourage your child from scratching or picking at them. In general, however, there is no need to keep him home from school.

Nosebleeds

Nosebleeds are quite common in school-age children and are usually not ominous, but the experience can be frightening for child and parent alike. If the blood drains to the back of the throat the child may also gag or vomit. A common cause of nosebleeds is nose picking. Nosebleeds are also common in the winter due to dry air. Colds and allergies can irritate the inside of the nose and may lead to a nosebleed. Anatomic concerns or problems with blood clotting are less common causes of nosebleeds.

Remain calm, have your child tilt her head slightly forward (not back), and teach her to pinch the lower, soft part of the nose closed and hold it firmly for ten minutes. After ten minutes, release the pressure and see if the bleeding has stopped; if not, repeat the process. If after another ten minutes there is still bleeding, call your pediatrician or go to the closest emergency department. Also call your pediatrician if you are concerned your child is losing too much blood or if there are other worrisome symptoms such as vomiting a substance that looks like coffee grounds.

Avoiding nose picking, using saline (salt water) nasal spray and a humidifier or vaporizer in the bedroom, and applying petroleum jelly to the inside of nostrils using your fingertip nightly can help prevent nosebleeds.

Sore Throat (Strep Throat, Tonsillitis)

Like colds, most sore throats are caused by viruses. Sore throats are often a companion to the common cold. When sore throats occur, your child may experience swelling and redness of the tissues in his throat and sometimes enlarged tonsils. He may also feel fatigued and run a fever. The pain in the throat can range from mild to burning, and swallowing can be very uncomfortable.

To ease your child's sore throat, have him drink plenty of clear fluids. Sucking on hard candy or throat lozenges can also help and is usually just as effective as more expensive over-the-counter throat sprays. A cool-mist humidifier or vaporizer can keep the throat moist and more comfortable. Contact your pediatrician if your child has difficulty swallowing because of severe throat pain or if he is having trouble breathing. Your physician may suggest acetaminophen or ibuprofen for pain relief and controlling any accompanying fever.

Even though sore throats are caused primarily by viruses, a minority are caused by streptococcal bacteria (strep throat). If your doctor suspects strep throat, he or she will recommend performing a rapid strep test or a throat culture, a quick procedure in which mucus is swabbed from the throat and analyzed in the laboratory. If strep is confirmed, antibiotics will be prescribed to prevent complications (the most serious of these is rheumatic fever, which can damage heart valves). These same antibiotics, however, are *not* effective for viral sore throats. When kids have a strep infection, they can return to school twenty-four hours after antibiotic treatment has started, as long as they are free of a fever.

Children who sleep with their mouths open often awaken with a sore throat. This discomfort usually disappears in a short time, particularly after the child has had something to drink. Using a humidifier while children sleep can reduce this problem.

Swimmer's Ear (*Otitis Externa*)

Swimmer's ear, also called *otitis externa*, is an inflammation of the skin of the external ear canal. It occurs when water gets into the ear—usually during swimming or bathing—and does not properly drain out. When that happens, the canal can become irritated and infected. Children with this condition will complain of itching or pain in the ear, the latter particularly when the head or the ear itself is moved. As the canal swells, hearing will decrease. The infected ear may ooze yellowish pus.

Your doctor will diagnose *otitis externa* after examining the ear canal with an otoscope. He or she may treat it with prescription ear drops. Sometimes you will need to insert a gauze wick into your child's ear to make sure the drops reach the site of the swelling. If it is needed, your physician will demonstrate this procedure. Also, try keeping your child's ear canal as dry as possible during the healing process; that means delaying washing and shampooing until the inflammation has disappeared.

Once a child has had a swimmer's ear infection, you should try to prevent future episodes. To help avoid them, your child should place drops in the ears after swimming—either an over-the-counter formula or a mixture of one half alcohol, one half white vinegar. Also, dry the ears with a towel immediately after swimming or bathing. Avoid cotton swabs, as these can be more harmful than helpful.

Swollen Glands

Glands, or lymph nodes, are a normal, healthy part of the body's immune system. Glands contain lymphocytes, which produce the antibodies that fight infections. Glands often get a little bigger when lymphocytes are mobilized to create more antibodies in response to an infection. It is healthy and appropriate for lymph nodes to enlarge and recede in response to routine infections, and they are often slightly tender to the touch in these situations. A typical scenario is a sore throat associated with swollen glands in the neck. Viral sore throats, as well as strep throat or other infections, can cause swollen glands that can be slightly tender to the touch.

Call your pediatrician if an enlarged lymph node is growing faster than expected, is increasingly warm or tender to the touch, or is associated with a fever above 101 degrees Fahrenheit. Rarely, if a gland is swollen for a longer amount of time (more than five days), if it is in a concerning location such as above the collarbone, or if there is a lack of other symptoms, the swelling may represent an abnormal growth and should be evaluated by a physician. Let your doctor know if there are any tooth problems or gum inflammation, if you have cats in the home, or if there have been recent animal scratches, insect or tick bites, or stings that may have become infected. If the lymph node itself has become infected, showing signs of warmth, tenderness, and swelling, it may require antibiotics and warm compresses. More severe cases may need surgical drainage.

~ 54 ~

Emergencies

PREPARATION IN ADVANCE of any actual emergencies will help everyone stay calm in the event that something happens, so that you can respond to the emergency appropriately. Have emergency phone numbers—including 911 and the number of your pediatrician's office—programmed into your phone. The Poison Help line at 800-222-1222 will direct your call to the nearest poison control center. Everybody should use the same number; keep the number posted prominently in your home and also program the number into your cellphones. Find out where the closest emergency room is located and the quickest route to get there. Also, ask your pediatrician

how she would like you to respond to emergencies, both during and after office hours.

When an emergency occurs, quickly assess the situation, use common sense, and decide whether to implement lifesaving procedures (such as CPR) immediately, call for an ambulance, or phone your pediatrician for advice. When dialing 911, explain your child's condition or injury as calmly as possible. Dialing from your cellphone is helpful because it will allow you access to your child and to speak to emergency personnel at the same time. When performing lifesaving maneuvers under instruction from the emergency personnel, turn your cellphone to speaker mode. Your child will need immediate attention if he has stopped breathing or if he has no pulse. He will also require emergency help if he has lost consciousness.

Anaphylaxis

See page 537.

Animal Bites

Most animal bites are by cats and dogs, but serious infections can come from the bites of many animals, domestic and wild. Human bites can also be serious. Whether the wound is a puncture or just a scratch, clean it with soap and water and keep it under running water for several minutes. Then wrap it in sterile gauze and call your pediatrician, who will monitor the wound for infection; signs of infection include swelling, redness, and tenderness.

In some cases your doctor may suggest a tetanus vaccine. In some instances, such as with a puncture wound that carries a high risk of infection, prophylactic antibiotics may be indicated. You also need to locate the animal that inflicted the wound; the animal may need to be quarantined to make sure it does not develop rabies. The psychological harm associated with an animal bite may be as serious as the physical wound itself. Once bitten—or even snapped at or growled at—by a dog, a child may develop a fear of dogs. For more on animal safety, see page 336.

If your child is bitten by a snake, your immediate task is to determine whether your child has been bitten by a poisonous snake. Call your doctor, poison center, or local emergency department and be prepared to describe what the snake looked like. Take a photo of the wound with your cellphone camera if you can. The appearance of the affected skin may change by the time you get to medical attention. Use basic wound care measures: wash the wound and apply a clean, dry bandage. Your child may need an injection of antivenom serum. Until you can get her to a hospital emergency department, don't give her anything to eat or drink, remove any jewelry, and try to keep the bitten region of her body lower than the heart. Do not attempt to suck the venom out of the wound; this is not effective and can increase the risk of infection in the wound. Only use a tourniquet (a constricting band) if instructed via 911 to do so. You might be instructed to use a tourniquet if long transport (more than thirty to sixty minutes) is anticipated; the bands should not cut off the pulse or the blood flow through the arteries, and should be loose enough to place a finger within. For insect stings and bites, see page 543.

Burns

In addition to fires, children suffer burns in a variety of ways, ranging from hot water scalds and sun exposure to chemical agents and electrical burns. Thermal burns from sun exposure are the most common types of burns, and while most cause only a temporary inconvenience, in the long term they have been found to be related to skin cancer. Children also suffer burns when they are using fireworks or playing with wires that are not properly insulated. There are three types of burns. *First-degree burns* are the least serious, causing redness and in some cases mild swelling of the skin; they usually heal in a week or two with no scarring. *Second-degree burns* result in redness, blistering, and a lot of swelling; the burn can ooze fluid, the pain can be severe, and some scarring may result. *Third-degree burns* are the most serious, injuring not only the surface skin but the deeper layers of skin as well. This can leave the skin often having a dry, leathery appearance, a loss of sensation, and a color that can range from black to pearly white.

Immediately after a burn has occurred, immerse the affected area in cool water. Do not use ice, but rather

When Is Your Child in an Emergency Situation?

A parent's instincts can help decide whether a child needs emergency attention. Here are some situations that generally require immediate attention:

- Severe cuts or lacerations

- A head injury accompanied by loss of consciousness or vomiting

- A very high fever in a child who is excessively sleepy or not normally responsive and has a headache, vomiting, or a stiff neck

- Severe burns of all types, including chemical and electrical burns, especially on the face

- Poisoning, caused by ingesting dangerous chemicals or medications

- Seizures lasting more than fifteen minutes, or any unexpected seizures

- A serious animal bite, particularly one that has caused a break in the skin

- Difficulty in breathing, or a cessation of breathing, including airway obstruction and choking

- Absence of a heartbeat and pulse

- Sudden onset of a severe headache

- Signs of shock, including pale, cold, clammy skin and a weak and rapid pulse

- An altered mental state: either a decrease in the level of consciousness or, conversely, uncontrollable agitated behavior

- A fracture (broken bone), which can look like a deformed or swollen arm or leg, after an injury

run the water over the burn, relieving the pain and cooling the area. Also, remove all clothing from the burned area, except for clothing stuck to the skin. Cover the injured area with a sterile gauze pad, applying it lightly if the burn is oozing. Do not apply grease, butter, or powder to the burn.

For chemical burns, flush the burned area immediately with large amounts of water. Do not waste precious time removing clothing before this flushing process begins; the clothing can be removed once flushing has started. Call 911 for emergency services while continuing to soak the child with water for ten to twenty minutes. Contact your pediatrician at once for all serious burns, as well as for any burns to the mouth, hands, or genitals. Your child may have to be hospitalized if she has suffered third-degree burns, or if a larger area of the body has been burned.

You can help prevent burns by installing smoke detectors in your home in all the rooms in which people sleep, as well as in the hallways outside the bedrooms. Also place detectors in the kitchen and the living room, with at least one on each level of the house. Make sure your home's water heater is set so the temperature at the faucet is no higher than 120 degrees Fahrenheit to prevent scalding burns.

Your family should practice fire drills regularly. Make sure everyone knows where to meet outside the house when the smoke alarm goes off. Remind your children to crawl to the exits if there is smoke in the room, staying below the smoke, where there is more oxygen. Also teach your kids to stop, drop, and roll on the ground if their clothing catches fire.

Cardiopulmonary Resuscitation (CPR)

CPR can save a child's life if he has stopped breathing or his heart has stopped beating. The American Academy of Pediatrics recommends that all parents and caregivers take a CPR and choking course to be prepared for an emergency; contact your local chapter of the American Heart Association or the American Red Cross to find certified courses in your community. Please refer to the Choking/CPR chart instructions opposite.

Choking happens when food or another object blocks air flow to the lungs. Choking can be a life-threatening emergency and requires a prompt response from parents and caregivers. Please refer to the Choking/CPR chart instructions opposite.

Cold and Heat Emergencies

If your child is exposed to extreme temperatures—usually for an extended period of time and without appropriate clothing or other protection—he could find himself in a life-threatening situation.

Hypothermia

Hypothermia develops when a child's temperature falls below normal due to exposure to cold. This condition often

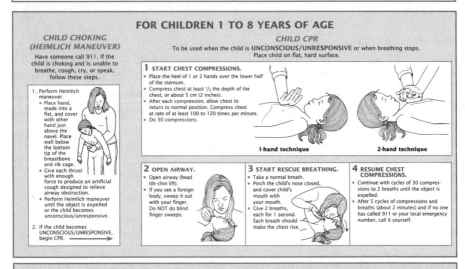

CHOKING/CPR

LEARN AND PRACTICE CPR (CARDIOPULMONARY RESUSCITATION).

IF ALONE WITH A CHILD WHO IS CHOKING...

1. SHOUT FOR HELP. 2. START RESCUE EFFORTS. 3. CALL 911 OR YOUR LOCAL EMERGENCY NUMBER.

START FIRST AID FOR CHOKING IF	DO *NOT* START FIRST AID FOR CHOKING IF
• The child cannot breathe at all (the chest is not moving up and down). • The child cannot cough or talk or looks blue. • The child is found unconscious/unresponsive. (Go to CPR.)	• The child can breathe, cry, or talk. • The child can cough, sputter, or move air at all. The child's normal reflexes are working to clear the airway.

FOR CHILDREN 1 TO 8 YEARS OF AGE

CHILD CHOKING (HEIMLICH MANEUVER)

Have someone call 911. If the child is choking and is unable to breathe, cough, cry, or speak, follow these steps.

1. Perform Heimlich maneuver.
   - Place hand, made into a fist, and cover with other hand just above the navel. Place well below the bottom tip of the breastbone and rib cage.
   - Give each thrust with enough force to produce an artificial cough designed to relieve airway obstruction.
   - Perform Heimlich maneuver until the object is expelled or the child becomes unconscious/unresponsive.
2. If the child becomes UNCONSCIOUS/UNRESPONSIVE, begin CPR. ➡

CHILD CPR

To be used when the child is **UNCONSCIOUS/UNRESPONSIVE** or when breathing stops.
Place child on flat, hard surface.

1 START CHEST COMPRESSIONS.
- Place the heel of 1 or 2 hands over the lower half of the sternum.
- Compress chest at least $^1/_3$ the depth of the chest, or about 5 cm (2 inches).
- After each compression, allow chest to return to normal position. Compress chest at rate of at least 100 to 120 times per minute.
- Do 30 compressions.

1-hand technique   2-hand technique

2 OPEN AIRWAY.
- Open airway (head tilt-chin lift).
- If you see a foreign body, sweep it out with your finger. Do NOT do blind finger sweeps.

3 START RESCUE BREATHING.
- Take a normal breath.
- Pinch the child's nose closed, and cover child's mouth with your mouth.
- Give 2 breaths, each for 1 second. Each breath should make the chest rise.

4 RESUME CHEST COMPRESSIONS.
- Continue with cycles of 30 compressions to 2 breaths until the object is expelled.
- After 5 cycles of compressions and breaths (about 2 minutes) and if no one has called 911 or your local emergency number, call it yourself.

If at any time an object is coughed up or the infant/child starts to breathe, stop rescue breaths and call 911 or your local emergency number.

Ask your pediatrician for information on choking/CPR instructions for children older than 8 years and for information on an approved first aid or CPR course in your community.

occurs when a child is playing outdoors in extremely cold weather without wearing proper clothing. As hypothermia sets in, the child may shiver and become lethargic and clumsy; his speech may become slurred and his body temperature will decline. Call 911 at once. Until help arrives, take the child indoors, remove any wet clothing, and wrap him in blankets or warm clothes. If his breathing or pulse stops, he will need mouth-to-mouth resuscitation or CPR.

Frostbite

Frostbite takes place when the skin and outer tissues become frozen. This condition tends to occur on extremities like the fingers, toes, ears, and nose, which may become pale, gray, and blistered. At the same time, the child may complain that his skin burns or has become numb. Bring the child indoors, where you should place the frostbitten parts of his body in warm (not hot) water; warm washcloths may be applied to a frostbitten nose, ears, and lips. Do not rub the frozen area. After a few minutes, dry and cover him with clothing or blankets. Give him something warm to drink. If the numbness continues for more than a few minutes, call your doctor.

Heatstroke

Heatstroke can occur when a child overexerts herself in very hot weather and becomes dehydrated. The mechanisms in the brain that control body temperature can stop working, and he may run a temperature of 105 degrees or higher. His skin will become hot, *dry* (not perspiring), and flushed. He may feel dizzy and nauseated, and experience stomach cramps and rapid breathing. You should move a child with heatstroke out of the sun, and call for emergency help (911) quickly. Take off his clothing and place him in a cool (not cold) bathtub. To help restore circulation, massage his arms, legs, and other body parts.

Your child should always increase his fluid intake in hot weather, especially while exercising. Encourage him to drink readily available liquids regularly, typically a cup of water for every twenty to thirty minutes the child has been outside. When your child participates in organized sports in the hot months of summer, he should dress in a minimal amount of loose-fitting clothing.

Cuts and Lacerations

All kids scrape their knees or elbows from time to time, often causing mild bleeding. However, when children suffer a serious cut or laceration, or profuse bleeding, this should be treated as an emergency. First, clean the wound with soap and water, even placing it under running water, which will allow you to examine the wound more closely and gauge the intensity of the bleeding. Next, your immediate task is to stop the bleeding. Apply a sterile gauze pad over the cut. If gauze is not available, use a clean handkerchief, towel, or shirt. Press forcefully with the palm of the hand until the bleeding subsides, and then keep the dressing on for a few extra minutes. If the gauze becomes saturated, put a new layer over the one that is there. Seek medical attention to determine if the laceration requires suturing in order to be closed and heal well.

If the bleeding is pulsating or spurting and continues this way for several minutes, it may be harder to stop. In that case, apply direct pressure with the palm of your hand and call 911. Large amounts of blood loss can cause your child to lapse into a state of shock. You can minimize the chances of shock by having your child lie down and elevate her feet a few inches until the emergency team arrives. If the cut is deep or its edges are rough, take your child to the emergency room. Wounds such as this almost always need emergency care.

Drowning

Drowning is a leading cause of death among children. Children older than 5 years old are most likely to drown in rivers and lakes, but this varies from one area of the country to another. Swimming lessons are invaluable; however, even strong swimmers can drown, so parents and caregivers must remain vigilant whenever children are in or near water. Even experienced swimmers should not swim alone; a watchful adult should always be present in case of emergency. In social situations such as a pool party, adults can take turns monitoring the kids and should avoid using phones, doing chores, carrying on conversations with others, and other distractions while being on watch. Home swimming pools need to be fenced on all four sides with a self-locking, self-latching gate. For any home by a pool or other body of water such as a lake, river, or creek, parents should learn CPR and keep safety equipment such as life preservers and a shepherd's crook ready at the water's edge, and use life preservers when boating.

In real life, drowning doesn't look the way it is represented on television and in the movies. If the child's head is low in the water, with mouth at water level, or tilted back with an open mouth, eyes closed or unable to focus, gasping, or if the child is trying to move and not making progress, help that child immediately.

If your child is involved in a drowning emergency, check for breathing first, and if she is not breathing, start CPR immediately (see page 600). If you have help, have the other person call 911 while you keep working. Do not stop CPR unless the child begins breathing on her own. Gagging or vomiting water is common in this situation. Afterward the child should see a physician for an exam, even if all seems well. Longer monitoring overnight in the hospital, to monitor for damage to the heart, lungs, or brain, may be warranted if she lost consciousness or if there are other concerns.

Eye Injuries

If a foreign substance is splashed in your child's eye, flush it gently with water for at least fifteen minutes. Call your pediatrician or Poison Help (800-222-1222) for additional recommendations. If your child's eye is injured or if it hurts, do not touch or rub the injured eye; do not apply medications. Gently place a soft covering over the painful eye (do not apply pressure) and seek medical attention promptly. If an object becomes stuck in the eye, do not try to remove it; take your child to an emergency room immediately.

Fainting

An episode of fainting, or syncope, requires consultation with your pediatrician, although brief periods of unconsciousness, while frightening, are usually not serious. Prior to fainting, a child may feel light-headed and nauseated; she will then become limp and fall to the floor. These episodes typically take place when there is a temporarily inadequate supply of blood and oxygen to the brain, often related to stress, fear, or overexertion. Hot weather, pain, an empty stomach, or a peculiar odor can also sometimes cause a child to faint. A classic example of fainting is an otherwise healthy child who has been standing too long in a warm room without having had anything to eat or drink for a while.

Generally, fainting spells last for just a minute or less (although to a parent it may seem like much longer), after which normal blood flow returns and the child regains consciousness. Until then, keep your child lying down with her feet slightly elevated. Some fainting episodes require immediate attention: Call 911 if your child remains unconscious for more than two minutes, has difficulty breathing, or shakes or jerks while unconscious. A weak pulse or shallow breathing requires emergency care.

At times children can hit their head when fainting; for more on head injuries, see page 604.

Fingertip Injuries

Children's fingers sometimes get caught in closing doors. If there is bleeding from the fingertip, wash gently with soap and water and cover the injury with a soft, sterile dressing. Apply a cold compress such as a bag of frozen peas to keep down the swelling. Call your pediatrician at once if there is ex-

cessive swelling, a deep cut, or a loose fingernail. Over the ensuing hours, contact your pediatrician if the swelling and pain worsen, if there is drainage from the injury, or if a fever develops. Pain from blood under a fingernail can be relieved by your child's doctor. If pain persists or if there is point tenderness over a bone, there may be a fracture.

First-Aid Guidelines

Please refer to the diagrams on pages 606 and 607 for more information.

Fractures and Sprains

If your child has a neck or back injury, do not move her, since this can cause serious additional harm. If an injured part of the body hurts or is swollen or deformed, or if moving it causes pain, there might be a fracture. Do not tape or splint an injured arm or leg. You can apply a cold compress (a bag of frozen peas is perfect for this) and call an ambulance or your pediatrician.

For more on sprains, see page 641.

Head Injury/Concussion

From playing with friends at a playground to competing on the soccer field, school-age kids will bump their heads from time to time. While most head injuries are minor, parents and caregivers should be aware of worrisome symptoms following a head injury that indicate the need for urgent medical attention. If a head bump occurs and your child is alert and responsive, apply a cold compress as needed and monitor your child's symptoms. If headache persists or gets worse, your child vomits more than two times, speech is slurred, vision is blurry, or your child is irritable or otherwise not acting like her usual self, call the pediatrician. If your child loses consciousness, call 911 immediately. If the head bump occurs during an athletic event, the child should not be allowed to return to play.

After a head injury an adult should monitor the child for the next twenty-four hours to see if symptoms develop. It is okay for your child to go to sleep; however, your pediatrician may recommend waking your child every three hours to make sure she responds appropriately to you. Avoid over-the-counter pain medications unless your pediatrician says it is okay. If your child does well with twenty-four hours of close observation, there should not be longer-term issues.

Some children develop persistent headaches, dizziness, irritability, and other symptoms following a head injury that may indicate that the child sustained a concussion. For more on concussion, see page 58.

Meningitis

Meningitis is a condition in which the fluid and tissues that cover the brain and spinal cord are inflamed. Children with meningitis fare better with early detection and treatment; some forms of bacterial meningitis progress quite rapidly and risk complications. Due to the success of modern-day vaccines that protect against several types of bacterial meningitis, in the twenty-first century most cases of meningitis are caused by viruses.

Typically viral meningitis has a less serious course than bacterial meningitis. There is no need for antibiotics with viral meningitis, and with supportive care, most children recover well. There are several types of bacterial meningitis that can be more serious than the viral types. With prompt diagnosis and initiation of treatment, most children with bacterial meningitis improve, but in some cases there can be complications such as hearing loss, seizures, learning difficulties, or even death. For this reason, call your pediatrician or go to the ER immediately if your child has a severe headache, stiff neck, fever, sensitivity to bright lights, vomiting, extreme sleepiness, or other worrisome signs. If meningitis is suspected, blood tests and a spinal tap (lumbar puncture) will be performed. A spinal tap involves inserting a sterile needle into the lower back to obtain a sample of spinal fluid, which can then be tested in the lab.

Vaccines are safe and effective, and can prevent several types of bacterial meningitis. The meningococcal vaccine is given to children at 11 years and 16 years of age. A meningococcal vaccine that covers type B is now available for teens entering the college years.

FIRST AID

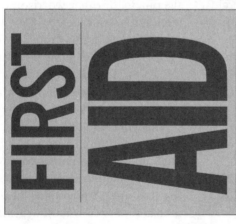

Call 911 or your local emergency number for a severely ill or injured child.

Call 1-800-222-1222 (Poison Help) if you have a poison emergency.

GENERAL

- Know how to get help.
- Make sure the area is safe for you and the child.
- When possible, personal protective equipment (such as gloves) should be used.
- Position the child appropriately if her airway needs to be opened or CPR (cardiopulmonary resuscitation) is needed. (Please see other side.)
- DO NOT MOVE A CHILD WHO MAY HAVE A NECK OR BACK INJURY (from a fall, motor vehicle crash, or other injury or if the child says his neck or back hurts) unless he is in danger.
- Look for anything (such as emergency medical identification jewelry or paperwork) that may give you information about health problems.

SKIN WOUNDS

Make sure the child is up to date for tetanus vaccination. Any open wound may need a tetanus booster even when the child is currently immunized. If the child has an open wound, ask the pediatrician if the child needs a tetanus booster.

Bruises Apply cool compresses. Call the pediatrician if the child has a crush injury, large bruises, continued pain, or swelling. The pediatrician may recommend acetaminophen for pain.

Cuts Rinse small cuts with water until clean. Use direct pressure with a clean cloth to stop bleeding and hold in place for 1 to 2 minutes. If the cut is not deep, apply an antibiotic ointment; then cover the cut with a clean bandage. Call the pediatrician or seek emergency care for large or deep cuts, or if the wound is wide open. For major bleeding, call for help (911 or your local emergency number). Continue direct pressure with a clean cloth until help arrives.

Scrapes Rinse with clean, running tap water for at least 5 minutes to remove dirt and germs. Do not use detergents, alcohol, or peroxide. Apply an antibiotic ointment and a bandage that will not stick to the wound.

Splinters Remove small splinters with tweezers; then wash until clean. If you cannot remove the splinter completely, call the pediatrician.

Puncture Wounds Do not remove large objects (such as a knife or stick) from a wound. Call for help (911 or your local emergency number). Such objects must be removed by a doctor. Call the pediatrician for all puncture wounds. The child may need a tetanus booster.

Bleeding Apply pressure with gauze over the bleeding area for 1 to 2 minutes. If still bleeding, add more gauze and apply pressure for another 5 minutes. You can also wrap an elastic bandage firmly over gauze and apply pressure. If bleeding continues, call for help (911 or your local emergency number).

EYE INJURIES

If anything is splashed in the eye, flush gently with water for at least 15 minutes. Call Poison Help (1-800-222-1222) or the pediatrician for further advice. Any injured or painful eye should be seen by a doctor. Do NOT touch or rub an injured eye. Do NOT apply medicine. Do NOT remove objects stuck in the eye. Cover the painful or injured eye with a paper cup or eye shield until you can get medical help.

CONVULSIONS, SEIZURES

If the child is breathing, lay her on her side to prevent choking. Call 911 or your local emergency number for a prolonged seizure (more than 5 minutes).

Make sure the child is safe from objects that could injure her. Be sure to protect her head. Do not put anything in the child's mouth. Loosen any tight clothing. Start rescue breathing if the child is blue or not breathing. (Please see other side.)

HEAD INJURIES

DO NOT MOVE A CHILD WHO MAY HAVE A SERIOUS HEAD, NECK, OR BACK INJURY. This may cause further harm.

Call 911 or your local emergency number right away if the child

- Loses consciousness
- Has a seizure (convulsion)
- Experiences clumsiness or inability to move any body part
- Has oozing of blood or watery fluid from ears or nose
- Has abnormal speech or behavior

Call the pediatrician for a child with a head injury and any of the following symptoms:

- Drowsiness
- Difficulty being awakened
- Persistent headache or vomiting

For any questions about less serious injuries, call the pediatrician.

POISONS

If the child has been exposed to or ingested a poison, call Poison Help at 1-800-222-1222. A poison expert is available 24 hours a day, 7 days a week.

Swallowed Poisons Any nonfood substance is a potential poison. Do not give anything by mouth or induce vomiting. Call Poison Help right away. Do not delay calling, but try to have the substance label or name available when you call.

Fumes, Gases, or Smoke Get the child into fresh air and call 911, the fire department, or your local emergency number. If the child is not breathing, start CPR and continue until help arrives. (Please see other side.)

Skin Exposure If acids, lye, pesticides, chemicals, poisonous plants, or any potentially poisonous substance comes in contact with a child's skin, eyes, or hair, brush off any residual material while wearing rubber gloves, if possible. Remove contaminated clothing. Wash skin, eyes, or hair with a large amount of water or mild soap and water. Do not scrub. Call Poison Help for further advice.

If a child is unconscious, becoming drowsy, having convulsions, or having trouble breathing, call 911 or your local emergency number. Bring the poisonous substance (safely contained) with you to the hospital.

STINGS, BITES, AND ALLERGIES

Stinging Insects Remove the stinger as soon as possible with a scraping motion using a firm item (such as the edge of a credit card). Put a cold compress on the bite to relieve the pain. If trouble breathing; fainting; swelling of lips, face, or throat; or hives over the entire body occurs, call 911 or your local emergency number right away. For hives in a small area, nausea, or vomiting, call the pediatrician. For spider bites, call the pediatrician or Poison Help (1-800-222-1222).

Have the pediatrician check any bites that become red, warm, swollen, or painful.

Animal or Human Bites Wash the wound well with soap and water. Call the pediatrician. The child may need a tetanus or rabies shot or antibiotics.

Ticks Use tweezers or your fingers to grasp as close as possible to the head of the tick and briskly pull the tick away from where it is attached. Call the pediatrician if the child develops symptoms such as a rash or fever.

Snake Bites Take the child to an emergency department if you are unsure of the type of snake or if you are concerned that the snake may be poisonous. Keep the child at rest. Do not apply ice. Loosely splint the injured area and keep it at rest, positioned at or slightly below the level of the heart. Identify the snake if you can do so safely. If you are not able to identify the snake but are able to kill it safely, take it with you to the emergency department for identification.

Allergy Swelling, problems breathing, and paleness may be signs of severe allergy. Call 911 or your local emergency number right away. Some people may have emergency medicine for these times. If possible, ask about emergency medicine they may have and help them administer it if necessary.

FEVER

Fever in children is usually caused by infection. It also can be caused by chemicals, poisons, medicines, an environment that is too hot, or an extreme level of overactivity.

Take the child's temperature to see if he has a fever. Most pediatricians consider any thermometer reading 100.4°F (38°C) or higher as a fever. However, the way the child looks and acts is more important than how high the child's temperature is.

Call the pediatrician right away if the child has a fever and

- Appears very ill, is unusually drowsy, or is very fussy
- Has other symptoms such as a stiff neck, a severe headache, severe sore throat, severe ear pain, an unexplained rash, repeated vomiting or diarrhea, or difficulty breathing
- Has a condition causing immune suppression (such as sickle cell disease, cancer, or chronic steroid use)
- Has had a first seizure but is no longer seizing
- Is younger than 3 months (12 weeks) and has a temperature of 100.4°F (38°C) or higher
- Has been in a very hot place, such as an overheated car

To make the child more comfortable, dress him in light clothing, give him cool liquids to drink, and keep him calm. The pediatrician may recommend fever medicines. Do NOT use aspirin to treat a child's fever. Aspirin has been linked with Reye syndrome, a serious disease that affects the liver and brain.

FRACTURES AND SPRAINS

If an injured area is painful, swollen, or deformed, or if motion causes pain, wrap it in a towel or soft cloth and make a splint with cardboard or other firm material to hold the arm or leg in place. Do not try to straighten. Apply ice or a cool compress wrapped in thin cloth for not more than 20 minutes. Call the pediatrician or seek emergency care. If there is a break in the skin near the fracture or if you can see the bone, cover the area with a clean bandage, make a splint as described above, and seek emergency care.

If the foot or hand below the injured part is cold or discolored (blue or pale), seek emergency care right away.

BURNS AND SCALDS

General Treatment First, stop the burning process by removing the child from contact with hot water or a hot object (for example, hot iron). If clothing is burning, smother flames. Remove clothing unless it is firmly stuck to the skin. Run cool water over burned skin until the pain stops. Do not apply ice, butter, grease, medicine, or ointment.

Burns With Blisters Do not break the blisters. Ask the pediatrician how to cover the burn. For burns on the face, hands, feet, or genitals, seek emergency care.

Large or Deep Burns Call 911 or your local emergency number. After stopping and cooling the burn, keep the child warm with a clean sheet covered with a blanket until help arrives.

Electrical Burns Disconnect electrical power. If the child is still in contact with an electrical source, do NOT touch the child with bare hands. Pull the child away from the power source with an object that does not conduct electricity (such as a wooden broom handle) only after the power is turned off. ALL electrical burns need to be seen by a doctor.

NOSEBLEEDS

Keep the child in a sitting position with the head tilted slightly forward. Apply firm, steady pressure to both nostrils by squeezing them between your thumb and index finger for 5 minutes. If bleeding continues or is very heavy, call the pediatrician or seek emergency care.

TEETH

Baby Teeth If knocked out or broken, apply clean gauze to control bleeding and call the pediatric or family dentist.

Permanent Teeth If knocked out, handle the tooth by the top and not the root (the part that would be in the gum). If dirty, rinse gently without scrubbing or touching the root. Do not use any cleansers. Use cold running water or milk. Place the tooth in egg white or coconut water or, if those are unavailable, milk, saline solution (1 teaspoon of table salt added to 8 ounces of water), or water, and transport the tooth with the child when seeking emergency care. If the tooth is broken, save the pieces in milk. Stop bleeding using gauze or a cotton ball in the tooth socket and have the child bite down. Call and go directly to the pediatric or family dentist or an emergency department.

FAINTING

Check the child's airway and breathing. If necessary, call 911 and begin rescue breathing and CPR. (Please see other side.)

If vomiting has occurred, turn the child onto one side to prevent choking. Elevate the feet above the level of the heart (about 12 inches).

Does your community have 911? If not, note the number of your local ambulance service and other important numbers below.

BE PREPARED: CALL 911
KEEP EMERGENCY NUMBERS BY YOUR TELEPHONE.

PEDIATRICIAN

PEDIATRIC OR FAMILY DENTIST

POISON HELP 1-800-222-1222

AMBULANCE

EMERGENCY DEPARTMENT

FIRE

POLICE

ADDRESS OF AND DIRECTIONS TO THE LOCATION

(FOR BABYSITTERS, CAREGIVERS)

American Academy of Pediatrics

DEDICATED TO THE HEALTH OF ALL CHILDREN®

Poisoning/Substance Use

While usually more common in children younger than 6 years of age, poisoning can occur at any age. You should suspect poisoning if your child has been handling an open or empty container of a medication or other potentially toxic substance, especially if he is not acting like himself. Signs to look for include unusual drooling, burns in the mouth, unexplained vomiting, abdominal cramping with no fever, breathing problems, excessive sleepiness, loss of consciousness, or other worrisome signs.

If you suspect your child has been exposed to poison or an inappropriate medication, call Poison Help or your pediatrician as soon as possible. In the United States and many of its territories, the Poison Help line at 800-222-1222 is available twenty-four hours a day. When in doubt call 911 instead. The next steps will depend on what the child has ingested or been exposed to. Poison Help can give specific instructions if you know the particular substance your child has ingested. If your child ingested part of a plant, take a picture of the plant with your phone if possible. If your child ingested medications or chemicals, it is helpful to take the bottle to the emergency department if your child needs to be seen.

Inhalants

When most people think of the term "drug use" they think of illicit or illegal substances; however, younger children may experiment with regular household items. School-age children as young as 5 or 6 may try inhalants, for example. Inhalants are easily found in the home and can be misused to get high. Inhalants can be deadly, even the first time they are tried. Parents should have open discussions with their kids to inform them of the risks and facts about inhalant abuse, which is also known as huffing, sniffing, or solvent abuse.

Inhalants include solvents, fuels, nitrous oxide, and volatile nitrites. Solvents are in most homes, may be liquid or aerosol, and include glues, felt-tip markers, paints, and disinfectants. Any products in pressurized spray cans, including hair spray or spray paint, can be abused. Fuels include gasoline and refrigerants. Nitrous oxide can be found in the steel cylinder of a whipped-cream dispenser. Volatile nitrites are found in air fresheners. Inhalant users sniff or huff the fumes using a rag soaked with the chemicals, or breathe in the fumes directly from the product cans.

Signs of inhalant abuse can be subtle, such as attitude changes or poor school performance. Parents should be alerted to behavior changes, anxiety, sores around the mouth, loss of appetite, or other worrisome signs. Even with the first use, inhalants can directly affect the heart, leading to abnormal heart rhythms and sudden death, or lead to permanent brain damage. Initially a user feels a brief stimulating feeling, followed by dizziness. Kids who use inhalants are at risk of progressing to other drugs.

Keep the doors of communication open with your kids. Teach your child healthy values and discuss the risks of drug use, including inhalants. Encourage your children to ask you questions, and listen to them while they talk. Develop strategies to combat peer pressure, and role-play scenarios in which your child may encounter peers experimenting with inhalants or other drugs. If you have concerns that your child is using inhalants or other drugs, consult with your pediatrician.

Seizures

See page 629.

Teeth

If a baby (primary) tooth is knocked out or broken, apply clean gauze to the gum to control the bleeding and call your dentist. If a permanent tooth is dislodged, rinse the tooth gently without handling the root. Then insert the tooth into its socket and hold it there on the way to the dentist's office; alternatively, transport the tooth in a glass of cold cow's milk. Time is important, so get your child into the dentist as soon as possible. If the tooth is broken, save the pieces, and gently clean the injured area with warm water. Apply a cold compress to reduce swelling, and go to the dentist at once.

~ 55 ~

Environmental Health

YOU MAY BE surprised that there are substances or items inside the home that could potentially harm your child. There can also be hazards found in the dust and dirt in or around your home and yard. The following are examples of environmental hazards found where children live and play, and what you can do to keep your children safe from harm.

Asbestos

Asbestos is a natural fiber that was often used for fireproofing, insulating, and soundproofing in schools, homes, and public buildings between the 1940s and 1970s.

Asbestos is only dangerous when it becomes crumbly. If that happens, asbestos fibers get into the air and are breathed into the lungs. Breathing in these fibers can cause chronic health problems, including a rare form of lung cancer. Asbestos can still be found in some older homes, often as insulation around pipes.

Schools are required by law to remove asbestos or make sure that children are not exposed to it. If you think there might be asbestos in your home, have a professional inspector check it out to be safe. Older homes should have a certified contractor help contain and remove the asbestos properly. Local health departments and regional offices of the Environmental Protection Agency (EPA) can provide the names of individuals and labs certified to inspect homes for asbestos. To locate the regional EPA office nearest to you, go to epa.gov/asbestos.

Carbon Monoxide

Carbon monoxide (CO) is a toxic gas that has no taste, no color, and no odor. It comes from appliances or heaters that burn gas, oil, wood, propane, or kerosene. Carbon monoxide poisoning is very dangerous. If left unchecked, exposure to CO can lead to memory loss, personality changes, brain damage, and death. When a child breathes carbon monoxide, it harms his blood's ability to transport oxygen. Although everyone is at risk for carbon monoxide poisoning, it is particularly dangerous for children, because they breathe faster and inhale more carbon monoxide per pound of body weight. Symptoms may include flu-like symptoms such as headache and nausea, shortness of breath, fatigue, confusion, and fainting.

It is important to make sure your home has proper carbon monoxide detectors. Make sure they are placed on each floor of your house, near bedrooms, and near the furnace. Remember to change the batteries so that the detector is always working properly. Have furnaces, wood stoves, fireplaces, and gas-fired water heaters, ovens, ranges, and clothes dryers checked and serviced each year.

To avoid carbon monoxide poisoning, remember:

■ Never leave a car running in an attached garage, even if the garage door is open.

■ Never use a charcoal grill inside the home or in a closed space.

■ Never use a gas oven to heat your home.

If you suspect carbon monoxide poisoning, call Poison Help at 800-222-1222, and call the fire department to check your home for carbon monoxide. See your doctor right away if more than one person in your house has flu-like symptoms (headache, fatigue, nausea) at the same time, especially if the symptoms go away when you leave the house.

Household Products

Many cleaning products give off dangerous fumes or leave residues. These products can be harmful if they are not thrown out properly (for example, if they are left in the garage). It is important to ensure proper ventilation of fumes when using these products. Open a window or the front door to allow fresh air in. Read the directions carefully for proper use of the product, and don't combine products. More importantly, store these products in a safe place where children can't reach. Bring empty containers to your local hazardous waste disposal center.

Lead

Lead exposure, a significant environmental problem, is of particular concern to children younger than 5 years of age. Lead is a metal that can be found in old houses or products from outside the United States. Your child can get lead in her body if she swallows lead dust, breathes lead vapors, or eats soil or paint chips that have lead in them. Lead poisoning can cause learning disabilities, behavioral problems, anemia, or damage to the brain and kidneys.

Lead is most often found in:

- Paint that is on the inside and outside of homes built before 1978

- Dust and chips from old paint

- Soil that has lead in it (particularly around older homes, businesses that used lead, or highways)

- Hobby materials such as paints, solders, fishing weights, and buckshot

- Dust from bullets and firing ranges

- Food stored in certain ceramic dishes (especially if dishes were made in another country)

- Ethnic spices from outside the United States

- Jewelry and cosmetics made outside of the United States

- Older painted toys and furniture such as cribs

- Tap water, especially in homes that have lead solder on pipes

- Mini-blinds manufactured outside the United States before July 1997

If your home was built before 1978, you need to test the paint for lead. Any

WHERE WE STAND

Lead may cause behavioral and cognitive problems to children even with low levels of exposure. While the effects from lead can be irreversible, proper nutrition and enrichment activities may help overcome these effects. The American Academy of Pediatrics supports primary prevention, including knowing about and fixing lead hazards before the child lives in the home. The pediatrician should ask questions about the risks of lead exposure; if a risk is found, a blood test should be done. Education about lead risks and fixing the hazards should be provided. Programs should be funded to assess and remove lead hazards from the environment.

lead must be safely removed; do not live in the home while it is being renovated. Unsafe repairs can increase your child's risk for exposure to lead. Check with your health department to see if the water in your area contains lead.

A child who has high lead levels may not look or act sick. The only way to know if your child has lead in her body is with a blood test. If you have any concerns, talk to your pediatrician for more information.

Mold

Mold grows almost anywhere where there is moisture, and can be found in any part of a home. It can grow in damp basements, bathrooms that are not ventilated, refrigerators, air conditioners, humidifiers, or carpet (especially if it gets wet). Children who live in moldy places are more likely to develop allergies, asthma, and other health problems. Always keep the surfaces in your home dry, throw away wet carpet, and use exhaust fans in the kitchen and bathroom to help keep the air dry. Keep air conditioners and humidifiers clean and in good working order.

Pesticides

Commercial pesticides are often used to reduce the amount of plant damage caused by pests. Children may be exposed to pesticides when they are playing on treated grass, or when eating treated plant foods that have not been washed. Children who live near farms may also be exposed to sprayed pesticides if the spray drifts into their area.

To minimize exposure to pesticides, try to keep children off wet grass after pesticides have been sprayed. Avoid using spray pesticides inside the home, and always wash fruits and vegetables well before eating.

~ 56 ~

Eyes

Eye Infections

Pinkeye (conjunctivitis) is an inflammation of the mucous membrane on the inner side of the eyelids. An affected child develops symptoms such as bright pink eyes and yellow-green pus that can make the eyelids stick together, particularly upon awakening in the morning. It is common and usually not a serious condition.

Viruses and allergies may be responsible for pinkeye. A number of different bacteria—including staphylococcus and streptococcus—can also cause conjunctivitis. Both the bacterial and viral infections are contagious, so make sure your child does not share towels, washcloths, and pillows with other family members. Careful hand-washing is the most important preventive measure.

Viral eye infections tend to clear up on their own in a few days. Your doctor may prescribe an antibiotic—either eye drops or an ointment—for bacterial conjunctivitis. Make sure your child uses the antibiotic for the prescribed period, even if the symptoms disappear. A good technique to administer eye drops to a school-age child is to have the child lie flat on a bed or couch with the eyes closed; place a drop or two of the medication on the inner corner of the eye, and when the child opens the eye and blinks, gravity helps the fluid work its way onto the eye surface. To eliminate crusted or sticky discharge, periodically wash the eyelids gently, using a clean washcloth soaked in warm water with the excess squeezed out. Keep your child home from school until her eyes no longer have a discharge.

Eye Injuries

See page 603.

Eyelid Problems

Two eyelid problems—chalazia and styes—are common but not serious. A chalazion is a cyst resulting from a blockage of an oil gland. A sty, or hordeolum, is a bacterial infection of the cells surrounding the sweat glands or hair follicles on the edge of the lid. Call your pediatrician regarding treatment of these conditions. Warm compresses applied directly to the eyelid for twenty or thirty minutes three or four times a day can help the chalazion or sty to clear. The doctor may want to examine your child before prescribing additional treatment, such as an antibiotic ointment or drops. Once your child has had a sty or chalazion, she may be more likely to get them again. When chalazia occur repeatedly, it's sometimes necessary to perform lid scrubs to reduce the bacterial colonization of the eyelids and open the oil gland pores.

Impetigo is a very contagious bacterial infection that may occur on the eyelid. Your pediatrician will advise you on how to remove the crust from the lid and then prescribe an eye ointment and oral antibiotics.

Vision Problems

Middle childhood is a common time for the recognition of vision problems, especially when children first have assigned seats in classrooms. Your child may tell you that he cannot read the board unless he squints or moves to a front-row seat. Less commonly, your child may complain that the words on the pages of books are blurry. All of these suggest a focusing problem and may call for an examination by an eye doctor. Talk to your pediatrician about having your child's vision checked at a well-child visit and getting a referral to an eye doctor if concerns persist.

Myopia, or nearsightedness, is the most common vision problem among school-age children, often developing between age 6 and adolescence. With this condition, the eyeball has an elongated shape; as a result, the child cannot clearly see distant objects.

Children with hyperopia, or farsightedness, have the opposite problem. Because of the shorter shape of their eyeballs, these children cannot clearly see objects that are close to them. Even distance vision can be blurred in farsighted children. Small amounts of hyperopia are normal in children and may not need correction.

Both of these conditions can be inherited. Myopia and hyperopia may require eyeglasses to correct the poor vision. Some children prefer contact lenses; because the lenses require diligent care, doctors recommend taking the child's developmental stage and level of personal responsibility into consideration to determine if contact lenses are appropriate. Laser surgery to correct myopia is not done until adulthood, when the eye has finished growing.

Some children also have an astigmatism, in which the front of the eye has an irregular curvature to it. As a result, the distorted vision may be similar to that seen when looking in a mirror with a wavy surface. Astigmatism is usually inherited, may be present at birth, and may remain little changed throughout life. Normally, the blur from astigmatism is corrected with glasses or contact lenses. Small amounts of astigmatism are common and often do not require correction.

Points to note about the eyes:

■ Even though visual difficulties can sometimes cause headache, this pain is most often associated with problems unrelated to the eyes.

■ If your child wears glasses and participates in competitive sports, the glasses should be secured in place by attaching a strap that connects the two earpieces and stretches behind the head. Also, special sports glasses are available.

■ Some optometrists recommend eye exercises to help treat learning disorders like dyslexia; however, controlled studies have failed to demonstrate any benefits from these eye exercises (or from wearing colored lenses).

~ 57 ~

Fever

FEVER IN AND of itself is not an illness; it is usually a sign that the body is fighting an illness or infection. Fevers are generally harmless. In fact, a fever can be considered a good sign that your child's immune system is working properly and that the body is making an effort to heal itself. Many of our body's immune factors work more efficiently at a higher body temperature. While it is important to look for the cause of a fever, the main reason to treat a fever is to help your child feel better if he is uncomfortable or has pain so he can get the rest he needs and stay hydrated.

Everyone has his or her own internal "thermostat" that regulates body temperature. A normal body temperature is around 98.6 degrees Fahrenheit, plus or minus about one degree. When the body detects an infection or other illness, the immune system responds by raising the body temperature to help fight the condition. Most pediatricians consider a temperature above 100.4 degrees Fahrenheit as indicative of a fever.

If your child has a fever, he may feel warm, appear flushed, or sweat more than usual. He may also be thirstier than usual. Some children are not particularly affected by a fever and continue to be playful and somewhat active. However, most will have symptoms of the illness that is causing the fever. Your child may have a painful ear, a sore throat, a rash, or a stomach-ache. These signs can provide important clues as to the cause of the fever, and you will want to call your pediatrician right away.

It is not always necessary for a child with a fever to see the doctor. It depends on the age of the child and other symptoms the child is experiencing.

Taking Your Child's Temperature

A digital thermometer is needed to tell how high the temperature is. Your child's temperature, along with other physical signs and symptoms, will help your pediatrician evaluate your child. For a school-age child, a digital oral thermometer can be used in the mouth to read the temperature. In general, axillary (taken by placing the thermometer in the armpit) temperatures are not as accurate as oral temperatures. In addition, temporal (forehead) and tympanic (ear) thermometers are not as accurate as oral temperatures.

If your child has a fever, he needs to take sips of fluid to prevent dehydration. If the fever has been present only a day or so and your child is for the most part comfortable and well hydrated, you don't need to bring the child to get medical care. Acetaminophen or ibuprofen will typically relieve discomfort and also lower a fever. Before giving your child any medicine, read the label to make sure that you are giving the right dose for his age and weight. If you are unsure, call your pediatrician's office and ask. Ice packs are not typically recommended, as they can make children quite uncomfortable and they won't really help anyway. If the fever has lasted longer than forty-eight hours, or if your child has not been acting like her usual self, has not urinated in over six hours, has other worrisome symptoms (such as a stiff neck, bad headache, vomiting, or diarrhea), or has had a seizure, call your pediatrician immediately.

~ 58 ~

Genital and Urinary Systems

Blood in the Urine (Hematuria)

Color changes in the urine can be upsetting to child and parent alike. Some foods (such as beets or red food dye) and medications can cause color changes in the urine. Urine that turns red, orange, or brown may indicate blood or hematuria. This may be caused by injury, inflammation, infection, or other underlying medical problems. If there is no clear cause for the color change, you should contact your pediatrician for further testing.

Protein in the Urine (Proteinuria)

The kidneys have an important job of filtering our body's blood. Occasionally protein may be lost in the urine, either due to a current infection or because of an underlying kidney issue. A lowered amount of protein in the blood results in symptoms such as swelling in the eyelids, legs, ankles, or abdomen, or the affected child's blood pressure may be elevated. The pediatrician can check a urine sample in the office to see if there is protein being lost in the urine.

Labial Adhesions

Occasionally the lips of skin (labia) that surround the vaginal opening may stick together, partially or completely covering the opening. Often there are no symptoms, but adhesions can lead to urinary issues and may cause a urinary tract infection. Frequently the adhesions resolve on their own, but contact your pediatrician for an evaluation if you have concerns. Your doctor may prescribe an estrogen-containing cream to help the adhesions resolve.

Urinary Tract Infections

Has your child complained of pain, burning, or stinging when she urinates? Does she seem to go to the bathroom more frequently than normal? Is the urine discolored? If so, she may have a urinary tract infection (UTI). These infections occur much more often in girls than boys, and they increase in frequency in middle childhood.

Urinary tract infections are caused by bacteria from the child's own body. Normally these bacteria are present on the skin or in the intestinal tract, and they can make their way to the urethra (the tube that carries off the urine from the bladder). However, when the bacteria travel along the urethra into the bladder, rather than being washed away during urination, they may attach to the bladder wall and infect the bladder or perhaps the kidney. Because the urethra in girls is much shorter than the urethra in boys, the bacteria have a shorter distance to go to reach the bladder, and so girls get more bladder and kidney infections.

When your pediatrician suspects a urinary tract infection, he or she will examine the child's urine with both a quick urinalysis test in the office and a culture of the urine specimen sent to the laboratory to identify the bacteria if present. If a urinary tract infection is diagnosed, your child should be placed on an antibiotic. Be sure she takes the full course of medication, even if her symptoms disappear before it is used up. Following a UTI, your doctor may suggest additional evaluations, including a repeat urine examination. A child with recurring UTIs may need imaging at some point, including ultrasound visualization of the kidneys or X-ray examination of urinary voiding.

In order to prevent urinary tract infections, children should be encouraged to drink plenty of liquids—six or more glasses of water a day. After going to the bathroom, children—especially girls—should pat dry, not rub, in a front-to-back motion to avoid contaminating the urethra with more bacteria. Also, girls should wear 100 percent cotton underpants (the moisture that accumulates with nylon panties can promote the growth of bacteria and cause UTIs) and alternate days when tights or leggings are worn with days with looser-fitting clothing for breathability. Do not use bubble baths, since their chemicals can be irritating and lead to urinary tract infections. Use a mild soap for bathing.

Wetting Problems or Enuresis

Bed-wetting is normal and very common among preschoolers, affecting 40 percent of children at age 3. It is much less frequent in school-age children, occurring in 20 percent of 5-year-olds, 10 percent of 6-year-olds, and 3 percent of 12-year-olds. During the middle years of childhood, parents may seek the assistance of their pediatrician in an effort to reduce or eliminate bed-wetting, or enuresis.

For a child to remain dry at night, his brain must keep a full bladder from emptying. A signal from a full bladder must be strong enough to awaken the child from sleep and send him to the toilet. It is a complex neurodevelopmental process for the bladder to send the signal, for the brain to receive it, and for the child to respond by awakening and using the toilet.

In the majority of cases of bed-wetting, the cause is delayed maturation of bladder control mechanisms, often related to the child's genetic background. These children are physically and psychologically normal. Emotional problems are an occasional cause of enuresis. For instance, a child who is overwhelmed with stress may develop enuresis, even though she was formerly dry at night. Children may develop enuresis in the context of a parental separation or divorce or with severe stressors like sexual or physical abuse.

Most school-age children who wet their beds have *primary enuresis*, meaning they have had this condition since birth and have never developed nighttime bladder control. These children often have a family history of this problem, and they seem to have inherited the tendency for developing nighttime bladder control at a later-than-average age. In most cases the child becomes dry at about the same age that his parent(s) did.

Sometimes parents pressure a child to develop nighttime bladder control before his body is ready to do so. These parents may view bed-wetting as a willful and oppositional act, and thus they may try coercing the child to change his behavior. As hard as he may try, the enuresis is beyond his voluntary control, and he may become discouraged, frustrated, or depressed because of his lack of success.

For the child who wets the bed, parents need to remain supportive and encouraging. They should be sensitive to the child's embarrassment or discomfort over this problem. The child may resist spending the night at a friend's house or going to summer camp and may be uncomfortable at the thought of his friends finding out about this condition. Parents can reassure the child that it is not his fault, and the problem *will* get better in time.

Reassure your child that the symptoms of enuresis will pass with age. Until that natural maturation process occurs, however, several techniques might help the situation.

1. **Protecting and changing the bed.** Until your child fully achieves bladder control, encase his mattress in a

plastic cover to protect it from becoming saturated, thus avoiding a permanent urine smell.

2. **Assuming responsibility.** You may wish to encourage your child to change his own linens when they are wet. This will show that he is taking responsibility for himself, and it will relieve him of the embarrassment of having to alert others in the family when he wets the bed. However, if others in the family don't have similar household tasks, your child may see this as punishment, and in that case it is not recommended.

3. **Waking the child during the night.** Sometimes parents wake a child to use the bathroom before they go to bed or have the child set an alarm clock to wake himself in the middle of the night in order to empty the bladder. For some children these strategies can be effective in preventing bed-wetting, but they do not teach the child to wake up when he has to urinate. They may be appropriate for a short period in younger children, but they are not considered a treatment for the problem of the child not waking up when he has to urinate at night.

4. **Use a bed-wetting alarm device.** If your child reaches age 7 or 8 and still is having little success at achieving nighttime dryness, you might try an alarm device. It senses the presence of urine and triggers a buzzer that awakens the child at the time the bed-wetting occurs. This device should be positioned on or close to the child's underwear so it will detect the wetness immediately and sound the alarm; upon awakening, the child should go to the bathroom and then reset the alarm before returning to sleep. These alarms are available at most pharmacies and usually cost from $65 to over $100. They provide a 60 to 90 percent cure rate when used consistently for a period of one to four months. They tend to be most helpful when children are starting to experience occasional dry nights, indicating that they are gradually developing some control on their own. Consultation with a pediatrician or psychologist experienced in treating bed-wetting may be helpful if you are having difficulty using an alarm device.

5. **Try bladder-stretching exercises.** If your child shows an interest in becoming actively involved in decreasing his bed-wetting, the bed-wetting alarm (described above) is the most effective intervention. In addition, bladder-stretching exercises may help some children. With these exercises the child practices holding his urine as long as possible during the waking hours when he has ready access to a toilet. (Weekends are easier than weekdays.) Whenever he feels the urge to go, he should wait an additional ten minutes or longer, until the bladder spasms stop. As he learns to resist and postpone the elimina-

tion of urine, he may enhance his bladder capacity and develop greater urine control.

6. **Eliminate all teasing and negative comments within the family about bed-wetting.** In particular, talk with siblings who are teasing a child who has not yet acquired this developmental skill. Parents do best when they completely ignore the occurrence of wet beds, and certainly they should avoid making it a part of regular conversations with the child.

If your child has primary enuresis, you might wish to discuss the problem with your pediatrician in order to understand it better and simply to be reassured that it is normal.

When a child develops enuresis after having been dry at night in the past, he should be evaluated by his physician. This may be a sign that the condition is disease-related or associated with psychological stress. In some cases, particularly if your child is exhibiting emotional strain because of his enuresis, your pediatrician may perform a physical examination, do a urinalysis, and review your child's entire developmental history.

The use of drugs to treat bed-wetting is controversial. Since primary enuresis typically resolves itself as the child matures, some doctors worry that reliance on medications may pose more risks (because of side effects) than benefits. On occasion, a drug called desmopressin may be prescribed. It is an antidiuretic hormone that reduces the amount of urine released by the kidneys. The medication is taken by mouth at bedtime and may relieve bed-wetting in some children. It is an expensive treatment best used for special circumstances such as overnights with friends or grandparents or attendance at summer camp.

When enuresis is due to stress or causes emotional distress, psychological intervention may be helpful to resolve the bed-wetting. Sometimes hypnosis is useful in giving children more control over nighttime wetting. Proponents of hypnosis as a treatment for bed-wetting have shown a cure rate of 75 to 80 percent. While hypnosis is known to be quite safe and often effective, its mechanism (that is, how it works) is unknown.

Fortunately, as each year passes, bed-wetting will decrease as the child's body matures; most children stop before adolescence.

~ 59 ~

Head, Neck, and Nervous System

Headaches

At one time or another, almost all children complain of a headache. In fact, the three most common recurring pain symptoms that pediatricians see in children are abdominal pain, chest pain, and headaches. While a headache that comes on suddenly may suggest a serious problem requiring prompt evaluation, headaches are most often a symptom of other problems. Your child may be feeling stress and tension. Or she may have a cold, the flu, or strep throat. Sometimes fevers and headaches occur at the same time, so if your child complains of head pain, check her temperature.

Some children experience a recurrent headache called migraine, which can begin in childhood. Migraines often run in families. Unlike headaches caused by tension, these are often accompanied by other symptoms. Children may have a premonition (an *aura*) that they will occur, or parents may notice their children acting differently before a headache begins. Often, the headache occurs along with nausea, vomiting, or visual disturbances. The head pain itself is typically throbbing or stabbing and may affect one or both sides of the front part of the head.

There may also be other unpleasant sensations in the head, including burning, tingling, aching, or squeezing. The child may prefer a darkened room and may find relief by lying down. Migraines tend to run in families. The head pain typically lasts for several hours or even overnight.

In diagnosing your child's headache, your pediatrician will look for an underlying disease or condition. For most types of headaches, rest, hydration, and pain medication such as acetaminophen or ibuprofen may be all that is necessary, along with treatment of the primary disorder. Depending on the type of headache, your doctor might also recommend prescription drugs or stress management techniques. If migraines occur more than two to three times a month—and particularly if they interfere with attending or functioning well in school—your doctor may prescribe medication as a preventive measure. The doctor may also suggest counseling to explore whether stress or emotional factors may be contributing to the headaches. Headaches should not be allowed to control home or school activities.

Meningitis

See page 605.

Motion Sickness

Motion sickness is quite common for school-age children. It occurs when the brain receives conflicting signals from the motion-detecting parts of the body: the inner ears, eyes, and nerves of the body. A car ride in which the body and ears detect motion but the eyes do not, or, conversely, watching fast action on a movie screen while the body and ears are still, can create this conflict, which results in a nauseous feeling. Queasiness can precede a cold sweat and possibly vomiting. Plane and boat rides are also known to precipitate motion sickness.

If your child becomes motion sick, stop the activity causing the issue, if you can. On a car ride, stop and walk around a bit. A light snack before the trip can help prevent symptoms. Distraction with music or conversation can help, as well as looking out the window at the horizon instead of at a screen or book in the lap.

There are over-the-counter medications that can help school-age kids with motion sickness, but consult with your pediatrician before using. Drowsiness and a dry mouth are common side effects of these medicines.

If your child has a feeling of motion sickness when not involved in an activity that would be expected to cause it, consult with your pediatrician, as these may be symptoms of issues other than motion sickness.

Mumps

Thanks to the mumps vaccine, mumps is much rarer than it was decades ago. These days you may hear in the news about clusters of mumps cases in a school or on a college campus. The mumps most often cause swelling and tenderness in the parotid glands (salivary glands located just above the jaw in front of the ear). Eating and drinking, especially acidic foods such as oranges, may cause pain due to the stimulation of the salivary glands. Fever, headache, and fatigue may occur, and in boys there may be testicular swelling.

The contagious period begins a day or two before the swelling is apparent, and the child will remain contagious about five days after the swelling has started. Not all kids develop the characteristic parotid swelling. Rest and fluids will help the child affected with mumps feel better. It is a virus, so antibiotics won't help. Speak with your pediatrician if you suspect mumps in your child, and certainly if her condition is getting worse. In most states, the mumps is a reportable illness—that is, doctors have an obligation to report cases of mumps to the local public health department in an effort to inform other healthcare providers and the community to be alert for symptoms and possible new cases, to reduce the spread.

Seizures and Epilepsy

Seizures are caused by abnormal electrical activity changes in the brain that causes temporary alterations in a child's movement, behavior, or consciousness. Some only last a few seconds, while others may last longer, requiring medical intervention to cease the symptoms. The area of the brain that is involved determines what the seizure will look like. The child may lose consciousness, have uncontrolled shaking of a single arm, a leg, or the entire body, have brief periods of staring, or stiffen. *Epilepsy* refers to when a person has a predisposition to recurring seizures.

There are generalized seizures and more focal seizures. *Generalized convulsive seizures* (formerly called grand mal) involve the whole body. They may begin with shaking of a specific area and then spread. *Absence seizures* (formerly called petit mal) are brief interruptions in awareness in which the child seems to stare off into space and is unresponsive. At times these episodes involve rapid eye blinking or lip smacking. *Focal seizures* are caused by abnormal electrical activity in a specific part of the brain and can involve stiffening or shaking of only one part of the body.

Most seizures stop on their own and do not necessarily need immediate medical treatment. The child should be laid on her side; make sure there is nothing in her mouth. Do not try to hold the child down or restrain the limbs. While the seizure may seem to last an eternity, watch the clock; if the seizure does not stop within five minutes, or if the child has difficulty breathing or is turning blue, call 911, making sure an adult stays with the child.

A fever can precipitate a seizure, especially for a child with a history of febrile seizures. These are more common in kids 6 months to 6 years of age, and are associated with the onset of a fever; it is common for the fever to be recognized only after the seizure happens. If there was no fever and this is the child's first seizure, your pediatrician will ask about a family history of seizures or any recent head injury. If you have a video of the seizure, your pediatrician may ask to see it. Testing includes blood tests, imaging, and possibly an electro-encephalogram (EEG), which examines the electrical activity of the brain. Consultation with a pediatric neurologist may be warranted, depending on your child's situation. If epilepsy is diagnosed, anticonvulsant medications may be required.

While seizures are frightening, they become less common as kids get older. If you need more information, ask your pediatrician or connect with the Epilepsy Foundation of America. Others may have misinformation about your child's diagnosis; educating your child's teachers, school, and friends will help your child feel better understood. Role-play various scenarios with your child so that he or she feels comfortable discussing the epilepsy with others when it is appropriate to do so.

~ 60 ~

Heart

Arrhythmias

The heart maintains a regular rhythm via an electrical circuit that runs through the muscles of the heart. It is normal and healthy for a child's heart rate to vary depending on the situation. Typically, a normal heart rhythm will speed up and slow down gradually. Fever, activity, pain, or crying can speed up the rate at which the heart is beating. Sinus arrhythmia is a *normal* variation in the heart rhythm where the heart rate speeds up as the child breathes in and slows down when the child breathes out.

Rhythm disorders can occur at any age, from infancy into adulthood. Premature beats are beats that cause an irregular rhythm by arriving earlier than expected. Usually premature beats by themselves do not require treatment. However, your pediatrician may order an ECG (electrocardiogram) to diagnose the type of premature beat. Your child may be referred to a pediatric cardiologist depending on the type of premature beat and how often they are occurring.

While tachycardia, a fast heart rate, can be normal (for example, a sinus tachycardia if your child is running or has a fever), there are some tachycardias that are not normal and are true rhythm disorders. Let the pediatrician know if your child has a sensation of a fast heartbeat when he is not exercising, if a fast heartbeat does not slow down gradually after he stops exercising, or if a fast heartbeat makes him feel dizzy or nauseated or if he passes out. Bradycardia is a slower-than-usual heart rate. Your pediatrician may order an ECG and recommend your child see a pediatric cardiologist to evaluate a problem with tachycardia or bradycardia.

Heart Murmur

A heart murmur is an extra noise of blood flow through the heart and can be heard when auscultating (listening to) the heart with a stethoscope. Heart murmurs are quite common in children. In fact, more than 50 percent of children may have an innocent (also called benign or functional) murmur. Innocent murmurs are caused by vibrations of normal flow through the heart. A typical innocent heart murmur may be detected during a routine checkup or when your child visits the doctor because of illness. It is not uncommon for an innocent heart murmur to sound louder at one checkup and then softer at another checkup. Usually no testing is needed if a murmur has the typical innocent sound quality and behavior, and children with innocent murmurs may fully participate in sports and activities. If there is a concern about the murmur—for example, if it is louder or has a different quality than expected for an innocent murmur—then your

doctor may recommend referral to a pediatric cardiologist. An echocardiogram (or ultrasound of the heart) may be performed to look at the structure and function of the heart.

Hypertension/High Blood Pressure

School-age children have their blood pressure checked at their annual health maintenance examinations (checkups) starting at the third birthday. High blood pressure (hypertension) is a common issue for adults; it can occur in children as well. Blood pressure is reported as two numbers: the top number (systolic pressure) is the higher pressure in the arteries when the heart pumps blood out to the body, and the bottom number (diastolic pressure) is the lower pressure present in the arteries when the heart relaxes. Hypertension is diagnosed if these numbers are consistently (on multiple measurements at different times) above the range expected for the child's age and sex. Overweight children are more likely to have hypertension. Your doctor will probably order tests to investigate whether there may be a kidney, heart, or endocrine problem causing the hypertension. Your doctor may also recommend referral to a pediatric hypertension or preventive cardiology specialist.

For more information on boosting kids' daily physical activity, see page 45. For more information on cholesterol screening, see page 40.

~ 61 ~

Immunizations

IMMUNIZATIONS, THE GREATEST public health advancement of the twentieth century, are a safe and effective way to prevent disease, disability, and death. For the individual child, the vaccine helps the body's immune system build antibodies specific to a particular illness, so that if the child comes into contact with the illness, the body can minimize its effects or prevent it from even causing any problems in the first place. For the greater community in which the vaccinated child lives, herd immunity (when more than 93 percent of the population has been vaccinated against the illness) helps not only to reduce the chances of encountering the illness but also to protect those who are too young or otherwise unable to receive a vaccine themselves (as an example, those with weak immune systems due to illness, treatment of cancer, or an organ transplant). Vaccines are safe and they work.

If you have questions about vaccines, such as what the side effects are, or what methods are in place to monitor for their ongoing safety, have a discussion with your pediatrician. There is a confusing amount of information available on the internet, and it is important to ensure that the information you read online is trustworthy, up-to-date, peer-reviewed (meaning that experts in the field agree), and founded on evidence-based

2017 Recommended Immunizations for Children from Birth Through 6 Years Old

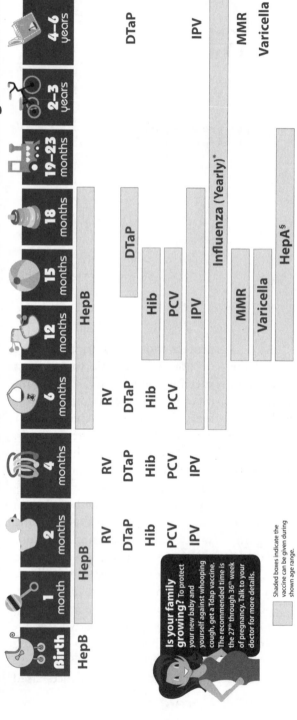

Vaccine	Birth	1 month	2 months	4 months	6 months	12 months	15 months	18 months	19–23 months	2–3 years	4–6 years
HepB	HepB	HepB			HepB						
RV			RV	RV	RV						
DTaP			DTaP	DTaP	DTaP		DTaP				DTaP
Hib			Hib	Hib	Hib	Hib					
PCV			PCV	PCV	PCV	PCV					
IPV			IPV	IPV	IPV						IPV
Influenza (Yearly)*					Influenza (Yearly)*						
MMR						MMR					MMR
Varicella						Varicella					Varicella
HepA§						HepA§					

Shaded boxes indicate the vaccine can be given during shown age range.

Is your family growing? To protect your new baby and yourself against whooping cough, get a Tdap vaccine. The recommended time is the 27th through 36th week of pregnancy. Talk to your doctor for more details.

NOTE:
If your child misses a shot, you don't need to start over, just go back to your child's doctor for the next shot. Talk with your child's doctor if you have questions about vaccines.

FOOTNOTES:
* Two doses given at least four weeks apart are recommended for children aged 6 months through 8 years of age who are getting an influenza (flu) vaccine for the first time and for some other children in this age group.

§ Two doses of HepA vaccine are needed for lasting protection. The first dose of HepA vaccine should be given between 12 months and 23 months of age. The second dose should be given 6 to 18 months later. HepA vaccination may be given to any child 12 months and older to protect against HepA. Children and adolescents who did not receive the HepA vaccine and are at high-risk, should be vaccinated against HepA.

If your child has any medical conditions that put him at risk for infection or is traveling outside the United States, talk to your child's doctor about additional vaccines that he may need.

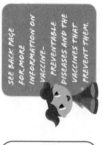

SEE BACK PAGE FOR MORE INFORMATION ON VACCINE-PREVENTABLE DISEASES AND THE VACCINES THAT PREVENT THEM.

For more information, call toll free
1-800-CDC-INFO (1-800-232-4636)
or visit
www.cdc.gov/vaccines/parents

U.S. Department of Health and Human Services
Centers for Disease Control and Prevention

American Academy of Pediatrics
DEDICATED TO THE HEALTH OF ALL CHILDREN™

AMERICAN ACADEMY OF FAMILY PHYSICIANS
STRONG MEDICINE FOR AMERICA

Vaccine-Preventable Diseases and the Vaccines that Prevent Them

Disease	Vaccine	Disease spread by	Disease symptoms	Disease complications
Chickenpox	Varicella vaccine protects against chickenpox.	Air, direct contact	Rash, tiredness, headache, fever	Infected blisters, bleeding disorders, encephalitis (brain swelling), pneumonia (infection in the lungs)
Diphtheria	DTaP* vaccine protects against diphtheria.	Air, direct contact	Sore throat, mild fever, weakness, swollen glands in neck	Swelling of the heart muscle, heart failure, coma, paralysis, death
Hib	Hib vaccine protects against *Haemophilus influenzae* type b.	Air, direct contact	May be no symptoms unless bacteria enter the blood	Meningitis (infection of the covering around the brain and spinal cord), intellectual disability, epiglottitis (life-threatening infection that can block the windpipe and lead to serious breathing problems), pneumonia (infection in the lungs), death
Hepatitis A	HepA vaccine protects against hepatitis A.	Direct contact, contaminated food or water	May be no symptoms, fever, stomach pain, loss of appetite, fatigue, vomiting, jaundice (yellowing of skin and eyes), dark urine	Liver failure, arthralgia (joint pain), kidney, pancreatic, and blood disorders
Hepatitis B	HepB vaccine protects against hepatitis B.	Contact with blood or body fluids	May be no symptoms, fever, headache, weakness, vomiting, jaundice (yellowing of skin and eyes), joint pain	Chronic liver infection, liver failure, liver cancer
Influenza (Flu)	Flu vaccine protects against influenza.	Air, direct contact	Fever, muscle pain, sore throat, cough, extreme fatigue	Pneumonia (infection in the lungs)
Measles	MMR** vaccine protects against measles.	Air, direct contact	Rash, fever, cough, runny nose, pinkeye	Encephalitis (brain swelling), pneumonia (infection in the lungs), death
Mumps	MMR**vaccine protects against mumps.	Air, direct contact	Swollen salivary glands (under the jaw), fever, headache, tiredness, muscle pain	Meningitis (infection of the covering around the brain and spinal cord), encephalitis (brain swelling), inflammation of testicles or ovaries, deafness
Pertussis	DTaP* vaccine protects against pertussis (whooping cough).	Air, direct contact	Severe cough, runny nose, apnea (a pause in breathing in infants)	Pneumonia (infection in the lungs), death
Polio	IPV vaccine protects against polio.	Air, direct contact, through the mouth	May be no symptoms, sore throat, fever, nausea, headache	Paralysis, death
Pneumococcal	PCV vaccine protects against pneumococcus.	Air, direct contact	May be no symptoms, pneumonia (infection in the lungs)	Bacteremia (blood infection), meningitis (infection of the covering around the brain and spinal cord), death
Rotavirus	RV vaccine protects against rotavirus.	Through the mouth	Diarrhea, fever, vomiting	Severe diarrhea, dehydration
Rubella	MMR** vaccine protects against rubella.	Air, direct contact	Children infected with rubella virus sometimes have a rash, fever, swollen lymph nodes	Very serious in pregnant women—can lead to miscarriage, stillbirth, premature delivery, birth defects
Tetanus	DTaP* vaccine protects against tetanus.	Exposure through cuts in skin	Stiffness in neck and abdominal muscles, difficulty swallowing, muscle spasms, fever	Broken bones, breathing difficulty, death

* DTaP combines protection against diphtheria, tetanus, and pertussis.
** MMR combines protection against measles, mumps, and rubella.

Last updated December 2016 • CS272886-E

INFORMATION FOR PARENTS | **2017 Recommended Immunizations for Children 7-18 Years Old**

Talk to your child's doctor or nurse about the vaccines recommended for their age.

	Flu *Influenza*	Tdap *Tetanus, diphtheria, pertussis*	HPV *Human papillomavirus*	Meningococcal MenACWY	Meningococcal MenB	Pneumococcal	Hepatitis B	Hepatitis A	Inactivated Polio	MMR *Measles, mumps, rubella*	Chickenpox *Varicella*
7-8 Years											
9-10 Years											
11-12 Years											
13-15 Years											
16-18 Years											
More information:	Preteens and teens should get a flu vaccine every year.	Preteens and teens should get one shot of Tdap at age 11 or 12 years.	All 11-12 year olds should get a 2-shot series of HPV vaccine at least 6 months apart. A 3-shot series is needed for those with weakened immune systems and those age 15 or older.	All 11-12 year olds should get a single shot of a quadrivalent meningococcal conjugate vaccine (MenACWY). A booster shot is recommended at age 16.	Teens, 16-18 years old, **may** be vaccinated with a MenB vaccine.						

These shaded boxes indicate when the vaccine is recommended for all children unless your doctor tells you that your child cannot safely receive the vaccine.

These shaded boxes indicate the vaccine is recommended for children with certain health or lifestyle conditions that put them at an increased risk for serious diseases. See vaccine-specific recommendations at www.cdc.gov/vaccines/pubs/ACIP-list.htm.

These shaded boxes indicate the vaccine should be given if a child is catching-up on missed vaccines.

This shaded box indicates the vaccine is recommended for children not at increased risk but who wish to get the vaccine after speaking to a provider.

U.S. Department of
Health and Human Services
Centers for Disease
Control and Prevention

CDC

American Academy of Pediatrics
DEDICATED TO THE HEALTH OF ALL CHILDREN™

AMERICAN ACADEMY OF FAMILY PHYSICIANS
STRONG MEDICINE FOR AMERICA

Vaccine-Preventable Diseases and the Vaccines that Prevent Them

Diphtheria (Can be prevented by Tdap vaccination)

Diphtheria is a very contagious bacterial disease that affects the respiratory system, including the lungs. Diphtheria bacteria can be passed from person to person by direct contact with droplets from an infected person's cough or sneeze. When people are infected, the bacteria can produce a toxin (poison) in the body that can cause a thick coating in the back of the nose or throat that makes it hard to breathe or swallow. Effects from this toxin can also lead to swelling of the heart muscle and, in some cases, heart failure. In serious cases, the illness can cause coma, paralysis, and even death.

Hepatitis A (Can be prevented by HepA vaccination)

Hepatitis A is an infection in the liver caused by hepatitis A virus. The virus is spread primarily person-to-person through the fecal-oral route. In other words, the virus is taken in by mouth from contact with objects, food, or drinks contaminated by the feces (stool) of an infected person. Symptoms can include fever, tiredness, poor appetite, vomiting, stomach pain, and sometimes jaundice (when skin and eyes turn yellow). An infected person may have no symptoms, may have mild illness for a week or two, may have severe illness for several months, or may rarely develop liver failure and die from the infection. In the U.S., about 100 people a year die from hepatitis A.

Hepatitis B (Can be prevented by HepB vaccination)

Hepatitis B causes a flu-like illness with loss of appetite, nausea, vomiting, rashes, joint pain, and jaundice. Symptoms of acute hepatitis B include fever, fatigue, loss of appetite, nausea, vomiting, pain in joints and stomach, dark urine, grey-colored stools, and jaundice (when skin and eyes turn yellow).

Human Papillomavirus (Can be prevented by HPV vaccination)

Human papillomavirus is a common virus. HPV is most common in people in their teens and early 20s. It is the major cause of cervical cancer in women and genital warts in women and men. The strains of HPV that cause cervical cancer and genital warts are spread during sex.

Influenza (Can be prevented by annual flu vaccination)

Influenza is a highly contagious viral infection of the nose, throat, and lungs. The virus spreads easily through droplets when an infected person coughs or sneezes and can cause mild to severe illness. Typical symptoms include a sudden high fever, chills, a dry cough, headache, runny nose, sore throat, and muscle and joint pain. Extreme fatigue can last from several days to weeks. Influenza may lead to hospitalization or even death, even among previously healthy children.

Measles (Can be prevented by MMR vaccination)

Measles is one of the most contagious viral diseases. Measles virus is spread by direct contact with the airborne respiratory droplets of an infected person. Measles is so contagious that just being in the same room after a person who has measles has already left can result in infection. Symptoms usually include a rash, fever, cough, and red, watery eyes. Fever can persist, rash can last for up to a week, and coughing can last about 10 days. Measles can also cause pneumonia, seizures, brain damage, or death.

Meningococcal Disease (Can be prevented by meningococcal vaccination)

Meningococcal disease is caused by bacteria and is a leading cause of bacterial meningitis (infection around the brain and spinal cord) in children. The bacteria are spread through the exchange of nose and throat droplets, such as when coughing, sneezing or kissing. Symptoms include sudden onset of fever, headache, and stiff neck. Meningococcal bacteria also cause blood infections. About one of every ten people who get the disease dies from it. Survivors of meningococcal disease may lose their arms or legs, become deaf, have problems with their nervous systems, become developmentally disabled, or suffer seizures or strokes.

Mumps (Can be prevented by MMR vaccination)

Mumps is an infectious disease caused by the mumps virus, which is spread in the air by a cough or sneeze from an infected person. A child can also get infected with mumps by coming in contact with a contaminated object, like a toy. The mumps virus causes swollen salivary glands under the ears or jaw, fever, muscle aches, tiredness, abdominal pain, and loss of appetite. Severe complications for children who get mumps are uncommon, but can include meningitis (infection of the covering of the brain and spinal cord), encephalitis (inflammation of the brain), permanent hearing loss, or swelling of the testes, which rarely results in decreased fertility.

Pertussis (Whooping Cough) (Can be prevented by Tdap vaccination)

Pertussis is caused by bacteria spread through direct contact with respiratory droplets when an infected person coughs or sneezes. In the beginning, symptoms of pertussis are similar to the common cold, including runny nose, sneezing, and cough. After 1-2 weeks, pertussis can cause spells of violent coughing and choking, making it hard to breathe, drink, or eat. This cough can last for weeks. Pertussis is most serious for babies, who can get pneumonia, have seizures, become brain damaged, or even die. About half of children under 1 year of age who get pertussis must be hospitalized.

Pneumococcal Disease (Can be prevented by pneumococcal vaccination)

Pneumonia is an infection of the lungs that can be caused by the bacteria called pneumococcus. This bacteria can cause other types of infections too, such as ear infections, sinus infections, meningitis (infection of the covering around the brain and spinal cord), and bacteremia (bloodstream infection). Sinus and ear infections are usually mild and are much more common than the more serious forms of pneumococcal disease. However, in some cases pneumococcal disease can be fatal or result in long-term problems, like brain damage and hearing loss. Pneumococcal disease spreads when people cough or sneeze. Many people have the bacteria in their nose or throat at one time or another without being ill—this is known as being a carrier.

Polio (Can be prevented by IPV vaccination)

Polio is caused by a virus that lives in an infected person's throat and intestines. It spreads through contact with the stool of an infected person and through droplets from a sneeze or cough. Symptoms typically include sore throat, fever, tiredness, nausea, headache, or stomach pain. In about 1% of cases, polio can cause paralysis. Among those who are paralyzed, about 2 to 10 children out of 100 die because the virus affects the muscles that help them breathe.

Rubella (German Measles) (Can be prevented by MMR vaccination)

Rubella is caused by a virus that is spread through coughing and sneezing. In children rubella usually causes a mild illness with fever, swollen glands, and a rash that lasts about 3 days. Rubella rarely causes serious illness or complications in children, but can be very serious to a baby in the womb. If a pregnant woman is infected, the result to the baby can be devastating, including miscarriage, serious heart defects, mental retardation and loss of hearing and eye sight.

Tetanus (Lockjaw) (Can be prevented by Tdap vaccination)

Tetanus is caused by bacteria found in soil, dust, and manure. The bacteria enters the body through a puncture, cut, or sore on the skin. When people are infected, the bacteria produce a toxin (poison) that causes muscles to become tight, which is very painful. Tetanus mainly affects the neck and belly. This can lead to "locking" of the jaw so a person cannot open his or her mouth, swallow, or breathe. Complete recovery from tetanus can take months. One to two out of 10 people who get tetanus die from the disease.

Varicella (Chickenpox) (Can be prevented by varicella vaccination)

Chickenpox is caused by the varicella zoster virus. Chickenpox is very contagious and spreads very easily from infected people. The virus can spread from either a cough, sneeze. It can also spread from the blisters on the skin, either by touching them or by breathing in these viral particles. Typical symptoms of chickenpox include an itchy rash with blisters, tiredness, headache and fever. Chickenpox is usually mild, but it can lead to severe skin infections, pneumonia, encephalitis (brain swelling), or even death.

Last updated on 01/10/2017 • CS278886-I

If you have any questions about your child's vaccines, talk to your healthcare provider.

medicine (meaning what the research shows). For more on evaluating the quality of medical and parenting information online, see page XXX.

Thanks to the success of vaccines, formerly prevalent viral and bacterial diseases are much less common today, leading some to question whether the vaccines are still necessary. They are still necessary because the illnesses still live within communities and globally; many vaccine-preventable illnesses are a simple plane ride away. A vaccine is a simple, safe, and effective way to prevent the illness.

Vaccines work very well; most childhood vaccines are 90 to 99 percent effective in preventing disease. If a vaccinated child does get the disease, the symptoms are usually milder, with less serious side effects, compared to a child who has not been vaccinated. Common side effects of vaccines include swelling or redness at the injection site, which usually resolves by the next day. A mild fever may arise that evening but usually resolves by itself.

Kids with certain health issues may need to adjust their immunization schedule. Kids who are under treatment for cancer, who are taking steroids for lung or kidney illness, or who have immune system problems should not receive vaccines made with live viruses. In order to protect these children, everyone else who is able to do so should be vaccinated in order to "cocoon" the child with herd immunity, meaning minimizing the chances of having the illness spread by contact with others.

What Vaccines Does Your Child Need?

In addition, refer to pages 633–637.

~ 62 ~

Musculoskeletal Problems

Arthritis

Arthritis, while often considered to be an adult issue, can affect kids as well. The progression and treatment of the arthritis depends on what type of arthritis it is.

Transient Synovitis (Inflammation) of the Hip

Transient synovitis (inflammation) of the hip is the most common type of arthritis in kids. Most commonly it develops suddenly following a viral infection such as a simple cold or upper respiratory infection. Kids between 2 and 10 years of age are most commonly affected, and the symptoms of groin and leg pain with limping typically resolve by themselves after a few days. Rest and anti-inflammatory medication such as ibuprofen can help the affected child feel better.

Bacterial Infection of the Joint

A bacterial infection of the joint is painful and often associated with a fever. When a lower extremity such as a leg is involved, the child may refuse to walk. Pain may be severe, and typically the hip is more comfortable flexed and out to the side. Contact your pediatrician quickly to begin treatment as soon as possible.

Lyme Disease

Lyme disease is an infection transmitted by a deer tick (a tiny, poppy-seed-sized tick, much smaller than the more common dog tick, which is sesame-seed-sized). The tick bite location forms a red mark surrounded by a ring, taking on the appearance of a target. Rash may spread elsewhere, and the child may develop flu-like symptoms, headache, fatigue, and body aches. Arthritis may develop weeks to months after the rash. Antibiotics are not warranted after every tick bite; however, if symptoms are concerning or a joint is involved, antibiotics and anti-inflammatory medications are recommended. Blood tests won't show Lyme disease until a few weeks or months later, after the initial infection. Prevention is the best strategy: when in wooded areas, wear long sleeves and pants, tuck pants into socks, and use insect repellent containing DEET. For more on tick bites, see page 640.

Juvenile Idiopathic Arthritis

Juvenile idiopathic arthritis (JIA; formerly termed rheumatoid arthritis) is the most common chronic (lasting longer than weeks or months) type of joint problem in kids. Not all kids are similarly affected. Common themes include stiffness, swelling, or pain involving one or more joints. A child's walking pattern may be affected. JIA symptoms may become evident between 3 and 6 years of age, or around puberty. Some types of JIA may affect the heart, lungs, or eyes, and it is extremely important to have a thorough eye examination because permanent damage may occur without symptoms. Treatment involves anti-inflammatory medication, exercise, physical therapy, and possibly prescription medications. A pediatric rheumatologist may be involved in the child's care.

Bowlegs and Knock-Knees

A child's walking pattern and leg appearance change as she grows from a toddler into a school-age child. Many kids have a bowlegged or knock-kneed appearance until the legs straighten at around 9 or 10 years of age. In most cases, bowlegs or knock-knees do not require special treatment, as they typically resolve by themselves. Generations ago, bracing or corrective shoes were used; consequently, grandparents or older relatives may suggest a visit to the doctor for an evaluation. Such interventions may actually do more harm than good, since most children outgrow the condition. If you feel the appearance is extreme, only one side is affected, or the child does not seem to be growing properly, talk with your pediatrician.

Flat Feet

Babies and toddlers usually have flat feet due to an age-appropriate fat pad that hides the arch. Typically, as the child reaches the school-age years, the arches become more apparent as the feet become less flexible. Flat feet are normal in children and in 15 percent of adults, and no treatment is recommended unless there is pain or disability. Arch supports, inserts, or orthotics are not indicated and will not promote the development of an arch. If a tight Achilles tendon (heel cord) is part of the issue, stretching exercises may help. Talk to your pediatrician if your child has foot pain, pressure sores, or stiffness of movement. Consultation with a pediatric orthopedic specialist may be warranted if there is pain or disability.

Intoeing

"Pigeon-toed" feet, or intoeing, is the term used to describe a walking pattern with the feet turned in. This is quite common and normal in children, may occur in one or both feet, and may run in families. For school-age children, intoeing is often due to an inward turning of the femur or thighbone (medial femoral torsion), and usually resolves by age 10. If you have concerns or your child has difficulty walking or running, speak with your pediatrician. Older generations used bracing, but more current research indicate that such devices do not correct the problem and actually cause more harm than good. Your primary care physician may enlist a pediatric orthopedic specialist if there are concerns.

Sprains

A sprain is defined as a stretching or tearing injury to a ligament (connective tissue that connects bones). Sprains are quite common in adults, but for younger kids, ligaments are actually stronger than bones, so any injury with swelling or deformity should be evaluated to ensure no fracture has occurred. Ankles, knees, and wrists are the more commonly sprained joints. Pain, swelling, or inability to walk or use the joint are all signs of a problem and warrant a call to the pediatrician and possible X-rays. Sprains benefit from RICE: rest, ice, compression (with an elastic bandage), and elevation (to minimize swelling).

~ 63 ~

Skin

Atopic Dermatitis/ Eczema

See page 540.

Fifth Disease (*Erythema Infectiosum*)

Schools can have outbreaks of fifth disease, also termed *erythema infectiosum,* in late winter or early spring. This common childhood illness is caused by a virus called parvovirus B19, and for most children it usually resolves on its own without significant issues. A hallmark feature of fifth disease is a "slapped cheek" appearance, with a bright red rash on the face. Of concern are pregnant women in their first trimester, as there can be complications for the developing fetus, or children with sickle cell or other hemolytic anemias, as the virus can cause a low blood count crisis; those individuals should seek medical attention if fifth disease is suspected.

For most children, the initial stages of fifth disease are accompanied by stuffy nose, sore throat, mild fever, or fatigue, similar to a simple cold. After about a week of these symptoms, the characteristic facial rash may appear, then spread in a lacy fashion to the chest, back, arms, and thighs. When the rash is present, the child is no longer contagious. Since the infection is caused by a virus, antibiotics won't help. Treatment is mainly supportive: acetaminophen may help a fever, and over-the-counter antihistamines may help with any itch associated with the rash.

Hair Loss (Alopecia)

In the school-age child, hair loss may be due to medications, a healing scalp injury, or a medical or nutritional problem. Tight braids or habitual hair twirling may pull the hairs out, resulting in a bald spot. Some children habitually pull hair out due to emotional stress; for more on this, see page 555. Less common is alopecia areata, an autoimmune condition in which one or more circular areas of hair are lost. More severe cases may require consultation with a pediatric dermatologist for evaluation and treatment options.

Head Lice

See page 488.

Impetigo

Impetigo, a common bacterial skin infection, can develop with any break in the skin, even irritation caused by blowing a runny nose. The infection can spread to other body parts and to others when the area is scratched. The typical appearance is an oozing rash with yellow crusting. If you suspect impetigo in your child, wash the area with soap and water, keep the area covered, and consult your pediatrician, as an antibiotic ointment is typically necessary. The child may return to school twenty-four hours after antibiotics are started.

MRSA Infections

MRSA (methicillin-resistant staphylococcus aureus) is a type of bacteria that has become more prevalent in the past couple of decades. While formerly more of an issue for hospitals and nursing homes, now it is found regularly in the community. It can cause skin and soft tissue infections and can be resistant to certain antibiotics. Consult with your pediatrician if your child has an area of the skin that is becoming more red, tender, and swollen, or is draining pus. The area may only need to be drained, or antibiotics may be required.

Pinworms

Pinworms, similar to head lice, cause emotional angst in families; however, they do not cause serious health concerns. Pinworms are typically spread by an infected child scratching his bottom, picking up an egg, and then transferring the egg to a surface that is then touched by another child, who then touches his mouth. The swallowed eggs then hatch and the pinworm lays more eggs at the anus. Nighttime itching in the anal area is common. Apply the sticky side of clear cellophane tape to the skin surrounding the anus and you may find the adult worms, which are whitish gray and threadlike.

An over-the-counter oral medication, repeated after a week, should treat the pinworms. Sometimes the entire family should be treated. Wash clothing and bedsheets to prevent reinfection.

Poison Ivy and Poison Oak

Most children who come in contact with poison ivy or poison oak will have the characteristic allergic reaction of red, itchy, blistering skin, often appearing in a streak or other pattern in which the child was physically exposed to the plant's oils. Avoiding poison ivy is easier than treating the reaction after exposure. Teach school-age children "leaves of three, let them be" and show them pictures of poison ivy and poison oak. Both have shiny green leaves clustered in groups of three with a red stem. Poison ivy is not contagious from person to person, but it is a good idea to wash with soap and water to remove as much of the allergen-containing oil as possible. Pets can carry and spread the oils.

Soaking in cool water and using hydrocortisone cream and oral antihistamines can relieve the itch. If the rash involves the face or groin, shows signs of infection (warmth and tenderness), or is difficult to control, talk with your pediatrician.

Ringworm

Ringworm is a common fungal skin infection in children and is spread by person-to-person contact. The characteristic rash is red, scaly, and round or oval in shape. The rash grows outward and becomes smooth in the center, hence the "ring" in the name. Ringworm is a common rash for those who wrestle as a sport, due to the skin-to-skin contact. Ringworm can be a single patch or several patches scattered throughout the body, including the scalp. Scalp involvement may lead to hair loss.

If there is only one patch on the body, the family can try an over-the-counter antifungal cream recommended by your pediatrician two or three times a day until it clears. If there are multiple patches present or the scalp is involved, check with your pediatrician, as an oral medication may be needed, possibly for a few weeks.

Scabies

Scabies are contagious mites (tiny insects) spread by skin-to-skin or clothing-to-skin contact. The rash, caused by mites burrowing into the skin, consists of itchy red bumps. The knees, elbows, armpits, and webbing of toes and fingers are often involved. A prescription medication will eradicate the mite, but usually the whole family should be treated, and clothing and bed linens should be washed and then dried in a hot dryer to heat and kill the mites and any eggs.

Sunburn

Exposure to the sun's ultraviolet rays, even on cloudy days, can cause skin damage in both the short run *and* the long run. Reflection of sunlight off sand, water, or snow, or the greater intensity of sunlight at higher altitudes, can increase a child's exposure. Long-term skin damage in children of any skin color can lead to cancer later in life. In the short term, a sunburn can cause red and painful skin, most uncomfortable in the first twenty-four hours. Apply cool compresses to help comfort your child; acetaminophen may help with the pain. In more severe sunburn cases, call your pediatrician because, in addition to blistering or body chills, there is a risk of infection or heatstroke.

Be aware that peak ultraviolet rays occur between 11:00 a.m. and 2:00 p.m. Use sunscreen with at least SPF 30; apply *before* going outside, and reapply every hour or two, especially if swimming or sweating. Wide-brimmed hats and lightweight long-sleeved shirts and pants will also block the sun's ultraviolet rays.

Tick Bites

There are different types of ticks: the larger, sesame-seed-sized dog ticks, and the smaller, poppy-seed-sized deer ticks, which are more concerning be-cause they may transmit diseases such as Lyme disease and Rocky Mountain spotted fever. Prevent tick bites with preparation before heading into wooded areas by wearing long sleeves and long pants that are tucked into the socks. Lighter-colored clothing makes it easier to find any ticks on the clothing. Use a DEET-containing insect repellent before heading outside. When returning from outside, check for ticks, including behind the child's ears and in the hair. Prompt identification and removal of ticks is helpful because the earlier the tick is identified, the more quickly it can be removed, minimizing the chance of an infection being transmitted.

To remove a tick, clean the area with a cotton ball soaked in alcohol, and then use tweezers to grasp the tick as close to the skin as possible to pull it up and out. You can put the tick into a sealed plastic bag for identification if you are not sure what type of tick it is. Monitor the location of the tick bite for any developing rash or problems over the next several days.

For more on Lyme disease, see page 640.

Warts

Warts are raised bumps on the skin caused by a human papilloma virus. They can happen anywhere, but can be painful and harder to treat if on the soles of the feet (called plantar warts). If left alone, the body's immune system eventually fights the virus and the wart will resolve; however, this may take a couple of years or longer. If they are unsightly or uncomfortable, there are over-the-counter salicylic acid solutions that can be applied nightly. Allow the solution to dry and then cover with a small patch of duct tape overnight. If this is not working, or if you have other concerns, check with your pediatrician, who may suggest freezing the wart or other treatments.

~ 64 ~

Sleep

FROM AGES 5 to 12, the average child requires an average of nine to twelve hours of sleep a night. Most of us, adults and kids alike, are not getting enough sleep; families can take specific steps to ensure that everyone gets a better night's sleep. Getting enough good-quality overnight sleep allows kids to learn in school with their full attention and play with energy. Proper sleep also strengthens the immune system to fight off illnesses more effectively, and boosts mood, relationships, and family harmony.

Good Sleep Habits

The term "oral hygiene" refers to how well we brush and care for our teeth. Similarly, the term "sleep hygiene" refers to specific steps families can take to promote quality sleep habits, and these steps are helpful for children and adults alike. How can your family employ good sleep hygiene choices to promote quality sleep of an appropriate length during the overnight hours?

The bedtime routine should be regular and relaxing. Whether it includes a nighttime bath, reading books together, cuddle time, or something else, try to do things in a similar order each night. The bedroom should be a media-free zone; glowing screens emit light of a specific wavelength that can interfere with quality sleep. Blackout curtains and white noise, even from a simple fan, can help promote sleep.

Most kids after the fifth birthday should avoid daytime naps, as naps cannot make up for inadequate nighttime sleep, and can also interfere with falling asleep restfully at bedtime in a timely manner. School-age children should avoid caffeinated beverages for many reasons, but especially to avoid caffeine's interference with quality sleep. Daily daytime exercise, especially outdoors in daylight and fresh air, can help promote a more restful overnight sleep.

Bedtime Challenges

During these middle childhood years, most children experience nightmares or other sleep issues from time to time. At times, sleep problems may have an emotional basis. For instance, insomnia (the inability to fall or stay asleep) can be caused by stress and anxiety. If a child is afraid of the dark or fearful of being alone at night, she may be unable to relax and go to sleep.

Does your child resist bedtime? Does he take several hours to settle down and go to sleep? Bedtime challenges can be caused by many factors:

- General problems with negative and oppositional behaviors, in which he has difficulty following rules and routines, including going to bed when he would rather keep playing.

- Separation anxiety. Some children have difficulty separating from their parents at bedtime.

- Too much media and screen time. The presence of a TV or other electronic devices in a child's bedroom will interfere with the ability to fall and stay asleep, as well as the quality of the sleep. The American Academy of Pediatrics recommends that all electronic devices be turned off at least thirty minutes before bedtime. For more on media use, see page 315.

- Wanting private time with parents when siblings are not around.

- Internal body clock. Many kids have a disturbance of the sleep-wake cycle. Your child may be an "owl," with a body clock set for falling asleep late at night and waking up in the late morning; or he may be a "lark," falling asleep early and waking up very early. Speak with your pediatrician about making gradual adjustments of your child's sleep-wake patterns to fit in with the family's daily schedule.

- Habits and learned behavior. Some children simply get used to being up late, when the household settles down and the pace slows.

- Attention deficit hyperactivity disorder (ADHD). These kids may have great difficulty settling down to sleep at bedtime. They, like all kids, should get plenty of exercise and activity during the day to help them settle better for overnight sleep. For more on ADHD, see page 558.

If sleep challenges such as these persist, talk with your pediatrician.

Sleep Talking

Sleep talking (or *somniloquy*) occurs quite frequently in school-age kids. During sleep, the child begins speaking, often unintelligibly and in a mumbling voice, and usually for no more than thirty seconds. Most episodes take place during nondreaming sleep. Treatment is rarely needed or prescribed.

Nightmares

Nightmares are common in middle childhood. In a typical episode a child will have a scary dream, filled with monsters or other frightening situations. She may awaken, become anxious, breathe heavily, and begin crying. Sometimes the experience is so scary that the child may resist going back to sleep, needing reassurance. Hug your child and speak calmly, reassuring her that it was only a bad dream. Often she will vividly describe the details of the scary dream in an effort to calm herself, helped along by her parents' comfort. She may also remember the dream the next day and want to discuss it further.

In most children nightmares occur only occasionally, usually in the early morning hours. Monitor your child's screen usage and ensure that media are age-appropriate, as exposure to violent or frightening images can contribute to nightmares. If they happen often—or if the same frightening dream recurs—talk to your physician about them. Nightmares seem to occur with increasing frequency during times of stress, so if these dreams are recurrent, evaluate the stress in your child's life.

Sleepwalking

Children between the ages of 5 and 12 frequently have at least one sleepwalking episode. This disorder (also called *somnambulism*) tends to affect boys more often than girls, and in a small number of children, episodes take place several nights a week. Sleepwalking usually occurs during the second or third hour of nighttime sleep. The child sits up and, without totally awakening, leaves his bed, usually walking awkwardly, with his eyes open and a blank look on his face.

For several minutes he may wander through the house, even opening doors along the way, but his actions are purposeless. If spoken to, he may seem to respond, but the words are usually unintelligible. He will probably return to his bed on his own and go back to normal sleeping, recalling nothing of this nighttime activity when he awakens in the morning.

If your child sleepwalks, you need to minimize his chances of hurting himself. Make sure he has a safe environment—that is, outside doors

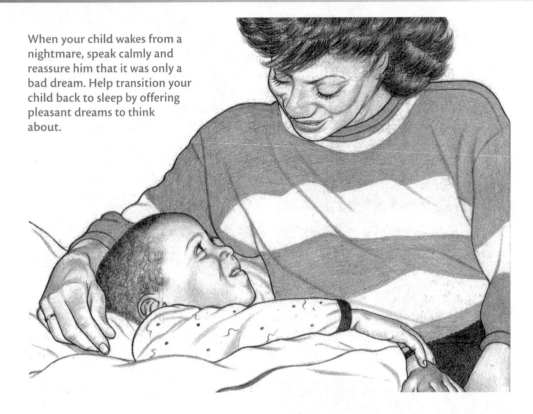

When your child wakes from a nightmare, speak calmly and reassure him that it was only a bad dream. Help transition your child back to sleep by offering pleasant dreams to think about.

should be locked so that he cannot leave the house, stairways should be blocked so he cannot walk up or down them, and hazardous objects should be moved to a less dangerous location. When you find him walking in his sleep, gently lead him back to bed. Sleepwalking tends to run in families. In most children sleepwalking disappears on its own, generally by early adolescence.

Night Terrors

Night terrors are a different phenomenon from nightmares and can be quite upsetting for a parent to watch. About 90 to 180 minutes after falling asleep, the affected child will abruptly sit up in bed, open his eyes, and scream loudly or cry out for help. For the next few minutes he may gasp, moan or mumble, thrash about, and seem to be in a confused, agitated state. His breathing and heart rate will accelerate significantly. He will be unresponsive to his parents' attempts at comforting him and may even push them away. These episodes can sometimes last for three to six minutes before the child rather quickly returns to a peaceful sleep, remembering nothing about it the next morning, and leaving parents baffled and terrorized—hence the name "night terrors."

Night terrors (or *pavor nocturnus*)

occur in a relatively small number of children (1 to 5 percent), taking place during a nondreaming, deep stage of sleep. As frightening as they may be for parents, they are *not* a reflection of a psychological disturbance. They are a normal, although infrequent, part of the body's transition between sleep states. Sometimes physical exhaustion can contribute to a child's having night terrors; as such, they are more likely to occur after an action-packed day. Most children outgrow night terrors without treatment. When possible, parents should work to maintain a good bedtime schedule, as an overtired child is more likely to have another episode. Parental patience and understanding are important, although these night terrors tend to be much more stressful for the parent than for the child.

Daytime Sleepiness

Some children are excessively sleepy during the daytime hours. The most frequent cause of daytime sleepiness is an insufficient amount of good-quality sleep at night. Parents should evaluate a child's overall sleep schedule and brainstorm ways to move bedtime earlier or otherwise increase total hours of overnight sleep. Daytime exercise and play outdoors can help reset a child's sleep-wake cycle and help him rest better overnight. Some medications can in-terfere with a child's normal daytime alertness.

Sleep apnea can cause daytime sleepiness. Children with sleep apnea briefly stop breathing at different times during the night due to an obstruction in the respiratory tract. For school-age children, this is often related to enlarged tonsils and adenoids, or to obesity. As the child instinctively gasps for breath, she awakens for a few moments, her normal breathing pattern returns, and she immediately goes back to sleep, probably with no recollection that this episode has occurred. Because these brief awakenings can occur dozens and even hundreds of times a night, the child is sleep-deprived, creating sleepiness the following day. Often these children will snore while asleep, a symptom of the obstruction of the respiratory tract. The underlying cause of this airway obstruction must be determined and treated to cure the apnea. Once it is relieved, the child can enjoy normal sleep again.

Children with *narcolepsy*, a rare condition, are overpowered by strong, uncontrollable urges to sleep. They may fall asleep immediately for several minutes to an hour at a time, often in inappropriate places like a classroom. Narcolepsy usually first occurs during adolescence and tends to run in families. Although it is a lifelong condition, it can usually be successfully treated with both behavioral modifications and medication.

INDEX

. . . .